# Your *Clinics* subscription just got better!

## You can now access the FULL TEXT of this publication online at no additional cost! Activate your online subscription today and receive...

- Full text of all issues from 2002 to the present
- Photographs, tables, illustrations, and references
- Comprehensive search capabilities
- Links to MEDLINE and Elsevier journals

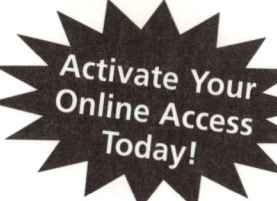

Activate Your Online Access Today!

Plus, you can also sign up for E-alerts of upcoming issues or articles that interest you, and take advantage of exclusive access to bonus features!

## To activate your individual online subscription:

1. Visit our website at **www.TheClinics.com**.

2. Click on "Register" at the top of the page, and follow the instructions.

3. To activate your account, you will need your subscriber account number, which you can find on your mailing label (note: the number of digits in your subscriber account number varies from six to ten digits). See the sample below where the subscriber account number has been circled.

**This is your subscriber account number**

```
**********************************************
FEB00   J0167   C7   (123456-89)

J.H. DOE, MD
531 MAIN ST
CENTER CITY, NY  10001-001
```

W0230065

4. That's it! Your online access to the most trusted source for clinical reviews is now available.

# the**clinics**.com

ELSEVIER

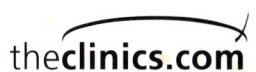

# RHEUMATIC DISEASE CLINICS OF NORTH AMERICA

## Systemic Lupus Erythematosus

GUEST EDITOR
Murray B. Urowitz, MD, FRCPC(C)

May 2005 • Volume 31 • Number 2

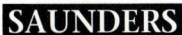

An Imprint of Elsevier, Inc.
PHILADELPHIA   LONDON   TORONTO   MONTREAL   SYDNEY   TOKYO

## W.B. SAUNDERS COMPANY
*A Division of Elsevier Inc.*

1600 John F. Kennedy Boulevard • Suite 1800 • Philadelphia, Pennsylvania 19103-2899

http://www.theclinics.com

**RHEUMATIC DISEASE**
**CLINICS OF NORTH AMERICA**     Volume 31, Number 2
**May 2005**                     ISSN 0889-857X
Editor: Barton Dudlick          ISBN 1-4160-2765-3

The ideas and opinions expressed in *Rheumatic Disease Clinics of North America* do not necessarily reflect those of the Publisher. The Publisher does not assume any responsibility for any injury and/or damage to persons or property arising out of or related to any use of the material contained in this periodical. The reader is advised to check the appropriate medical literature and the product information currently provided by the manufacturer of each drug to be administered to verify the dosage, the method and duration of administration, or contraindications. It is the responsibility of the treating physician or other health care professional, relying on independent experience and knowledge of the patient, to determine drug dosages and the best treatment for the patient. Mention of any product in this issue should not be construed as endorsement by the contributors, editors, or the Publisher of the product or manufacturers' claims.

*Rheumatic Disease Clinics of North America* (ISSN 0889-857X) is published quarterly by Elsevier Inc. Corporate and editorial offices: 1600 John F. Kennedy Boulevard, Suite 1800, Philadelphia, PA 19103-2899. Accounting and circulation offices: 6277 Sea Harbor Drive, Orlando, FL 32887-4800. Periodicals postage paid at Orlando, FL 32862, and additional mailing offices. Subscription prices are USD 180 per year for US individuals, USD 290 per year for US institutions, USD 90 per year for US students and residents, USD 214 per year for Canadian individuals, USD 350 per year for Canadian institutions, USD 240 per year for international individuals, USD 350 per year for international institutions and USD 120 per year for Canadian and foreign students/residents. To receive student/resident rate, orders must be accompanied by name of affiliated institution, date of term, and the *signature* of program/residency coordinator on institution letterhead. Orders will be billed at individual rate until proof of status received. Foreign air speed delivery is included in all *Clinics* subscription prices. All prices are subject to change without notice. POSTMASTER: Send address changes to *Rheumatic Disease Clinics of North America*, W.B. Saunders Company, Periodicals Fulfillment, Orlando, FL 32887-4800. **Customer Service: 800-654-2452 (USA). From outside of the USA, call (+1) 407-345-4000. E-mail: hhspcs@harcourt.com.**

*Reprints.* For copies of 100 or more of articles in this publication, please contact the Commercial Reprints Department, Elsevier Inc., 360 Park Avenue South, New York, New York, 10010-1710; Tel.: (+1) 212-633-3813, Fax: (+1) 212-462-1935, and E-mail: reprints@elsevier.com.

*Rheumatic Disease Clinics of North America* is covered in *Index Medicus, Current Contents/ Clinical Medicine, Science Citation Index, ISI/BIOMED,* and *EMBASE/Excerpta Medica.*

Printed in the United States of America.

# GUEST EDITOR

**MURRAY B. UROWITZ, MD, FRCPC(C),** Professor, Medicine, University of Toronto; and Director, Centre of Prognosis Studies in the Rheumatic Diseases, Toronto Western Hospital, Toronto, Ontario, Canada

# CONTRIBUTORS

**SASHA BERNATSKY MD, MSc,** Research Fellow, Division of Clinical Epidemiology, Montreal General Hospital, Quebec, Canada

**JILL P. BUYON, MD,** Professor, Medicine, Division of Rheumatology, Department of Medicine, New York University School of Medicine; and Department of Rheumatic Diseases and Molecular Medicine, Hospital for Joint Diseases, New York, New York

**ROBERT M. CLANCY, PhD,** Research Associate Professor, Division of Rheumatology, Department of Medicine, New York University School of Medicine; and Department of Rheumatic Diseases and Molecular Medicine, Hospital for Joint Diseases, New York, New York

**CHRISTINE A. CLARK, BSc,** Research Associate, Division of Rheumatology, Department of Medicine, University of Toronto Faculty of Medicine, Toronto, Ontario, Canada

**ANN CLARKE MD, MSc,** Associate Professor, Division of Clinical Epidemiology, Montreal General Hospital, Quebec, Canada

**ANDREA DORIA, MD,** Division of Rheumatology, Department of Medical and Surgical Science, University of Padua, Padua, Italy

**OLGA DVORKINA, MD,** Assistant Professor, Medicine, State University of New York–Downstate Medical Center, Brooklyn, New York

**ELLEN M. GINZLER, MD, MPH,** Professor, Medicine, State University of New York–Downstate Medical Center, Brooklyn, New York

**DAFNA D. GLADMAN, MD, FRCP(C),** Co-Director, University of Toronto Lupus Clinic, Toronto Western Hospital; and Professor, Medicine, University of Toronto, Toronto, Ontario, Canada

**JOHN G. HANLY, MD, MRCPI, FRCPC,** Head, Division of Rheumatology; and Director, Arthritis Center of Nova Scotia, Queen Elizabeth II Health Sciences Centre, Dalhousie University, Halifax, Nova Scotia, Canada

**JOHN B. HARLEY, MD, PhD,** Professor, James McEldowney Chair in Immunology, and George Lynn Cross Research Professor, Department of Medicine, University of Oklahoma Health Sciences Center; and United States Department of Veterans Affairs Medical Center, Oklahoma City, Oklahoma

**CARL A. LASKIN, MD,** Associate Professor, Division of Rheumatology, Department of Medicine, University of Toronto Faculty of Medicine, Toronto, Ontario, Canada

**CHIN LEE, MD,** Instructor, Medicine, Division of Rheumatology, Feinberg School of Medicine, Northwestern University, Chicago, Illinois

**PIER L. MERONI, MD,** Allergy and Clinical Immunology Unit, Department of Internal Medicine, IRCCS Instituto Auxologico Italiano, University of Milan, Milan, Italy

**SWAPAN K. NATH, PhD,** Assistant Member, Department of Arthritis and Immunology, Oklahoma Medical Research Foundation, Oklahoma City, Oklahoma

**MANDANA NIKPOUR, MBBS, FRACP,** Geoff Carr Lupus Fellow, University of Toronto Lupus Clinic, Toronto Western Hospital, Toronto, Ontario, Canada

**MICHELLE PETRI, MD, MPH,** Professor, Medicine, Johns Hopkins University School of Medicine, Baltimore, Maryland

**ROSALIND RAMSEY-GOLDMAN, MD, DrPH,** Professor, Medicine, Division of Rheumatology, Department of Medicine, Feinburg School of Medicine, Northwestern University, Chicago, Illinois

**ANDREA L. SESTAK, MD, PhD,** Research Assistant Member, Department of Arthritis and Immunology, Oklahoma Medical Research Foundation, Oklahoma City, Oklahoma

**YANIV SHERER, MD,** Department of Medicine B, Sackler Faculty of Medicine, Center for Autoimmune Diseases, Chaim Sheba Medical Center, Tel-Aviv University, Tel-Hashomer, Israel

**YEHUDA SHOENFELD, MD,** Head, Department of Medicine B, Sackler Faculty of Medicine, Center for Autoimmune Diseases, Chaim Sheba Medical Center, Tel-Aviv University, Tel-Hashomer, Israel

**KAREN A. SPITZER, BSc,** Clinical Trials Coordinator, Division of Rheumatology, Department of Medicine, University of Toronto Faculty of Medicine, Toronto, Ontario, Canada

**MURRAY B. UROWITZ, MD, FRCPC(C),** Professor, Medicine, University of Toronto; and Director, Centre of Prognosis Studies in the Rheumatic Diseases, Toronto Western Hospital, Toronto, Ontario, Canada

# CONTENTS

The authors focus on the emerging role of new modalities for noninvasive assessment of vascular health in patients who have SLE and offer a strategy for screening and management of those at risk of CAD. The article concludes with a discussion on the important questions that remain to be answered and future directions for research.

## Inflammation and Accelerated Atherosclerosis: Basic Mechanisms

Andrea Doria, Yaniv Sherer, Pier L. Meroni, and Yehuda Shoenfeld

This article summarizes knowledge of the pathogenic mechanisms in autoimmune rheumatic diseases as risk factors for accelerated atherosclerosis. The studies described support a role for immunologic–inflammatory mechanisms in the pathogenesis of atherosclerosis. This immunologic–inflammatory state is evident in many autoimmune diseases, but also in the general population lacking an overt autoimmune disease. The ability to immunomodulate atherosclerosis (currently only experimental) should lead to future research into the mechanisms and treatment of atherosclerosis, the leading cause of death in the Western world.

## Osteoporosis in Systemic Lupus Erythematosus Mechanisms

Chin Lee and Rosalind Ramsey-Goldman

Osteoporosis is a potentially preventable condition frequently encountered in patients who have systemic lupus erythematosus (SLE). Bone loss in SLE is heterogeneous and likely a multifactorial process involving both traditional and lupus-related risk factors. Recognizing potential contributors to bone loss in the SLE patient may allow for earlier detection of osteoporosis and optimize bone health. This article reviews the current epidemiologic information available on osteoporosis and fracture data in SLE and discusses evaluation and management strategies pertinent to patients who have lupus.

## Exploring the Links Between Systemic Lupus Erythematosus and Cancer

Sasha Bernatsky, Rosalind Ramsey-Goldman, and Ann Clarke

For decades, concern has been mounting that individuals with systemic lupus erythematosus (SLE) have increased susceptibility to cancer. Recent data confirm that certain cancers, particularly hematologic, occur more frequently in SLE than in the general population. Numerous pathogenic mechanisms are possible, but hypotheses remain largely speculative. In particular, data are inadequate on how cancer risk in SLE may be related to medication exposures. To evaluate the impact of medication exposures on cancer risk in SLE, cooperative efforts of Systemic Lupus International Collaborating Clinics and Canadian Network for Improved Outcomes in Systemic Lupus are currently in progress. This should provide much-needed insight into the pathogenesis of the association between cancer and SLE.

# FORTHCOMING ISSUES

# RECENT ISSUES

---

## THE CLINICS ARE NOW AVAILABLE ONLINE!

Access your subscription at:
http://www.theclinics.com

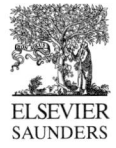

Rheum Dis Clin N Am 31 (2005) xi–xii

RHEUMATIC
DISEASE CLINICS
OF NORTH AMERICA

ELSEVIER
SAUNDERS

Preface

# Systemic Lupus Erythematosus

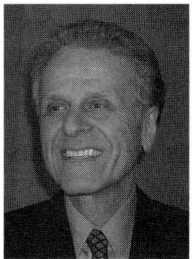

Murray B. Urowitz, MD, FRCPC(C)
*Guest Editor*

Our knowledge of the clinical presentation, etiology, pathogenesis, and treatment of systemic lupus erythematosus grows exponentially every few years. It is now 5 years since the *Rheumatic Disease Clinics of North America* has devoted an issue to this topic, and much new knowledge has been accumulated. We have attempted in these 11 articles to highlight some of this new information.

In articles by Urowitz and Gladman; Petri; Laskin; Hanly; and Buyon and Clancy, advances in our understanding of some of the clinical presentations of the basic disease are covered. The article by Sestak, Nath, and Harley reviews our understanding of the genetic predisposition to systemic lupus erythematosus. Ginzler and Dvorkina summarize the newer approaches to therapy. Nikpour, Urowitz, and Gladman cover newer atherosclerotic presentations; Doria, Sherer, Meroni, and Shoenfeld atherosclerosis; Lee and Ramsey-Goldman osteoporosis; and Bernatsky, Ramsey-Goldman, and Clarke malignancy occurring as a consequence of the disease itself (inflammation) or its therapy (steroids and cytotoxic drugs).

In each article, the investigators have brought us their contributions in the context of recent advances in their area. The issue can therefore serve as a resource for all students, clinicians, trainees, and researchers of this disease.

doi:10.1016/j.rdc.2005.01.012                    *rheumatic.theclinics.com*

Murray B. Urowitz, MD, FRCPC(C)
*Centre of Prognosis Studies in the Rheumatic Diseases*
*Toronto Western Hospital*
*399 Bathurst Street*
*Toronto, ON*
*Canada M5T 2S8*
*E-mail address:* m.urowitz@utoronto.ca

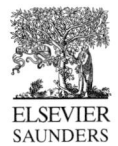

ELSEVIER
SAUNDERS

RHEUMATIC
DISEASE CLINICS
OF NORTH AMERICA

Rheum Dis Clin N Am 31 (2005) 211–221

# Contributions of Observational Cohort Studies in Systemic Lupus Erythematosus: The University of Toronto Lupus Clinic Experience

Murray B. Urowitz, MD, FRCPC(C)[a,b,*],
Dafna D. Gladman, MD, FRCP(C)[a,c]

[a]University of Toronto, Toronto, ON, Canada
[b]Centre of Prognosis Studies in the Rheumatic Diseases, Toronto Western Hospital,
Toronto, ON, Canada
[c]University of Toronto Lupus Clinic, Toronto Western Hospital, Toronto, ON, Canada

In 1996, the US Preventive Services Task Force [1] suggested that there were gradings for types of evidence that could qualify as evidence-based medicine. These grades depended on research design. The highest grade was reserved for evidence obtained from at least one properly executed randomized controlled trial. The task force also suggested, however, that evidence obtained from well-designed controlled trials without randomization, or evidence obtained from well-designed cohort or case-controlled studies qualified for the next level of evidence-based medicine. As Dr. Feinstein previously suggested, randomized trials alone cannot serve as the basic foundation for science in clinical management. Rather the resolution of future issues in clinical management would have to come from "analysis of events and observations that occur in non-experimental circumstances during the interaction of nature, people, technologic artifacts, and clinical practitioners" [2]. To make valid conclusions from these observations required a rigorous approach to clinical measurements, a clinical

* Corresponding author. Centre of Prognosis Studies in the Rheumatic Diseases, Toronto Western Hospital, 399 Bathurst Street, 1E 409 East Wing, Toronto, ON M5T 2S8, Canada.
  E-mail address: m.urowitz@utoronto.ca (M.B. Urowitz).

scientific approach he termed Clinimetrics, and the appropriate handling of these required measures with appropriate statistical analysis [2]. Well-done observational cohort studies today fulfill these requirements. This approach has been used successfully with important derived output for several rheumatologic diseases. Observation cohort research has been especially fruitful in those areas less amenable to study by randomized controlled trials such as prognosis studies, risk factors for specific outcomes, prognostic factors for outcome, and clinical laboratory correlations. These studies also can confirm in practice with a heterogeneous population of patients, the results of randomized controlled trials performed in a homogenous population of patients.

This article uses the University of Toronto Lupus Cohort to illustrate the benefits of observational cohort studies in generating important new knowledge in chronic disease such as systemic lupus erythematosus (SLE).

## Methods

### Setting

The University of Toronto Lupus clinic is located at the Centre for Prognosis Studies in The Rheumatic Diseases at the Toronto Western Hospital, Toronto, Ontario. The Lupus Clinic was established in 1970 to provide care for patients who have SLE, to study clinical laboratory correlations in this disease, and to better understand long-term outcomes of the disease [3].

### Assessments

To produce valid observations, it was important to standardize means of assessment of patients and the disease, and of recording these observations. Some assessment approaches were in existence, but many had to be developed. Patients are seen at regular intervals (2 to 6 months apart) regardless of medical condition to better describe the disease and its effects. Because some patients could not be seen at prescribed intervals, the authors have developed a mechanism to trace patients lost to follow-up. The 10% lost-to-follow-up rate did not affect major long-term outcome studies [4].

### Protocol

A data collection protocol was developed to include all known clinical and laboratory features of SLE. Each item was defined in a glossary based on existing accepted definitions where available, and newly derived definitions where necessary.

*Training*

The protocol was to be completed by the directors of the clinic or physician-trainees rotating through the Lupus Clinic. To assure standardization of assessments, training sessions were held with each set of trainees.

*Instruments*

As there was no universally accepted method to determine disease activity status including the authors' Lupus Activity Criteria Count (LACC) [5], the authors assembled a group of lupologists and methodologists in 1985 to develop the SLE Disease Activity Index (SLEDAI) [6]. SLEDAI was derived through computer modeling of assessments of 1400 case scenarios by experts, and it was found to have face and content validity and reproducibility by experts and novices, and it could measure change over time [7,8]. SLEDAI was revised in 2000 (SLEDAI-2K) to reflect reality in clinical trials [9]. To describe disease activity over time, the adjusted mean SLEDAI (AMS) was developed and validated [10,11]. At the conference to develop the SLEDAI it was determined that to describe outcome in patients who have SLE it was necessary to include an assessment of damage and quality of life in addition to disease activity. Therefore, the Systemic Lupus International Collaborating Clinic/American College of Rheumatology damage index (SLICC/ACR DI) was developed and validated [12,13]. The short form–36 (SF-36) was adopted as the quality of life measure in patients who have SLE [14].

## Results

Using the Lupus Clinic database, the authors have been able to make several observations with respect to clinical manifestations, clinical–laboratory correlation studies, prognosis and outcome studies, organ-specific outcome studies, risk factor studies, and therapeutic studies that have contributed new information to understanding of this disease.

## Clinical observations

Based on the observations of skin manifestations of patients who have SLE in the authors' clinic, several different nail changes associated with the disease were identified [15]. The authors' description of neuropsychiatric lupus highlighted the importance of lupus headache, a severe headache unresponsive to narcotic analgesics as a manifestation of central nervous system (CNS) lupus [16] and showed that single photon emission computerized tomography scanning of the brain could identify patients who have neuropsychiatric lupus requiring therapeutic interventions [17].

The authors also identified several patients who had liver disease associated with active SLE not requiring specific therapy [18]. They demonstrated that thrombocytopenia may have two presentations in SLE, one occurring in the presence of active disease and requiring aggressive therapy, and the other occurring as an isolated feature not requiring aggressive intervention [19]. The authors' pregnancy studies challenged traditional concepts of the inadvisability of pregnancy during SLE, indicating that pregnant patients who have SLE who enter pregnancy with inactive disease have no greater rates of flares than nonpregnant SLE patients [20].

**Prognosis/Outcome studies**

In 1974, the authors first described the bimodal mortality pattern in SLE [21], showing that early mortality in SLE is associated with lupus disease activity and infection, whereas late mortality is associated with atherosclerotic complications [22]. Subsequent studies from the authors' cohort confirmed this pattern in the clinic, in postmortem studies and compared with the Ontario population [23–25].

The authors recently described a prevalence of 13.2% of arterial and venous events (AVE) in their total cohort of 1087 patients who had SLE [26]. These included 24 patients who had myocardial infarction (MI), 76 who had angina, 7 who had transient ischemic attack (TIA), 25 who had stroke, 22 who had peripheral vascular disease (PVD), and 3 who suffered sudden death. A multivariate analysis of risk factors for AVE revealed significance for two lupus-related factors, vasculitis and neuropsychiatric disease, and the total number of coronary artery disease (CAD) risk factors. A similar analysis in an inception cohort, patients presenting to clinic within 1 year of disease onset, identified a similar prevalence (12.5%) in 541 patients. Again, risk factors for AVE included neuropsychiatric disease and vasculitis as disease-related factors, and smoking history. In the Toronto Risk Factor Study, which included 250 patients who had SLE and 250 healthy controls, although patients who had SLE and AVE had more CAD risk factors than healthy controls, there was no difference between SLE patients who did or did not have AVE with regards to both CAD risk factors and disease-related factors over 22.6 months [27]. Thus, these studies show that AVEs are common among patients who have SLE and are associated with disease-related and CAD-related risk factors. Therefore, all modifiable factors should be addressed in this patient population.

Although control of lupus has improved survival [28], prolonged complete remission, defined as 5 years without clinical or laboratory evidence of active disease and on no treatment, has remained elusive, occurring in 1.7% of the patients [29,30]. Even if the definition of complete remission was relaxed to 1 year, only 6.5% of the patients achieved such remission. When remission was defined more broadly as prolonged clinical quiescence but allowing serologic abnormalities, or even allowing for antimalarial therapy to these definitions, prolonged 5-year remission was rare, occurring in only eight additional patients.

## Organ-specific outcome

### Osteonecrosis (avascular necrosis)

In a study of the 744 patients recorded in the Lupus Clinic database, 95 (12.8%) were documented to have osteonecrosis [31]. The joints most commonly affected were the hips and knees, often in a bilateral distribution. Most of the patients (70.5%) had two or more joints affected, while less than a third of the patients had osteonecrosis in only one joint. Independent risk factors for the development of osteonecrosis included glucocorticosteroid use, the presence of arthritis, and the use of cytotoxic medications [32]. The authors recently reported that early, more intensive corticosteroid therapy in SLE patients may be a determining factor in the future development of osteonecrosis [33].

## Renal disease

In a study of 148 renal biopsies in patients who had SLE, the authors documented that there was frequently discordance between clinical features of renal disease and biopsy results [34]. This study showed that there were patients who had proliferative lupus nephritis who had had no evidence of clinical renal disease and that patients who had minimal renal lesion could have important clinical evidence of renal disease. These findings confirmed the necessity for renal biopsy in patients who have SLE. A recent study demonstrated that isolated hematuria or sterile pyuria is associated with active renal and nonrenal disease activity [35].

The role for renal biopsy was emphasized further in a study of 123 patients whose biopsies were performed after entry into the clinic and who were followed for a period of time following the biopsy. In patients who have normal serum creatinine, proliferative and chronic lesions on biopsy were shown to be predictive for mortality and end-stage renal disease [36,37]. The authors then evaluated the role of repeat renal biopsy [38]. The reasons for performing a repeat renal biopsy vary, but increasing proteinuria is the predominant reason. Renal morphology can change over time, not only in terms of World Health Organization class, but in terms of chronicity and activity indices. Although activity tends to decrease over time, there is accrual of damage and increase in the chronicity index. A single renal biopsy may not be sufficient to manage lupus nephritis throughout the course of the patient's disease.

An analysis of the authors' patients who developed refractory renal disease revealed that patient compliance was a significant factor in the progression to renal insufficiency and renal failure [39].

## Neuropsychiatric lupus

Patients who have SLE often complain of cognitive impairment, even in the absence of active disease. The authors performed neurocognitive studies in patients who had inactive SLE compared with healthy controls. Neurocognitive dysfunction was documented in 43% of SLE patients compared with 19% of healthy controls. SLEDAI greater than 10 at first presentation to the Lupus Clinic and previous vasculitis were associated with neurocognitive dysfunction, but previous CNS disease, renal disease, renal damage, or atherosclerotic complications were not. Neurophysiologic studies at the time of the assessment were not predictive of neurocognitive dysfunction.

A subsequent study of neurocognitive assessments of offspring of patients who have SLE compared with age- and sex-matched children revealed that offspring of patients who have SLE demonstrate abnormalities on neuropsychologic testing in the learning and memory and behavioral domains [40].

## Clinical laboratory correlation studies

A major initiative in the establishment of the University of Toronto Lupus Clinic was to evaluate the relationship between clinical and laboratory features. Prevailing dogma suggested that the presence of anti-DNA antibodies predicted subsequent lupus disease activity. In 1979, the authors demonstrated that 12% of their SLE clinic cohort had serologically active but clinically quiescent disease [41]. This was confirmed by a larger study [42].

The authors further identified another group of SLE patients who had clinical activity in the absence of serologic abnormalities [43]. They were unable to identify factors that could be used to separate concordant from discordant patients before the eventual course of the individual patients was observed.

## Therapeutic trials where randomized controlled trials are difficult or unethical

The authors sought to identify the effect of hormone replacement therapy in SLE. In a nested case control study, they were able to demonstrate that hormone replacement therapy was not associated with increased risk of flares in patients who had SLE [44].

To investigate the clinical observation that smoking cessation led to improvement in refractory cutaneous lupus, the authors performed a retrospective cohort study from the University of Toronto Lupus Clinic. Patients who had either acute discoid or subacute cutaneous lupus onset less than 6 months who received antimalarial therapy for their cutaneous lesions were selected. The smoking group consisted of 17 regular smokers, while the nonsmoking group consisted of 19 individuals who never smoked during the study period. The cutaneous eruption resolved completely in 3 of 17 smokers versus 9 of 17 non-smokers after 6 months of antimalarial therapy ($P < 0.035$) and 3 of 16 smokers and 9 of 17 nonsmokers at 12 months ($P < 0.046$). There was no significant change in the mean steroid dose or SLEDAI in either group. Smoking appears to decrease the efficacy of antimalarial therapy in cutaneous lupus.

## Discussion

In the past, observational cohort studies typically used historical controls or administrative databases. Recent longitudinal observational cohort studies use appropriate Clinimetrics as defined by Feinstein through consistent, reproducible processes of observation and expression [2]. Based on rigorous definition of case ascertainment, clinical observation, and recording, the data included in these observational cohorts are valid. The analytic approach to this data uses modern principles of design also used in randomized controlled trials, including specific inclusion criteria, case–control design, adjustments for differences at baseline, and appropriate statistical methodology. Therefore, data derived from such studies can generate new knowledge reliably.

In the authors' cohort, using these principles of data derivation and analysis, the authors have been able to describe new clinical features, outcomes, and prognostic factors and investigate therapies. This has allowed the authors to make clinical observations not immediately obvious with individual patient observations such as nail changes, thrombocytopenia, and liver enzyme abnormalities. Occasionally, clinical observations made in isolation such as flare in lupus during pregnancy can lead to erroneous conclusions such as pregnancy causing SLE flares. Careful case control studies clarified the situation, however, revealing that there was no difference in flare rates between pregnant and nonpregnant SLE patients. Similar conclusions have been reached by others [45].

Being able to follow patients sequentially over a long period according to a standardized protocol also allows a more accurate description of outcome and prognosis. Such follow-up first revealed in 1974 the unexpected finding of accelerated atherosclerosis as a major cause of mortality in SLE [21,22]. This finding subsequently has been demonstrated in other observational cohorts, and today, the study of prevalence, risk factors, and pathogenic mechanisms for atherosclerosis in SLE is the major endeavor in many centers around the world [25,46].

In assessing remission in SLE, several centers have described remissions of limited duration such as 1 year in a significant percentage of patients [47]. In the authors' longitudinal cohort study, they have shown that meaningful remission of 3 to 5 years is quite unusual; therefore continuous long-term monitoring of patients is essential [30].

Although specific organ outcomes are a focus of study for many centers, risk factors for these outcomes can be ascertained most reliably from studies of prospectively collected risk factor data. Thus, the authors have been able to show that not only are steroids the most important risk factor for osteonecrosis but that it is high-dose steroids given early in the therapy of lupus that is the determining risk factor [32,33].

Similarly, the authors' studies of over 123 kidney biopsies that related disease manifestations and outcomes have helped establish the prognostic value of renal histology for mortality and end-stage renal disease. The observation that renal biopsy was particularly useful in patients who had normal serum creatinine helped explain the apparent discrepancy in the literature regarding the value of biopsies in different studies, as some of these studies included patients who had renal insufficiency [48].

Although neurocognitive dysfunction is a well-known feature of active SLE [49,50], the authors have been able to demonstrate a more than twofold increase in neurocognitive dysfunction in patients who had inactive SLE compared with normal controls. They have determined the importance of high burden of disease at presentation and previous vasculitis as important risk factors. This was only possible as risk factors were collected prospectively.

Several investigators have shown that serologic abnormalities, elevated levels of anti-DNA antibodies, or low complement levels are associated with or predict disease flare [51–53]. It now can be shown that a significant percentage of prospectively followed patients are clinically and serologically discordant, either serologically active clinically quiescent (SACQ) or clinically active serologically quiescent (CASQ). The authors, however, were unable to identify factors that could be used to separate concordant from discordant patients before the eventual course of the individual patients was observed. This suggests that serologic monitoring of SLE patients would be useful only if followed longitudinally and frequently to first identify the concordance status of the patient, and then incorporate this information into subsequent clinical decisions. In future longitudinal studies of this issue, discordant patients should be identified and separated out from analyses of concordance.

Although efficacy of newer therapies awaits the results of randomized controlled trials, important observations on currently used therapies can be made in nested case controlled studies in patients followed in prospective cohorts on and off the therapy of interest. Thus, it has been shown that hormone replacement therapy was not associated with increased flares in SLE and that antimalarial therapy effectiveness in cutaneous SLE is decreased in smokers compared with nonsmokers.

In conclusion, long-term observational cohort studies have made important contributions to knowledge of SLE, its clinical presentation, outcome, and response to therapy. Fostering such research in individual clinics such as the authors' clinic, or in multicenter collaborative clinics such as the SLICC is a worthy endeavor.

## References

[1] Preventive Services Task Force. Guide to clinical preventive services: report of the US Preventive Services Task Force. 2nd edition. Baltimore (MD): Williams and Wilkins; 1996.

[2] Feinstein AR. An additional basic science for clinical medicine: IV. The development of Clinimetrics. Ann Intern Med 1983;99(6):843–8.

[3] Lee P, Urowitz MB, Bookman AAM, et al. SLE: a review of 110 cases with particular reference to lupus nephritis, CNS manifestations, infections. Aseptic necrosis and prognosis. Q J Med 1977;46:1–32.

[4] Gladman DD, Koh DR, Urowitz MB, et al. Lost to follow-up study in SLE. Lupus 2000;9:363–7.

[5] Urowitz MB, Gladman DD, Tozman ES, et al. Lupus activity criteria count. J Rheumatol 1984; 11:783–7.

[6] Bombardier C, Gladman DD, Urowitz MB, et al. The development and validation of the SLE Disease Activity Index (SLEDAI). Arthritis Rheum 1992;35:630–40.

[7] Gladman DD, Goldsmith CH, Urowitz MB, et al. Sensitivity to change of 3 systemic lupus erythematosus disease activity indices: international validation. J Rheumatol 1994;21:1468–71.

[8] Hawker G, Gabriel S, Bombardier C, et al. A reliability study of SLEDAI: a disease activity index for systemic lupus erythematosus (SLE). J Rheumatol 1993;20:657–60.

[9] Gladman DD, Ibañez D, Urowitz MB. SLE Disease Activity Index 2000. J Rheumatol 2002;29: 288–91.

[10] Ibanez D, Urowitz MB, Gladman DD. Summarizing disease features over time: I. Adjusted mean SLEDAI derivation and application to an index of disease activity in lupus. J Rheumatol 2003; 30:1977–82.

[11] Ibáñez D, Urowitz MB, Gladman DD. Disease activity over time (adjusted mean SLEDAI) predicts mortality and damage in SLE.

[12] Gladman D, Ginzler E, Goldsmith C, et al. The development and initial validation of the SLICC/ACR damage index for SLE. Arthritis Rheum 1996;39:363–9.

[13] Gladman D, Urowitz MB, Goldsmith C, et al. The reliability of the SLICC/ACR damage index for SLE. Arthritis Rheum 1997;40:809–13.

[14] Gladman DD, Urowitz M, Fortin P, et al. Systemic Lupus Erythematosus International Collaborating Clinics (SLICC) Conference on Assessment of Lupus Flare and Quality of Life Measures in SLE (workshop report). J Rheumatol 1996;23:1953–5.

[15] Urowitz MB, Gladman DD, Chalmers A, Ogryzlo MA. Nail lesions in systemic lupus erythematosus. J Rheumatol 1978;5:441–7.

[16] Abel T, Gladman DD, Urowitz MB. Neuropsychiatric lupus. J Rheumatol 1980;7:325–33.

[17] Kovacs JAJ, Urowitz MB, Gladman DD, et al. Single photon emission computerized tomography (SPECT) in neuropsychiatric SLE (NPSLE). J Rheumatol 1995;22:1247–53.

[18] Miller MH, Urowitz MB, Gladman DD, et al. The liver in systemic lupus erythematosus. Q J Med 1984;53:401–9.

[19] Miller MH, Urowitz MB, Gladman DD. The significance of thrombocytopenia in systemic lupus erythematosus. Arthritis Rheum 1983;26:1181–6.

[20] Urowitz MB, Gladman DD, Farewell VT, et al. Lupus and pregnancy studies. Arthritis Rheum 1993;36:1392–7.

[21] Bookman AAM, Urowitz MB, Koehler BE, et al. The bimodal pattern of mortality in systemic lupus erythematosus (SLE) [abstract]. J Rheumatol 1974;1:57.

[22] Urowitz MB, Bookman AAM, Koehler BE, et al. The bimodal mortality in systemic lupus erythematosus. Am J Med 1976;60:221–5.

[23] Rubin L, Urowitz MB, Gladman DD. Mortality in SLE. The bimodal pattern revisited. Q J Med 1985;55:87–98.

[24] Abu-Shakra M, Urowitz MB, Gladman DD, et al. Mortality studies in systemic lupus erythematosus. Results from a single centre. I. Causes of death. J Rheumatol 1995;22:1259–64.

[25] Bruce IN, Gladman DD, Urowitz MB. Premature atherosclerosis in SLE. Rheum Dis Clin North Am 2000;26:257–78.

[26] Urowitz MB, Ibáñez D, Gladman DD. Atherosclerotic vascular events (AVE) in a single large lupus cohort: prevalence and risk factors. Arthritis Rheum 2004;50(Suppl 9):S594.

[27] Urowitz MB, Gladman DD, Ibáñez I. Atherosclerotic vascular events in a risk factor study from a single center: prevalence and risk factors. Arthritis Rheum 2004;50(Suppl 9):S594.

[28] Urowitz MB, Gladman DD, Abu-Shakra M, et al. Mortality studies in systemic lupus erythematosus. Results from a single centre. III. Improved survival over 24 years. J Rheumatol 1997;24:1061–5.

[29] Tozman E, Urowitz MB, Gladman DD. Prolonged complete remission in SLE. Ann Rheum Dis 1982;41:39–40.

[30] Urowitz MB, Feletar M, Bruce IN, et al. Prolonged remission in systemic lupus erythematosus. J Rheumatol, in press.

[31] Gladman DD, Chaudhry-Ahluwalia V, Ibanez D, et al. Outcomes of symptomatic osteonecrosis in 95 patients with systemic lupus erythematosus. J Rheumatol 2001;28(10):2226–9.

[32] Gladman DD, Urowitz MB, Chaudhry-Ahluwalia V, et al. Predictive factors for symptomatic osteonecrosis in systemic lupus erythematosus. J Rheumatol 2001;28:761–5.

[33] Prasad R, Ibanez D, Gladman DD, et al. Corticosteroid dose in early SLE is a determining factor for avascular necrosis: a nested case control study of inception patients. Arthritis Rheum 2004;50:4090.

[34] Gladman DD, Urowitz MB, Cole E, et al. Kidney biopsy in SLE I: clinical–morphologic correlations. Q J Med 1989;73:1125–33.

[35] Rahman P, Gladman DD, Ibanez D, et al. Significance of isolated hematuria and isolated pyuria in systemic lupus erythematosus. Lupus 2001;10:418–23.

[36] McLaughlin J, Gladman DD, Urowitz MB, et al. Renal biopsy in SLE. II: Survival analyses according to biopsy results. Arthritis Rheum 1991;34:1268–73.

[37] McLaughlin JR, Bombardier CB, Farewell VT, et al. Kidney biopsy in systemic lupus erythematosus. III. Survival analysis controlling for clinical and laboratory variables. Arthritis Rheum 1994;37:559–67.

[38] Bajaj S, Albert L, Gladman DD, et al. Serial renal biopsy in systemic lupus erythematosus. J Rheumatol 2000;27:2822–6.

[39] Bruce IN, Gladman DD, Urowitz MB. Factors associated with refractory renal disease in patients with SLE: the role of patient nonadherence. Arthritis Care Res 2000;13:406–8.

[40] Bruto V, Urowitz MB, Gladman DD, et al. Neurocognitive abnormalities in offspring of mothers with SLE. Arthritis Rheum 2003;48(Suppl 9):S182.

[41] Gladman DD, Urowitz MB, Keystone EC. Serologically active clinically quiescent SLE— a discordance between clinical and serological features of SLE. Am J Med 1979;66:210–5.

[42] Walz-Leblanc B, Gladman DD, Urowitz MB, et al. Serologically active clinically quiescent SLE. J Rheumatol 1994;21:2239–41.

[43] Gladman DD, Hirani N, Ibañez D, et al. Clinically active serologically quiescent (CASQ) SLE. J Rheumatol 2003;30:1960–2.

[44] Kreidstein SH, Urowitz MB, Gladman DD, et al. Hormone replacement therapy in SLE. J Rheumatol 1997;24:2149–52.

[45] Lockshin MD, Reinitz E, Druzin ML, et al. Lupus pregnancy. Case control prospective study demonstrating absence of lupus exacerbation during or after pregnancy. Am J Med 1984;77: 893–8.

[46] Urowitz MB, Ibanez D. All SLICC members. Systemic Lupus International Collaborating Clinics (SLICC) inception cohort registry to study risk factors for atherosclerosis. Arthritis Rheum 2004;50(Suppl 9):S594.

[47] Drenkard C, Villa AR, Garcia-Padilla C, et al. Remission of systemic lupus erythematosus. Medicine (Baltimore) 1996;75:88–98.

[48] Golbus J, McCune WJ. Lupus nephritis. Classification, prognosis, immunopathogenesis, and treatment. Rheum Dis Clin North Am 1994;20:213–42.

[49] Denburg SD, Denburg JA, Carbotte RM, et al. Cognitive deficits in systemic lupus erythematosus. Rheum Dis Clin North Am 1993;19:815–31.

[50] Hanly JG, Fisk JD, Sherwood G, et al. Clinical course of cognitive dysfunction in systemic lupus erythematosus. J Rheumatol 1994;21(10):1825–31.

[51] Schur PH, Sandson J. Immunologic factors and clinical activity in lupus erythematosus. N Engl J Med 1968;278:533–8.

[52] Lightfoot Jr RW, Hughes GRV. Significance of persisting serologic abnormalities in SLE. Arthritis Rheum 1976;19:837–43.
[53] Ter Borg EJ, Horst G, Hummel EJ, et al. Measurement of increases in anti-double-stranded DNA antibody levels as a predictor of disease exacerbation in systemic lupus erythematosus: a long-term, prospective study. Arthritis Rheum 1990;33:624–43.

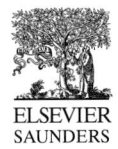

RHEUMATIC
DISEASE CLINICS
OF NORTH AMERICA

ELSEVIER
SAUNDERS

Rheum Dis Clin N Am 31 (2005) 223–244

# Genetics of Systemic Lupus Erythematosus: How Far Have We Come?

Andrea L. Sestak, MD, PhD[a],*, Swapan K. Nath, PhD[a],
John B. Harley, MD, PhD[b,c]

[a]Department of Arthritis and Immunology, Oklahoma Medical Research Foundation,
825 South 13th Street, MS 24, Oklahoma City, OK 73003, USA
[b]Department of Medicine, University of Oklahoma Health Sciences Center,
Oklahoma City, OK 73003, USA
[c]United States Department of Veterans Affairs Medical Center, Oklahoma City, OK, USA

Systemic lupus erythematosus (SLE) is a complex autoimmune disorder characterized by production of autoantibodies and tissue deposition of immune complexes. Evidence of a genetic component arises from the observation of familial clustering [1] and increased concordance in monozygotic twins (greater than 20%) compared with dizygotic twins and other full siblings (2%–5%) [2,3]. The search for genes predisposing to complex traits, like SLE, can be divided into two broad strategies: the hypothesis-driven candidate gene association analysis and genome-wide linkage studies. Association studies usually target a single gene, chosen at the investigator's discretion from over 25,000 known. The frequency of a genetic variant usually is tested in sets of cases and matched controls, and the evidence for association comes in the form of a significant difference in allele or genotype frequency. This evidence is strengthened tremendously if the finding can be repeated in an independent set of samples. The polymorphism causing genetic association with a candidate gene may identify

Supported by the US Department of Veterans Affairs and the National Institutes of Health (AR49272, AR048928, AI24717, AR42460, AR12253, AR049084, RR020143, RR015577, AI31584, AR48940, AI54117, AI053747, DE15223, and RR14467), an unrestricted educational grant from Abbott Laboratories, and by the Mary Kirkland Foundation.

* Corresponding author.
E-mail address: sestaka@omrf.ouhsc.edu (A.L. Sestak).

doi:10.1016/j.rdc.2005.01.005                          *rheumatic.theclinics.com*

the actual disease-causing gene, although often it instead is a marker very close (in genomic terms) to the responsible gene.

Linkage, the first step in reverse genetics, is fundamentally a statistical process testing for the coinheritance of genetic markers (such as DNA polymorphisms) with the disease phenotype in families with multiple affected members. Consistent coinheritance of the marker with the disease in many families indicates that it is in close proximity to the actual disease gene, and may be linked. Linkage studies use a set of markers to take an overview of the entire genome, and follow-up studies then try to define the peak regions and narrow them down to a single gene. Results of recent work in linkage and association will be discussed in this article.

## Genome-wide linkage studies in systemic lupus erythematosus

*Study design*

There are several different study designs with variable ascertainment approaches that have been used for genome-wide scanning to identify novel susceptibility loci for SLE. Study designs may involve sibling pairs, which may or may not have parents available, or small and large pedigrees with several generations. There are several genome scans by the four major scientific groups (located in California, Oklahoma, Minnesota, and Sweden), revealing many loci spread across the genome.

## Need for replication and confirmation

Replication of initial linkage signals from independent samples is an important and crucial step toward distinguishing between the true positive effects and the false-positive results [4]. The basis of all scientific research is hypothesis testing and validation of results by independent researchers. Independent replication is viewed typically as the sine qua non for accepting a hypothesis. Despite some recent successes for locating the genes in complex diseases, however, large studies of complex diseases have been difficult to replicate, especially, when genetic effects are weak and possibly context-dependent (eg, incidence may vary by sex, ethnicity, or precision of diagnosis), even with a reasonably large sample [5,6]. A recent review of the linkage findings of 31 complex human diseases based on whole genome scan concluded that genetic localization of most susceptibility loci is still imprecise and difficult to replicate [7]. This is caused in part by the inability to measure the precise underlying phenotype, low power from inadequate sample sizes, genetic heterogeneity, inaccurate genetic model, and statistical methods employed in analysis.

## Major systemic lupus erythematosus linkage findings

At least 30 different genomic locations have been identified with various degrees of significance using Lander-Kruglyak criteria [4]. Not surprisingly, linkages to many loci ordinarily are not replicated across different population groups and study sites [8,9]. Among the identified linkages, there are 8 SLE susceptibility regions that also have been replicated independently using lupus phenotype only. These are 1q23, 2q34, 2q37, 4p16, 6p21, 11p13, 12q24, and 16q13 [8–35]. An example of a linkage that is established [21] and confirmed [22,23] is the effect at 4p16, which is linked to SLE in European Americans and is shown in Fig. 1. All such key regions identified by at least two independent groups of pedigrees are summarized in Table 1. Each of the linkages is detected best in families from a single ethnicity or racial group. Some of these linked regions also were linked in other autoimmune diseases, suggesting that the same genes can be involved in related disorders. Three genes are identified in linkage intervals and are thought to explain the linkages: MHC-DR in 6p21 [26], FcγRIIA and FcγRIIIA for 1q23 [11–15], and PDCD-1 in 2q37 [18–20].

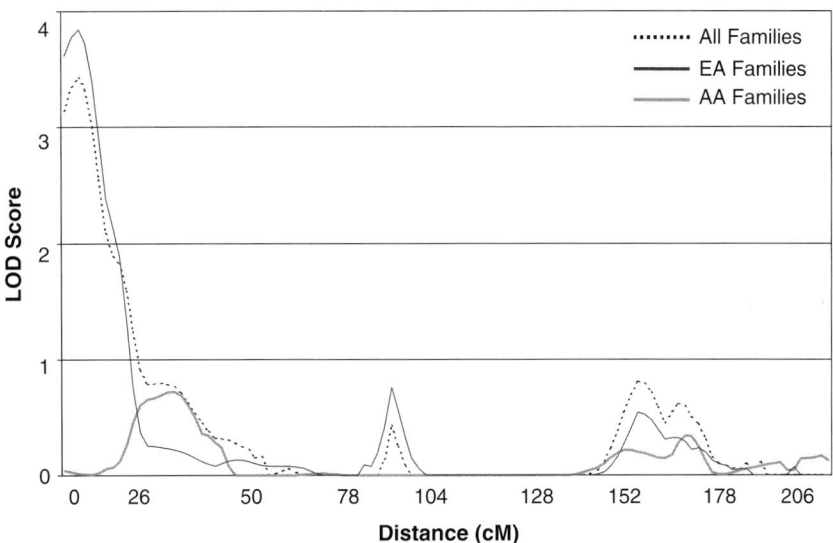

Fig. 1. Evidence of linkage at 4p16. The logarithm of the odd (LOD) scores were calculated for a genome-wide scan of 120 multiplex SLE pedigrees using the affected relative pair (ARP) method. A peak of 3.84 was found in European-American families on chromosome 4, between 0 and 26 centiMorgans. Although the linkage is still strong when all families are considered together (LOD = 3.44), African-American pedigrees make a minimal contribution at this locus. This linkage was confirmed in a second cohort containing 76 European-American multiplex pedigrees, with LOD = 2.3 at the same peak marker, D4s3007. (*Adapted from* Gray-McGuire C, Moser KL, Gaffney PM, et al. Genome scan of human systemic lupus erythematosus by regression modeling: evidence of linkage and epistasis at 4p16-15.2. Am J Hum Genet 2000;67(6):1460–9; with permission.)

Table 1
Confirmed linkage regions in systemic lupus erythematosus

| Cytogenetic location | Investigators | Study type | Associated gene | Population (stratification)[a] | Ref. |
|---|---|---|---|---|---|
| 1q23 | OK | Extended pedigrees | FcγRIIA, FcγRIIIA | AA, EA | [10–15] |
| 2q34 | OK | Extended pedigrees | — | AA (nephritis) | [16,17] |
| 2q37 | UU | Extended pedigrees | PDCD-1 | EM | [18–20] |
| 4p16 | OK | Extended pedigrees | — | EA | [21–23] |
| 5p15 | OK | Extended pedigrees | — | EA, AA, HIS (multiplex RA) | [24,25] |
| 6p11–p21 | MN | Sib-pairs, simplex | HLA-DR | EA | [26] |
| 10q22 | OK | Extended pedigrees | — | EA (nephritis) | [16,17] |
| 11q14 | OK | Extended pedigrees | — | AA (hemolytic anemia) | [27,28] |
| 12q24 | OK | Extended pedigrees | — | HIS EA | [29] |
| 16q13 | MN OK SU | Sib-pairs, extended pedigrees, trios | OAZ | EA, AA, HIS, Ch | [30–33] |
| 17p12–q11 | OK | Extended pedigrees | — | EA (vitiligo), Arg | [34,35] |

*Abbreviations:* AA, African-American; Arg, Argentine; Ch; Chinese; EA, European-American; EM, European-Mexican; HIS, Hispanic; MN, University of Minnesota; OK, Oklahoma Medical Research Foundation; SU, Shanghai Second Medical University; UU, Uppsala University.

[a] Stratification criteria are presented in parenthesis. Multiplex RA families had at least two members who were once told by a physician that they had RA.

Each of these candidate genes embraces some degree of uncertainty or controversy, however.

## Sources of complexity in systemic lupus erythematosus and probable solution for finding linkage

Systemic lupus erythematosus is a complex or polygenic autoimmune disease. Similar to studying other complex diseases, genome scans for SLE susceptibility genes suffer from low power to detect the small true-positive linkage effects. Causes of this include relatively small study populations, effects that are small in magnitude, and common causative alleles with low penetrance. These problems are compounded by the genetic heterogeneity of the phenotype, as suggested by the varied clinical manifestations. It is theoretically possible, for example, for two affected individuals to have completely different sets of criteria fulfilled. The authors suspect that multiple disease pathways exist in lupus, each of which may be caused in part by a distinct set of genes, and that understanding the genetic of lupus will be like peeling an onion, with each new layer of genetic understanding revealing another new level of genetic interaction and complexity.

Identifying genes that tend to be shared by family members—particularly by affected individuals—is a means of identifying genetically homogeneous subgroups of families. One method for improving the homogeneity of a sample is to separate multiplex families into subgroups that increase the homogeneity of the phenotype (eg, by a common clinical covariate). The rationale behind this method of grouping of families is to achieve a sample of families with a high degree of genetic and clinical homogeneity. Stratification by clinical symptoms could lead to increased power to detect linkage if phenotypic heterogeneity is the result of genetic heterogeneity [36–39]. Repeatedly testing subgroups, however, is likely to generate false-positive results. For this reason, confirmation in an independent group with the same stratification criteria is important.

## Major findings using pedigree stratification approach

This approach has been applied successfully to the Oklahoma collection. Linkage to 10q22.3 (SLEN1) and 2q34–q35 (SLEN2) was detected and confirmed in families with at least one SLE affected with renal involvement [16,17]. A linkage at 11p15.3 (SLEN3) was detected in pedigrees multiplex for SLE with nephritis, but this has not been confirmed. A possible SLE susceptibility gene SLER1 was identified at 5p15.3 in families with European American origin, in which at least two members reported rheumatoid arthritis (RA) [24]. The SLER1 has been confirmed in 88 additional pedigrees [25]. Previously, this region also was found to be in epitasis with SLEB3 at 4p15 [21]. Another SLE susceptibility locus, SLEH1, was detected at 11q14 to be linked in pedigrees with at least one SLE patient with hemolytic anemia [27]. This was confirmed later [28].

## Effect of stratification

Type-I errors are more likely to increase in the stratification-based analysis because more possibilities are tested. Moreover, the testing of several different parametric models (based on different penetrances), along with one or more nonparametric models further increase the likelihood of finding a false-positive result. This is a case of multiple testing problems, where many partially dependent tests were performed. A simulation-based approach may be applied to assess the significance of any linkage findings from subsets of stratified pedigrees. In this case, sets of $n$ pedigrees were randomly selected from the total available pedigrees 10,000 times (sampling with replacement). The logarithm of the odd (LOD) score was calculated at the peak marker for each sampling to determine an empirical distribution of the 10,000 LOD scores for the subset size $n$. Therefore, this gives the empirical $P$ value for $n$ initially selected pedigrees from the observed LOD score distribution. A similar approach was taken with the linkages at 5p15.3 and 11q14, with pedigrees stratified by RA and hemolytic anemia, respectively [24,27].

The following evidence demonstrates another example of finding a linkage using the pedigree stratification approach. The authors reported a SLE susceptibility locus, SLEV1, on 17p13 [34]. Linkage was found from the genome scan using 16 families multiplex for SLE, where at least one SLE patient also was reported to have vitiligo. Vitiligo is an autoimmune dermatologic disorder characterized by characteristic patches of cutaneous hypopigmentation [35]. This locus had remained undetected until the authors stratified the SLE families for the presence of at least one vitiligo case. The stratification of these few SLE families is thought to have increased genetic homogeneity, making SLEV1 detectable in these families.

Spritz et al [36] subsequently performed a genome scan for searching vitiligo susceptibility gene in multiplex vitiligo families. Along with two other susceptibility loci, they found significant evidence of linkage at 7p13, confirming SLEV1. Furthermore, they showed that the SLEV1 was concentrated in families stratified by other (nonvitiligo) autoimmune diseases in family members. They suggest, therefore, that the linkage to SLEV1 in these families indicates that SLEV1 confers susceptibility to a broader range of autoimmune diseases.

Recently, Johansson et al [40] performed a genome scan for searching SLE susceptibility genes on multiplex families collected from Argentina and detected a significant evidence of linkage at 52.78 cM (17q11). They also found suggestive evidence of linkage to marker at 17p12, 14 cM from SLEV1. The evidence of linkage to this second marker was increased with the nonparametric model free linkage analysis. If the linkage to this region from the three independent studies [34,36,39,40] is not a false-positive result, (and with this level of replication the authors suspect that it must be a true positive linkage), then this must be an important candidate susceptibility region, which may contain one or more putative susceptibility genes for autoimmune disease.

## Association studies

The availability of high-throughput single nucleotide polymorphism (SNP) typing has enabled several investigators to explore the association of various candidate genes with SLE. The literature in this area, mostly in the form of single reports, has surged dramatically over the last 5 years. Some of these association studies were initiated based on linkage data and others on the basis of gene function or association in other diseases. Firm conclusions regarding the role of any single gene, however, are difficult to obtain. There are two major confounding variables: linkage disequilibrium and ethnic background. There is great interest in finding genetic risk factors, and data have been published on at least 30 different collections of SLE patients, some partially overlapping, all of varying sizes and ethnic backgrounds. Different strategies for matching controls, for defining clinical subtypes, and for analysis of the resulting data have made this literature particularly cumbersome and difficult to interpret. The authors suspect that the literature will be that much more complicated over the next decade, before the robust effects can be identified.

## Association work related to linkage results: 6p21 and major histocompatibility

Linkage disequilibrium is most obviously a confounding factor in studies of genes in the major histocompatibility (MHC) region. These would include not only the class I and II MHC proteins themselves but also minor histocompatibility antigens, tumor necrosis factor (TNF)-α and β, TAP1 and TAP2, and complement components C4 and C2. Not only are these genes in the same genomic neighborhood, but some haplotypes in this region (eg, the one containing DR3) also do not appear to recombine randomly as often as rules of inheritance would predict. This means that a phenomenon called linkage disequilibrium (LD), where the alleles at one locus tend to be transmitted with the alleles of another locus extend over a greater genomic distance than is usual. Additionally, all of these particular candidate genes have natural variants, each of which may be potentially important in autoimmune pathogenesis. To confound the issue even further, more than one variation at more than one gene may play a role in disease risk. Before work is completed, all of the variants of all of the genes will be studied, although the interpretation of these results likely will be complicated. Although work in the MHC region began long before the first genome scan, and indeed, MHC associations in families who have SLE were appreciated in the early 1970s [41], it is gratifying that the linkage in this region was confirmed [26].

The only known single-gene mutations that cause SLE are in the early components of the complement family, and two members of this family are located in the MHC region, C2 and C4, making them obvious targets for investigation. The most common single-gene deficiency in SLE patients is for complement component C2 [42]. It has been estimated that C2 deficiency occurs in 1 out of 10,000 individuals [43] and that nearly one-third of the deficient patients will develop SLE [44]. Two studies have concluded that MHC genes are not responsible for the phenotype in C2-deficient patients [45,46], but the mild phenotype and female predominance are likely caused by other genetic influences that remain to be explained.

There are two homologs of the C4 gene in the MHC region, C4A and C4B. Deficiency of all four alleles (both copies of C4A and C4B) has been shown to cause severe SLE and susceptibility to infection [36], but this condition is quite rare [32]. Deletion of only the C4A allele (also known as C4A*Q0, or C4 null) has been associated with disease risk [47], but C4A*Q0 is in linkage disequilibrium with DR3 [48], an MHC haplotype strongly associated with autoantibody production and SLE in its own right [8].

Several other genes of potential functional importance in autoimmunity also lie within the MHC region. TNF-β has been studied less well than some candidates, but the results are positive to date [49–52]. The relationship to MHC is unclear, however, since a Chinese group found no relationship to MHC type [49]; a Korean group found association with DR2 [50], and a larger German study determined that TNF-β was a risk factor but only when added to a haplotype containing DR3 [51]. There also has been some interest in the transporters of antigen processing (TAP) genes in this region, but the results are mostly negative [53–56]. Although there was some association with disease in a Columbian cohort [57], MHC was not tested, and the only other positive study found association with DR3, also [58]. A British study involving whites and African-Caribbeans determined that most of the TAP2 effect was mediated through linkage disequilibrium with DR3, and that association with disease in these two ethnic groups was weak and with the opposite alleles [56], increasing the likelihood that these findings are an artifact.

The −308A variant of TNF-α (also known as TNF2) has been the subject of dozens of studies, but the ultimate role of this mutation remains unclear. Part of the difficulty in interpretation lies in the linkage disequilibrium of this variant with HLA-B8, C4A*Q0, DR3 [59]. Because these variants tend to be inherited as a unit, researchers can argue that any of the variants are causative of disease. Of course, it is possible that they are all correct, and a combination of effects could be the true risk factor. In summary, although it is clear that there are multiple strong genetic influences on disease emanating from the MHC region, it remains to be established how many genes are involved, how they act, and which ones they are beyond HLA-DR2 and complete deficiencies of C4 and C2.

## Association work arising from other linkages

The search for genes in the 1q23 linkage interval [10,11] has led to an interest in the receptors for immunoglobulin that are encoded there. There are three distinct but closely related classes of FcγR in people: FcγRI (CD64), FcγRII (CD32), and FcγRIII (CD16). They have different affinities for IgG and its subclasses. Most are stimulatory (eg, FcγRIIA, FcγRIIIA, FcγRIIIB, and FcγRIIC), while at least one is inhibitory (FcγRIIB). Those encoded on 1q23 include FcγRIIA, FcγRIIB, FcγRIIIA, and FcγRIIIB. The Arginine variant at amino acid position 131 of FcγRIIA (or R131) is associated with SLE, particularly in African Americans [12], while FcγRIIIA-F176 is associated with SLE in European-derived peoples and other ethnic groups [11]. A gene–dose effect with FcγRIIA-R131 for the risk of SLE also was identified in a meta-analysis [13], with the risk of SLE increasing with the number of R alleles (RR > RH > HH). The data are also convincing that FcγRIIIA-F176 is a risk factor for lupus nephritis [14].

Of all of the known and confirmed genetic linkages in SLE, PDCD-1 was the first gene that was identified by using the reverse genetic approach [18]. The PDCD-1 association is presumed to explain the 2q37 linkage found in Scandinavian pedigrees. This association is found in European-derived peoples and has been replicated [19]. This association does not appear to be present in

African Americans. A confirmatory study has found association in PDCD-1 in Spanish cases of lupus, but with an inverted allele distribution [20]. This is an extremely confounding result. A weak explanation for the contradiction has been offered, that a combination of a crossover and linkage disequilibrium operates between the marker and the causative polymorphism to generate this result. Evidence for this has not been generated.

An association with poly-ADP-ribose polymerase (PARP) in 124 US families of varying ethnic backgrounds was presented as an explanation for the 1q41–q42 linkage [60,61]. This finding could not be confirmed in a cohort of 171 French white cases and controls [62] or in a consortium of groups who combined their collections to explore this polymorphism [63].

The best evidence for association in the 16q12–q13 region linked to SLE in the Chinese is in OAZ [24], a zinc-finger protein implicated in signal transduction, but this result remains unconfirmed. Studies in the mouse indicate that OAZ and PARP interact in the TGF-$\beta$ (transforming growth factor-$\beta$) response pathway [64].

## Association testing based on gene function

### Complement

Because many SLE patients have low levels of circulating complement, genes in the complement family are obvious candidates for causing disease. With seeming paradox, deficiencies of the early components of the complement pathway lead to autoimmune disease [42]. Perhaps the most powerful single gene deficiency associated with SLE is C1q, which unlike C2 and C4, is located outside of the HLA antigen linkage region. In a study of Turkish kindreds, over 90% of homozygous C1q–deficient patients developed a severe SLE phenotype at an early age, although there are only about 40 known cases [65].

Mannose binding lectin (MBL) has a similar function to C1q in the alternate pathway for complement activation, making C1q a logical target for further investigation. The contribution to the risk of SLE by the genetic variance at MBL is small. Although there are no known patients completely deficient for MBL, a common polymorphism found in most ethnic groups is associated with decreased circulating levels of MBL [66]. As of this writing, there are 15 published studies on MBL in SLE; roughly half show association. Overall, meta-analysis favors a role for polymorphisms that impair production of MBL in increased disease risk across all ethnic groups (Young Ho Lee, PhD, unpublished data, 2004).

### Interleukins

As with other candidate genes, reports of associations in the interleukin (IL) family are scattered and varied. There have been mixed reports on the effects of

Table 2
Interleukins and related genes in association with systemic lupus erythematosus

| Gene | Population of origin | [Ref.] Supporting association | Against association |
|------|---------------------|------------------------------|---------------------|
| IL1RA | White | [69,70] | [50–52] |
| — | Asian | [68] | — |
| — | Mixed American | [67] | — |
| IL4 | Asian | — | [83] |
| IL4R | Asian | [83] | — |
| IL6 | White | [84] | [85] |
| IL8 | African-American | [82] | — |
| IL10 | White | [71,76,77] | [78] |
| — | African-American | [74] | — |
| — | Mexican or Mexican-American | [75] | [79] |
| — | Asian | — | [80] |

*Abbreviations:* IL1RA, IL-1 receptor antagonist; IL4R, IL-4 receptor.

polymorphisms in the IL-1 receptor antagonist, with four positive [67–70] and three negative reports [71–73], mostly in European-derived populations from various regions. Unfortunately, no firm conclusions can be drawn (Table 2).

Work on the IL-10 gene SNPs seems more promising, with most reports in support of an effect [74–80]. Meta-analysis supports a strong linkage in this region, particularly in European-derived populations [77]. Indeed, IL-10 has been reported to be elevated in the first-degree relatives of SLE patients [81]. Final confirmation of this association and the mechanism of action for IL-10 alleles remain to be determined.

Single reports of an IL-8 risk allele in African Americans and [82] and an IL-4 receptor risk haplotype in the Japanese [83] remain to be confirmed. Mini-satellites in the promoter region of IL-6 have been associated with disease in one US collection and may lead to increased production of IL-6 [84]. A German population tested −176GC, another IL-6 promoter polymorphism, and found no association with disease [85], but this mutation was not associated significantly in the United States study, either [84]. IL-6 continues to hold potential as a risk factor.

*Other cytokines and receptors*

High levels of interferon-γ (IFN-γ) are produced by peripheral blood mononuclear cells (PBMCs) from patients with active SLE [86]. In one study of IFN-γ, a CA repeat in the first intron was not associated with disease [87]. The Val14Met variant of the IFN-γ receptor 1 has been associated with disease in a Japanese population, and cells bearing this variant did not upregulate HLA-DR to the same extent [88]. This functional shift toward Th2 cells may be significant in disease pathogenesis, but the finding remains to be confirmed. In this same population, a mutation in the IFN-γ receptor 2 acted synergistically with Val14Met to increase risk of SLE [89]. The M196R mutation in RNFRII, which is a

receptor for TNF-α, has been shown to cause increased IL-6 production following TNF-α stimulation [90]. Following the initial positive report of association
of 196R with SLE in 105 Japanese patients [90], this association was unconfirmed in several subsequent studies, including one in a Japanese group [91].

*Genes related to apoptosis*

In some animal models of autoimmune disease, impairment of apoptosis leads
to proliferation of autoreactive cells and promotion of disease [92]. The most
obvious correlation of animal models and human SLE is the Fas/FasL system,
which is defective in the MRL/lpr mouse [93] and in the human disease autoimmune lymphoproliferative syndrome, ALPS [94,95]. In general, however, Fas
polymorphisms are not associated with SLE [96,97]. Polymorphisms of the Fas
ligand are rare, race-specific, and only weakly associated with disease [98,99].

An association with Bcl-2 was found in the Chinese [100] and in Mexican
Americans [101], but it was unconfirmed in three other studies [71,101,102].
There are single reports of APRIL [103] and BLyS [104] associated with SLE
in Japanese subjects, but these also are unconfirmed. A rare mutation of DNaseI
was found in a Japanese SLE pedigree [105] but was not demonstrated in a
subsequent population study [106].

*Other immune system genes*

CTLA4 has been examined by many groups because it was associated with
increased risk of autoimmune thyroid disease and diabetes [107]. SLE subjects
have higher levels of soluble CTLA4 than controls, but the mechanism behind
this increase is unknown [108]. Most published studies looking for association
of SLE with a particular CTLA4 genotype are negative [71,75,108–112], and
even the four positive studies do not agree on a causative mutation [98–101].
Japanese [113] and Slovakian cohorts [114] were found to associate disease with
the +49G/G variant. Studies of a Korean cohort found association of disease
with the −1722 TT genotype [115] but not with the +49 or two other variants.
A Spanish group confirmed association with the −1722 genotype but found that
the T allele was instead protective for disease [116]. Clearly, more work remains
to be done to define the genetic effects of CTLA-4.

Of the remaining immune system genes, C-reactive protein (CRP) is perhaps
the most promising. In a study of 586 British families, promoter polymorphisms were found to correlate with the lower basal levels of CRP associated
with SLE, and with antinuclear antibody production and disease risk [117]. The
number of CA repeats in the 3'UTR of CD40 ligand was found to correlate
with disease risk in a Spanish cohort [118], but this finding has not been
replicated in a second population.

Other unconfirmed associations are with Ro/SSA1 in African Americans [119]
and osteopontin [120]. A CD19 polymorphism causing decreased transcription
has been associated with SLE in the Japanese [121] but was not confirmed in

an Italian cohort [71]. Three studies have failed to find correlation with MCP1 [122–124], although one of them found increased incidence of the AA allele in lupus nephritis [124]. Additional unconfirmed immune system genes associated with SLE include T-cell receptors $\alpha$ [125], $\beta$ [126], and $\zeta$ [127], and the immunoglobulin heavy and light chains [128–131].

*Hormones and receptors*

Given the preponderance of SLE in women, hormones are thought to play an important role in disease risk. Estrogen receptor polymorphisms were not found to be associated with disease in two studies, the first in 40 Greek subjects [132] and the second in 245 Chinese subjects [133]. Conflicting results have been put forth for prolactin, which was associated with SLE in a British study [134] but was not confirmed in an Italian cohort [135]. To date, there is no strong genetic association to explain the gender bias in SLE.

The vitamin D receptor genotype has been studied in two small Asian groups, but again with conflicting results. Ozaki first reported association of the BsmI RFLP with SLE and increased risk of nephritis in Japanese subjects [136]. Huang initially confirmed this association with SLE in 47 Chinese subjects [137] but later reported no association with a second mutation in the vitamin D receptor (at FokI) in a slightly larger overlapping group of 52 [138].

*Enzymes*

Naturally occurring variants in metabolic enzymes have been proposed to play a role in risk of SLE. Perhaps the effects of certain environmental triggers (such as UV exposure, medications, or hair dyes) might be enhanced in individuals carrying such variants. The evidence supporting this contention is limited. For example, glutathione S-transferase null alleles have been found in three different ethnic groups, but despite an association with autoantibody production [139], they are not associated with risk of SLE [140]. Mixed evidence exists for nitric oxide synthetase 2, which was associated in an African-American cohort [141] but was not confirmed in a Spanish study [142]. A deletion of 21-hydroxylase is part of an extended haplotype containing C4 null, HLA-B8, and HLA-DR3; consequently, one cannot be certain which, if any, of these variations is responsible for the increased risk [143]. The slow acetylator NAT2 phenotype, which causes impaired metabolism of hydralazine and other drugs, has been implicated in a German cohort of 106 subjects [144], but excluded as a risk factor for SLE in two larger white cohorts (209 [145] and 243 cases [146]).

Angiotensin-converting enzyme (ACE) also has been studied widely in SLE, but again, the results are mixed. One of the largest studies, involving 644 subjects and their parents in a transmission disequilibrium design (TDT), concluded that the ID genotype was associated with SLE in European Americans and that another variant (CT) was associated with nephritis in non-whites [147].

Two other studies of European-derived subjects found increased incidence of DD in disease [148,149], but the authors' work [150] and an Israeli study [151] found no association. DD has been reported to be lower than expected in African Americans who have SLE [152]. In three Asian populations, there was no association with SLE risk [153–155], but the D allele was protective for renal disease in Japanese and Chinese populations [153,154]. Perhaps further studies will reveal interacting genes that explain these findings.

Enzymes of the clotting cascade have been examined for their role in risk of thrombotic complications of SLE. Although there is a single case report of a prothrombin variant in a lupus patient with a deep vein thrombosis, a sibling homozygous for the same mutation had no autoimmune disease [156]. Two Chinese groups found an association of the 4G/5G variant of plasminogen activator inhibitor-1 with nephritis risk, although neither group found a significant difference between SLE subjects and controls [157,158]. No association of PAI-1 with SLE was found in a Spanish cohort, nor was there any correlation with the antiphospholipid (APL) syndrome or risk of thrombosis [159]. Platelet GPIIb/IIIb polymorphisms were associated weakly with APL in two cohorts without increasing risk of thrombosis appreciably [160]. To date, there is no strong genetic association to explain either APL or thrombosis risk.

**Summary**

Work on the genetic components of SLE is an evolving area of active scientific inquiry. Over the last 10 years, considerable progress has been made, defining several linkage regions that contain risk genes and discovering several genetic associations. Work will continue to identify the polymorphisms and risk haplotypes within these linkage regions. No doubt, many more cohorts of cases and controls will be examined for polymorphisms in genes of functional interest. Very soon the community of investigators performing this work will identify more of these risk alleles and move into cross-typing of subject cohorts. The most exhilarating and frustrating aspects of this are bound to be the many attempts to confirm and correlate genetic associations found in other groups. Defining the robust and reproducible association is an indispensable and necessary first step toward integrated model building. It has been appreciated for some time now that no single gene will be strongly predictive of disease risk in SLE, but it remains entirely unknown how the many SLE risk genes must interact to produce an immune system predisposed to self-destruction in this particularly pernicious way. A simple additive model where multiple risk-associated genetic polymorphisms lead to an accumulation of risk may not be sufficient to explain the genetic interactions at work, and only concerted efforts to refine the currently conflicting data can resolve the nature of these genetic interactions. It is not only possible but in fact likely that some genes will associate with SLE only in the context of other genes. Although geographic origins and ethnic identification only roughly reflect the actions of those other genes, they are apparently required temporary way stations on the progression toward a comprehensive description of the genetic architecture of SLE. Out of this growing pile of puzzle pieces understanding of the nature of the genetic forces at work in this autoimmune disease will improve progressively.

## Addendum

This is a rapidly advancing field, so it should not be a surprise that over a dozen new genetic associations have been published since manuscript submission. These important new papers include studies of large samples for polymorphisms in PTPN22 [161] and TYK2 and IRF5 [162] that await further confirmation. TYK2 is of particular interest, as it lies within a previously established region of linkage at 19p13 with European-American pedigrees stratified by anti-dsDNA [163].

## References

[1] Sestak AL, Shaver TS, Moser KL, et al. Familial aggregation of lupus and autoimmunity in an unusual multiplex pedigree. J Rheumatol 1999;26(7):1495–9.

[2] Deapen D, Escalante A, Weinrib L, et al. A revised estimate of twin concordance in systemic lupus erythematosus. Arthritis Rheum 1992;35(3):311–8.

[3] Reichlin M, Harley JB, Lockshin MD. Serologic studies of monozygotic twins with systemic lupus erythematosus. Arthritis Rheum 1992;35(4):457–64.

[4] Lander E, Kruglyak L. Genetic dissection of complex traits: guidelines for interpreting and reporting linkage results. Nat Genet 1995;11(3):241–7.

[5] Risch N, Merikangas K. The future of genetic studies of complex human diseases. Science 1996;273(5281):1516–7.

[6] Risch N. Searching for genes in complex diseases: lessons from systemic lupus erythematosus. J Clin Invest 2000;105(11):1503–6.

[7] Altmuller J, Palmer LJ, Fischer G, et al. Genome-wide scans of complex human diseases: true linkage is hard to find. Am J Hum Genet 2001;69:936–50.

[8] Kelly JA, Moser KL, Harley JB. The genetics of systemic lupus erythematosus: putting the pieces together. Genes Immun 2002;3(Suppl 1):S71–85.

[9] Tsao BP. The genetics of human systemic lupus erythematosus. Trends Immunol 2003;24(11): 595–602.

[10] Moser KL, Neas BR, Salmon JE, et al. Genome scan of human systemic lupus erythematosus: evidence for linkage on chromosome 1q in African-American pedigrees. Proc Natl Acad Sci U S A 1998;95(25):14869–74.

[11] Edberg JC, Langefeld CD, Wu J, et al. Genetic linkage and association of Fc gamma receptor IIIA (CD16A) on chromosome 1q23 with human systemic lupus erythematosus. Arthritis Rheum 2002;46(8):2132–40.

[12] Salmon JE, Millard S, Schachter LA, et al. Fc gamma RIIA alleles are heritable risk factors for lupus nephritis in African-Americans. J Clin Invest 1996;97(5):1348–54.

[13] Karassa FB, Trikalinos TA, Ioannidis JP. Role of the Fc gamma receptor IIa polymorphism in susceptibility to systemic lupus erythematosus and lupus nephritis: a meta-analysis. Arthritis Rheum 2002;46(6):1563–71.

[14] Karassa FB, Trikalinos TA, Ioannidis JP. The Fc gamma RIIIA-F158 allele is a risk factor for the development of lupus nephritis: a meta-analysis. Kidney Int 2003;63(4):1475–82.

[15] Magnusson V, Johanneson B, Lima G, et al. SLE Genetics Collaboration Group. Both risk alleles for Fc gamma RIIA and Fc gamma RIIIA are susceptibility factors for SLE: a unifying hypothesis. Genes Immun 2004;5(2):130–7.

[16] Quintero-del-Rio AI, Kelly JA, Kilpatrick J, et al. The genetics of systemic lupus erythematosus stratified by renal disease: linkage at 10q22.3 (SLEN1), 2q34–35 (SLEN2), and 11p15.6 (SLEN3). Genes Immun 2002;3(Suppl 1):S57–62.

[17] Quintero-del-Rio AI, Kelly JA, Garriott CP, et al. SLEN2 (2q34–35) and SLEN1 (10q22.3) replication in systemic lupus erythematosus stratified by nephritis. Am J Hum Genet 2004; 75:346–8.

[18] Prokunina L, Castillejo-Lopez C, Oberg F, et al. A regulatory polymorphism in PDCD1 is associated with susceptibility to systemic lupus erythematosus in humans. Nat Genet 2002; 32(4):666–9.

[19] Prokunina L, Gunnarsson I, Sturfelt G, et al. The systemic lupus erythematosus-associated PDCD1 polymorphism PD1.3A in lupus nephritis. Arthritis Rheum 2004;50(1):327–8.

[20] Lindqvist AK, Steinsson K, Johanneson B, et al. A susceptibility locus for human systemic lupus erythematosus (hSLE1) on chromosome 2q. J Autoimmun 2000;14(2):169–78.

[21] Gray-McGuire C, Moser KL, Gaffney PM, et al. Genome scan of human systemic lupus erythematosus by regression modeling: evidence of linkage and epitasis at 4p16–15.2. Am J Hum Genet 2000;67(6):1460–9.

[22] Kelly JA, Sestak AL, Kilpatrick J, et al. Confirmation of susceptibility loci at 1q22–23, 4p16–15 and 11p13 in pedigrees multiplex for systemic lupus erythematosus. Arthritis Rheum 2003;48:S225.

[23] Sestak AL, Kelly JA, Gray-McGuire C, et al. Confirmation of the 4p16 Linkage to SLE. Arthritis Rheum 2003;48:3648.

[24] Namjou B, Nath SK, Kilpatrick J, et al. Stratification of pedigrees multiplex for systemic lupus erythematosus and for self-reported rheumatoid arthritis detects a systemic lupus erythematosus susceptibility gene (SLER1) at 5p15.3. Arthritis Rheum 2002;46(11):2937–45.

[25] Nath SK, Namjou B, Garriott CP, et al. Linkage analysis of SLE susceptibility: confirmation of SLER1 at 5p15.3. Genes Immun 2004;5:209–14.

[26] Graham RR, Ortmann WA, Langefeld CD, et al. Visualizing human leukocyte antigen class II risk haplotypes in human systemic lupus erythematosus. Am J Hum Genet 2002;71(3):543–53.

[27] Kelly JA, Thompson K, Kilpatrick J, et al. Evidence for a susceptibility gene (SLEH1) on chromosome 11q14 for systemic lupus erythematosus (SLE) families with hemolytic anemia. Proc Natl Acad Sci U S A 2002;99(18):11766–71.

[28] Kelly JA, Shadfar S, Kaufman KM, et al. Confirmation and localization of SLEH1 on 11q14 in African-American pedigrees with hemolytic anemia and multiplex for SLE. Abstracts for Lupus 2004:S258.

[29] Nath SK, Quintero-Del-Rio AI, Kilpatrick J, et al. Linkage at 12q24 with systemic lupus erythematosus (SLE) is established and confirmed in Hispanic and European-American families. Am J Hum Genet 2004;74(1):73–82.

[30] Gaffney PM, Kearns GM, Shark KB, et al. A genome-wide search for susceptibility genes in human systemic lupus erythematosus sib-pair families. Proc Natl Acad Sci U S A 1998; 95(25):14875–9.

[31] Gaffney PM, Ortmann WA, Selby SA, et al. Genome screening in human systemic lupus erythematosus: results from a second Minnesota cohort and combined analyses of 187 sib-pair families. Am J Hum Genet 2000;66(2):547–56.

[32] Nath SK, Namjou B, Hutchings D, et al. Systemic lupus erythematosus (SLE) and chromosome 16: confirmation of linkage to 16q12–13 and evidence for genetic heterogeneity. Eur J Hum Genet 2004;12:668–72.

[33] Feng XB, Shen N, Chen SL, et al. Susceptibility gene of systemic lupus erythematosus in 16q12 in Chinese cohort. Zhonghua Yi Xue Yi Chuan Xue Za Zhi 2003;20(1):27–30.

[34] Nath SK, Kelly JA, Namjou B, et al. Evidence for a susceptibility gene, SLEV1, on chromosome 17p13 in families with vitiligo-related systemic lupus erythematosus. Am J Hum Genet 2001;69(6):1401–6.

[35] Halder RM, Nootheti PK. Ethnic skin disorders overview. J Am Acad Dermatol 2003; 48(Suppl 6):S143–8.

[36] Spritz RA, Gowan K, Bennett DC, et al. Novel vitiligo susceptibility loci on chromosomes 7 (AIS2) and 8 (AIS3), confirmation of SLEV1 on chromosome 17, and their roles in an autoimmune diathesis. Am J Hum Genet 2004;74(1):188–91.

[37] Kidd KK, Ott J. Power and sample size in linkage studies. Cytogenet Cell Genet 1984;37: 510–1.

[38] Ott J. Analysis of human genetic linkage. 3rd edition. Baltimore (MD): Johns Hopkins University Press; 1999.

[39] Leal SM, Ott J. Effects of stratification in the analysis of affected-sib-pair data: benefits and costs. Am J Hum Genet 2000;66:567–75.

[40] Johansson CM, Zunec R, Garcia MA, et al. Chromosome 17p12-q11 harbors susceptibility loci for systemic lupus erythematosus. Hum Genet 2004;115:230–8.

[41] Grumet FC, Coukell A, Bodmer JG, et al. Histocompatibility (HL-A) antigens associated with systemic lupus erythematosus. A possible genetic predisposition to disease. N Engl J Med 1971;285:193–6.

[42] Sullivan KE, Winkelstein JA. Genetically determined deficiencies of the complement system. In: Ochs H, Smith C, Puck J, editors. Primary immunodeficiency diseases: a molecular and genetic approach. New York: Oxford University Press; 1999. p. 397–416.

[43] Sullivan KE, Petri MA, Schmeckpeper BJ, et al. Prevalence of a mutation-causing C2 deficiency in systemic lupus erythematosus. J Rheumatol 1994;21(6):1128–33.

[44] Agnello V. Association of systemic lupus erythematosus and SLE-like syndromes with hereditary and acquired complement deficiency states. Arthritis Rheum 1978;21(Suppl 5):S146–52.

[45] Johnson CA, Densen P, Hurford Jr RK, et al. Type I human complement C2 deficiency. A 28-base pair gene deletion causes skipping of exon 6 during RNA splicing. J Biol Chem 1992;267(13):9347–53.

[46] Truedsson L, Alper CA, Awdeh ZL, et al. Characterization of type I complement C2 deficiency MHC haplotypes. Strong conservation of the complotype/HLA-B-region and absence of disease association due to linked class II genes. J Immunol 1993;151(10):5856–63.

[47] Hauptmann G, Tappeiner G, Schifferli JA. Inherited deficiency of the fourth component of human complement. Immunodefic Rev 1988;1(1):3–22.

[48] Hartung K, Baur MP, Coldewey R, et al. Major histocompatibility complex haplotypes and complement C4 alleles in systemic lupus erythematosus. Results of a multicenter study. J Clin Invest 1992;90(4):1346–51.

[49] Zhang J, Ai R, Chow F. The polymorphisms of HLA-DR and TNF B loci in northern Chinese Han nationality and susceptibility to systemic lupus erythematosus. Chin Med Sci J 1997;12(2): 107–10.

[50] Kim HY, Lee SH, Yang HI, et al. TNFB gene polymorphism in patients with systemic lupus erythematosus in Korean. Korean J Intern Med 1995;10(2):130–6.

[51] Bettinotti MP, Hartung K, Deicher H, et al. Polymorphism of the tumor necrosis factor β gene in systemic lupus erythematosus: TNFβ-MHC haplotypes. Immunogenetics 1993;37(6):449–54.

[52] Wang Y, Zhang Y, Zhu S. The association of susceptibility of SLE and the gene polymorphism of TNF. Zhonghua Yi Xue Za Zhi 1998;78(2):111–4.

[53] Kanagawa S, Morinobu A, Koshiba M, et al. Association of the TAP2*Bky2 allele with presence of SS-A/Ro and other autoantibodies in Japanese patients with systemic lupus erythematosus. Lupus 2003;12(4):258–65.

[54] Takeuchi F, Nakano K, Nabeta H, et al. Polymorphisms of the TAP1 and TAP2 transporter genes in Japanese SLE. Ann Rheum Dis 1996;55(12):924–6.

[55] Davies EJ, Donn RP, Hillarby MC, et al. Polymorphisms of the TAP2 transporter gene in systemic lupus erythematosus. Ann Rheum Dis 1994;53(1):61–3.

[56] Ocal L, Russell K, Beynon H, et al. Genetic analysis of TAP2 in systemic lupus erythematosus patients from two ethnic groups. Br J Rheumatol 1996;35(6):529–33.

[57] Correa PA, Molina JF, Pinto LF, et al. TAP1 and TAP2 polymorphisms analysis in northwestern Colombian patients with systemic lupus erythematosus. Ann Rheum Dis 2003;62(4):363–5.

[58] Martin-Villa JM, Martinez-Laso J, Moreno-Pelayo MA, et al. Differential contribution of HLA-DR, DQ, and TAP2 alleles to systemic lupus erythematosus susceptibility in Spanish patients: role of TAP2*01 alleles in Ro autoantibody production. Ann Rheum Dis 1998; 57(4):214–9.

[59] Wilson AG, Gordon C, di Giovine FS, et al. A genetic association between systemic lupus erythematosus and tumor necrosis factor alpha. Eur J Immunol 1994;24(1):191–5.

[60] Tsao BP, Cantor RM, Kalunian KC, et al. Evidence for linkage of a candidate chromosome 1 region to human systemic lupus erythematosus. J Clin Invest 1997;99(4):725–31.

[61] Tsao BP, Cantor RM, Grossman JM, et al. PARP alleles within the linked chromosomal region are associated with systemic lupus erythematosus. J Clin Invest 1999;103(8):1135–40.

[62] Delrieu O, Michel M, Frances C, et al. Poly(ADP-ribose) polymerase alleles in French Caucasians are associated neither with lupus nor with primary antiphospholipid syndrome. GRAID Research Group. Group for Research on Auto-Immune Disorders. Arthritis Rheum 1999;42(10):2194–7.

[63] Criswell LA, Moser KL, Gaffney PM, et al. PARP alleles and SLE: failure to confirm association with disease susceptibility. J Clin Invest 2000;105(11):1501–2.

[64] Ku MC, Stewart S, Hata A. Poly(ADP-ribose) polymerase 1 interacts with OAZ and regulates BMP-target genes. Biochem Biophys Res Commun 2003;311(3):702–7.

[65] Berkel AI, Birben E, Oner C, et al. Molecular, genetic and epidemiologic studies on selective complete C1q deficiency in Turkey. Immunobiology 2000;201:347–55.

[66] Crosdale DJ, Ollier WE, Thomson W, et al. Mannose binding lectin (MBL) genotype distributions with relation to serum levels in UK Caucasoids. Eur J Immunogenet 2000;27(3): 111–7.

[67] Parks CG, Cooper GS, Dooley MA, et al. Systemic lupus erythematosus and genetic variation in the interleukin 1 gene cluster: a population-based study in the southeastern United States. Ann Rheum Dis 2004;63(1):91–4.

[68] Huang CM, Wu MC, Wu JY, et al. Interleukin-1 receptor antagonist gene polymorphism in Chinese patients with systemic lupus erythematosus. Clin Rheumatol 2002;21(3):255–7.

[69] Tjernstrom F, Hellmer G, Nived O, et al. Synergetic effect between interleukin-1 receptor antagonist allele (IL1RN*2) and MHC class II (DR17,DQ2) in determining susceptibility to systemic lupus erythematosus. Lupus 1999;8(2):103–8.

[70] Blakemore AI, Tarlow JK, Cork MJ, et al. Interleukin-1 receptor antagonist gene polymorphism as a disease severity factor in systemic lupus erythematosus. Arthritis Rheum 1994; 37(9):1380–5.

[71] D'Alfonso S, Rampi M, Bocchio D, et al. Systemic lupus erythematosus candidate genes in the Italian population: evidence for a significant association with interleukin-10. Arthritis Rheum 2000;43(1):120–8.

[72] Heward J, Allahabadia A, Gordon C, et al. The interleukin-1 receptor antagonist gene shows no allelic association with three autoimmune diseases. Thyroid 1999;9(6):627–8.

[73] Danis VA, Millington M, Huang Q, et al. Lack of association between an interleukin-1 receptor antagonist gene polymorphism and systemic lupus erythematosus. Dis Markers 1995;12(2): 135–9.

[74] Gibson AW, Edberg JC, Wu J, et al. Novel single nucleotide polymorphisms in the distal IL-10 promoter affect IL-10 production and enhance the risk of systemic lupus erythematosus. J Immunol 2001;166(6):3915–22.

[75] Mehrian R, Quismorio Jr FP, Strassmann G, et al. Synergistic effect between IL-10 and bcl-2 genotypes in determining susceptibility to systemic lupus erythematosus. Arthritis Rheum 1998;41(4):596–602.

[76] Eskdale J, Wordsworth P, Bowman S, et al. Association between polymorphisms at the human IL-10 locus and systemic lupus erythematosus. Tissue Antigens 1997;49(6):635–9.

[77] D'Alfonso S, Giordano M, Mellai M, et al. Association tests with systemic lupus erythematosus (SLE) of IL-10 markers indicate a direct involvement of a CA repeat in the 5′ regulatory region. Genes Immun 2002;3(8):454–63.

[78] Crawley E, Woo P, Isenberg DA. Single nucleotide polymorphic haplotypes of the interleukin-10 5′ flanking region are not associated with renal disease or serology in Caucasian patients with systemic lupus erythematosus. Arthritis Rheum 1999;42(9):2017–8.

[79] Alarcon-Riquelme ME, Lindqvist AK, Jonasson I, et al. Genetic analysis of the contribution of IL10 to systemic lupus erythematosus. J Rheumatol 1999;26(10):2148–52.

[80] Mok CC, Lanchbury JS, Chan DW, et al. Interleukin-10 promoter polymorphisms in southern Chinese patients with systemic lupus erythematosus. Arthritis Rheum 1998;41(6):1090–5.

[81] Llorente L, Richaud-Patin Y, Couderc J, et al. Dysregulation of interleukin-10 production in relatives of patients with systemic lupus erythematosus. Arthritis Rheum 1997;40(8):1429–35.

[82] Rovin BH, Lu L, Zhang X. A novel interleukin-8 polymorphism is associated with severe systemic lupus erythematosus nephritis. Kidney Int 2002;62(1):261–5.

[83] Kanemitsu S, Takabayashi A, Sasaki Y, et al. Association of interleukin-4 receptor and interleukin-4 promoter gene polymorphisms with systemic lupus erythematosus. Arthritis Rheum 1999;42(6):1298–300.

[84] Linker-Israeli M, Wallace DJ, Prehn J, et al. Association of IL-6 gene alleles with systemic lupus erythematosus (SLE) and with elevated IL-6 expression. Genes Immun 1999;1(1):45–52.

[85] Schotte H, Schluter B, Rust S, et al. Interleukin-6 promoter polymorphism (–174 G/C) in Caucasian German patients with systemic lupus erythematosus. Rheumatology (Oxford) 2001;40(4):393–400.

[86] Csiszar A, Nagy G, Gergely P, et al. Increased interferon-gamma (IFN-gamma), IL-10 and decreased IL-4 mRNA expression in peripheral blood mononuclear cells (PBMC) from patients with systemic lupus erythematosus (SLE). Clin Exp Immunol 2000;122(3):464–70.

[87] Lee JY, Goldman D, Piliero LM, et al. Interferon-gamma polymorphisms in systemic lupus erythematosus. Genes Immun 2001;2(5):254–7.

[88] Tanaka Y, Nakashima H, Hisano C, et al. Association of the interferon-gamma receptor variant (Val14Met) with systemic lupus erythematosus. Immunogenetics 1999;49(4):266–71.

[89] Nakashima H, Inoue H, Akahoshi M, et al. The combination of polymorphisms within interferon-gamma receptor 1 and receptor 2 associated with the risk of systemic lupus erythematosus. FEBS Lett 1999;453:187–90.

[90] Morita C, Horiuchi T, Tsukamoto H, et al. Association of tumor necrosis factor receptor type II polymorphism 196R with systemic lupus erythematosus in the Japanese: molecular and functional analysis. Arthritis Rheum 2001;44(12):2819–27.

[91] Takahashi M, Hashimoto H, Akizuki M, et al. Lack of association between the Met196Arg polymorphism in the TNFR2 gene and autoimmune diseases accompanied by vasculitis including SLE in Japanese. Tissue Antigens 2001;57(1):66–9.

[92] Wakeland EK, Wandstrat AE, Liu K, et al. Genetic dissection of systemic lupus erythematosus. Curr Opin Immunol 1999;11(6):701–7.

[93] Nose M, Nishihara M, Kamogawa J, et al. Genetic basis of autoimmune disease in MRL/lpr mice: dissection of the complex pathological manifestations and their susceptibility loci. Rev Immunogenet 2000;2(1):154–64.

[94] Rieux-Laucat F, Le Deist F, Fischer A. Autoimmune lymphoproliferative syndromes: genetic defects of apoptosis pathways. Cell Death Differ 2003;10(1):124–33.

[95] Wu J, Wilson J, He J, et al. Fas ligand mutation in a patient with systemic lupus erythematosus and lymphoproliferative disease. J Clin Invest 1996;98(5):1107–13.

[96] Cascino I, Ballerini C, Audino S, et al. Fas gene polymorphisms are not associated with systemic lupus erythematosus, multiple sclerosis and HIV infection. Dis Markers 1998;13(4):221–5.

[97] Huang QR, Manolios N. Investigation of the -1377 polymorphism on the Apo-1/Fas promoter in systemic lupus erythematosus patients using allele-specific amplification. Pathology 2000;32(2):126–30.

[98] Wu J, Metz C, Xu X, et al. A novel polymorphic CAAT/enhancer-binding protein beta element in the FasL gene promoter alters Fas ligand expression: a candidate background gene in African-American systemic lupus erythematosus patients. J Immunol 2003;170(1):132–8.

[99]  Huang QR, Danis V, Lassere M, et al. Evaluation of a new Apo-1/Fas promoter polymorphism in rheumatoid arthritis and systemic lupus erythematosus patients. Rheumatology (Oxford) 1999;38(7):645–51.

[100] Wu H, Shen N, Gu Y, et al. Association between Bcl-2 gene polymorphism with systemic lupus erythematosus. Zhonghua Yi Xue Za Zhi 2002;82(7):467–70.

[101] Johansson C, Castillejo-Lopez C, Johanneson B, et al. Association analysis with microsatellite and SNP markers does not support the involvement of BCL-2 in systemic lupus erythematosus in Mexican and Swedish patients and their families. Genes Immun 2000;1(6):380–5.

[102] Huang QR, Morris D, Manolios N. Evaluation of the BCL-2 gene locus as a susceptibility locus linked to the clinical expression of systemic lupus erythematosus (SLE). Rheumatol Int 1996;16(3):121–4.

[103] Koyama T, Tsukamoto H, Masumoto K, et al. A novel polymorphism of the human APRIL gene is associated with systemic lupus erythematosus. Rheumatology (Oxford) 2003;42(8): 980–5.

[104] Kawasaki A, Tsuchiya N, Fukazawa T, et al. Analysis on the association of human BLYS (BAFF, TNFSF13B) polymorphisms with systemic lupus erythematosus and rheumatoid arthritis. Genes Immun 2002;3(7):424–9.

[105] Yasutomo K, Horiuchi T, Kagami S, et al. Mutation of DNASE1 in people with systemic lupus erythematosus. Nat Genet 2001;28(4):313–4.

[106] Liu MF, Wang CR, Fung LL. No evidence of mutation in exon 2 of DNAse1 gene in Chinese patients with systemic lupus erythematosus. Lupus 2004;13(2):142–3.

[107] Vaidya B, Pearce S. The emerging role of the CTLA-4 gene in autoimmune endocrinopathies. Eur J Endocrinol 2004;150(5):619–26.

[108] Liu MF, Wang CR, Chen PC, et al. Increased expression of soluble cytotoxic T-lymphocyte-associated antigen-4 molecule in patients with systemic lupus erythematosus. Scand J Immunol 2003;57(6):568–72.

[109] Matsushita M, Tsuchiya N, Shiota M, et al. Lack of a strong association of CTLA-4 exon 1 polymorphism with the susceptibility to rheumatoid arthritis and systemic lupus erythematosus in Japanese: an association study using a novel variation screening method. Tissue Antigens 1999;54(6):578–84.

[110] Heward J, Gordon C, Allahabadia A, et al. The A-G polymorphism in exon 1 of the CTLA-4 gene is not associated with systemic lupus erythematosus. Ann Rheum Dis 1999;58(3):193–5.

[111] Liu MF, Wang CR, Lin LC, et al. CTLA-4 gene polymorphism in promoter and exon-1 regions in Chinese patients with systemic lupus erythematosus. Lupus 2001;10(9):647–9.

[112] Lee YH, Kim YR, Ji JD, et al. Polymorphisms of the CTLA-4 exon 1 and promoter gene in systemic lupus erythematosus. Lupus 2001;10(9):601–5.

[113] Ahmed S, Ihara K, Kanemitsu S, et al. Association of CTLA-4 but not CD28 gene polymorphisms with systemic lupus erythematosus in the Japanese population. Rheumatology (Oxford) 2001;40(6):662–7.

[114] Pullmann Jr R, Lukac J, Skerenova M, et al. Cytotoxic T lymphocyte antigen 4 (CTLA-4) dimorphism in patients with systemic lupus erythematosus. Clin Exp Rheumatol 1999;17(6): 725–9.

[115] Hudson LL, Rocca K, Song YW, et al. CTLA-4 gene polymorphisms in systemic lupus erythematosus: a highly significant association with a determinant in the promoter region. Hum Genet 2002;111:452–5.

[116] Fernandez-Blanco L, Perez-Pampin E, Gomez-Reino JJ, et al. A CTLA-4 polymorphism associated with susceptibility to systemic lupus erythematosus. Arthritis Rheum 2004;50(1): 328–9.

[117] Russell AI, Cunninghame Graham DS, et al. Polymorphism at the C-reactive protein locus influences gene expression and predisposes to systemic lupus erythematosus. Hum Mol Genet 2004;13(1):137–47.

[118] Citores MJ, Rua-Figueroa I, Rodriguez-Gallego C, et al. The dinucleotide repeat polymorphism in the 3'UTR of the CD154 gene has a functional role on protein expression and is associated with systemic lupus erythematosus. Ann Rheum Dis 2004;63(3):310–7.

[119] Tsugu H, Horowitz R, Gibson N, et al. The location of a disease-associated polymorphism and genomic structure of the human 52-kDa Ro/SSA locus (SSA1). Genomics 1994;24(3):541–8.

[120] Forton AC, Petri MA, Goldman D, et al. An osteopontin (SPP1) polymorphism is associated with systemic lupus erythematosus. Hum Mutat 2002;19(4):459.

[121] Kuroki K, Tsuchiya N, Tsao BP, et al. Polymorphisms of human CD19 gene: possible association with susceptibility to systemic lupus erythematosus in Japanese. Genes Immun 2002; 3(Suppl 1):S21–30.

[122] Tucci M, Barnes EV, Sobel ES, et al. Strong association of a functional polymorphism in the monocyte chemoattractant protein 1 promoter gene with lupus nephritis. Arthritis Rheum 2004; 50(6):1842–9.

[123] Kim HL, Lee DS, Yang SH, et al. The polymorphism of monocyte chemoattractant protein-1 is associated with the renal disease of SLE. Am J Kidney Dis 2002;40(6):1146–52.

[124] Aguilar F, Gonzalez-Escribano MF, Sanchez-Roman J, et al. MCP-1 promoter polymorphism in Spanish patients with systemic lupus erythematosus. Tissue Antigens 2001;58(5):335–8.

[125] Tebib JG, Alcocer-Varela J, Alarcon-Segovia D, et al. Association between a T-cell receptor restriction fragment length polymorphism and systemic lupus erythematosus. J Clin Invest 1990;86(6):1961–7.

[126] Morito F, Hiida M, Ohta A, et al. Genetic analysis of systemic lupus erythematosus: association with a T cell receptor restriction fragment length polymorphism in Japanese patients. Intern Med 1992;31(8):998–1003.

[127] Nambiar MP, Enyedy EJ, Warke VG, et al. T cell signaling abnormalities in systemic lupus erythematosus are associated with increased mutations/polymorphisms and splice variants of T cell receptor zeta chain messenger RNA. Arthritis Rheum 2001;44(6):1336–50.

[128] Yang PM, Olsen NJ, Siminovitch KA, et al. Possible deletion of a developmentally regulated heavy-chain variable region gene in autoimmune diseases. Proc Natl Acad Sci U S A 1990; 87(20):7907–11.

[129] Whittingham S, Mathews JD, Schanfield MS, et al. HLA and Gm genes in systemic lupus erythematosus. Tissue Antigens 1983;21(1):50–7.

[130] Kumar A, Martinez-Tarquino C, Maria-Forte A, et al. Immunoglobulin heavy chain constant-region gene polymorphism in systemic lupus erythematosus. Arthritis Rheum 1991;34(12): 1553–6.

[131] Queiroz RG, Tamia-Ferreira MC, Carvalho IF, et al. Association between EcoRI fragment-length polymorphism of the immunoglobulin lambda variable 8 (IGLV8) gene family with rheumatoid arthritis and systemic lupus erythematosus. Braz J Med Biol Res 2001;34(4):525–8.

[132] Kassi EN, Vlachoyiannopoulos PG, Moutsopoulos HM, et al. Molecular analysis of estrogen receptor alpha and beta in lupus patients. Eur J Clin Invest 2001;31(1):86–93.

[133] Liu ZH, Cheng ZH, Gong RJ, et al. Sex differences in estrogen receptor gene polymorphism and its association with lupus nephritis in Chinese. Nephron 2002;90(2):174–80.

[134] Stevens A, Ray D, Alansari A, et al. Characterization of a prolactin gene polymorphism and its associations with systemic lupus erythematosus. Arthritis Rheum 2001;44(10):2358–66.

[135] Mellai M, Giordano M, D'Alfonso S, et al. Prolactin and prolactin receptor gene polymorphisms in multiple sclerosis and systemic lupus erythematosus. Hum Immunol 2003;64(2): 274–84.

[136] Ozaki Y, Nomura S, Nagahama M, et al. Vitamin-D receptor genotype and renal disorder in Japanese patients with systemic lupus erythematosus. Nephron 2000;85(1):86–91.

[137] Huang CM, Wu MC, Wu JY, et al. Association of vitamin D receptor gene BsmI polymorphisms in Chinese patients with systemic lupus erythematosus. Lupus 2002;11(1):31–4.

[138] Huang CM, Wu MC, Wu JY, et al. No association of vitamin D receptor gene start codon fok 1 polymorphisms in Chinese patients with systemic lupus erythematosus. J Rheumatol 2002; 29(6):1211–3.

[139] Ollier W, Davies E, Snowden N, et al. Association of homozygosity for glutathione-S-transferase GSTM1 null alleles with the Ro + /La- autoantibody profile in patients with systemic lupus erythematosus. Arthritis Rheum 1996;39(10):1763–4.

[140] Tew MB, Ahn CW, Friedman AW, et al. Systemic lupus erythematosus in three ethnic groups. VIII. Lack of association of glutathione S-transferase null alleles with disease manifestations. Arthritis Rheum 2001;44(4):981–3.

[141] Oates JC, Levesque MC, Hobbs MR, et al. Nitric oxide synthase 2 promoter polymorphisms and systemic lupus erythematosus in African-Americans. J Rheumatol 2003;30(1):60–7.

[142] Lopez-Nevot MA, Ramal L, Jimenez-Alonso J, et al. The inducible nitric oxide synthase promoter polymorphism does not confer susceptibility to systemic lupus erythematosus. Rheumatology (Oxford) 2003;42(1):113–6.

[143] Goldstein R, Arnett FC, McLean RH, et al. Molecular heterogeneity of complement component C4-null and 21-hydroxylase genes in systemic lupus erythematosus. Arthritis Rheum 1988; 31(6):736–44.

[144] von Schmiedeberg S, Fritsche E, Ronnau AC, et al. Polymorphisms of the xenobiotic-metabolizing enzymes CYP1A1 and NAT-2 in systemic sclerosis and lupus erythematosus. Adv Exp Med Biol 1999;455:147–52.

[145] Zschieschang P, Hiepe F, Gromnica-Ihle E, et al. Lack of association between arylamine N-acetyltransferase 2 (NAT2) polymorphism and systemic lupus erythematosus. Pharmacogenetics 2002;12(7):559–63.

[146] Cooper GS, Treadwell EL, Dooley MA, et al. N-acetyl transferase genotypes in relation to risk of developing systemic lupus erythematosus. J Rheumatol 2004;31(1):76–80.

[147] Parsa A, Peden E, Lum RF, et al. Association of angiotensin-converting enzyme polymorphisms with systemic lupus erythematosus and nephritis: analysis of 644 SLE families. Genes Immun 2002;3(Suppl 1):S42–6.

[148] Prkacin I, Novak B, Sertic J, et al. Angiotensin-converting enzyme gene polymorphism in patients with systemic lupus. Acta Med Croatica 2001;55(2):73–6.

[149] Pullmann Jr R, Lukac J, Skerenova M, et al. Association between systemic lupus erythematosus and insertion/deletion polymorphism of the angiotensin converting enzyme (ACE) gene. Clin Exp Rheumatol 1999;17(5):593–6.

[150] Kaufman KM, Kelly J, Gray-McGuire C, et al. Linkage analysis of angiotensin-converting enzyme (ACE) insertion/deletion polymorphism and systemic lupus erythematosus. Mol Cell Endocrinol 2001;177:81–5.

[151] Molad Y, Gal E, Magal N, et al. Renal outcome and vascular morbidity in systemic lupus erythematosus (SLE): lack of association with the angiotensin-converting enzyme gene polymorphism. Semin Arthritis Rheum 2000;30(2):132–7.

[152] Tassiulas IO, Aksentijevich I, Salmon JE, et al. Angiotensin I converting enzyme gene polymorphisms in systemic lupus erythematosus: decreased prevalence of DD genotype in African American patients. Clin Nephrol 1998;50(1):8–13.

[153] Akai Y, Sato H, Iwano M, Kurumatani N, Kurioka H, Kubo A, et al. Association of an insertion polymorphism of angiotensin-converting enzyme gene with the activity of lupus nephritis. Clin Nephrol 1999;51(3):141–6.

[154] Guan T, Liu Z, Chen Z. Angiotensin-converting enzyme gene polymorphism and the clinical pathological features and progression in lupus nephritis. Zhonghua Nei Ke Za Zhi 1997;36(7): 461–4.

[155] Uhm WS, Lee HS, Chung YH, et al. Angiotensin-converting enzyme gene polymorphism and vascular manifestations in Korean patients with SLE. Lupus 2002;11(4):227–33.

[156] Sivera P, Bosio S, Bertero MT, et al. G20210A homozygosity in antiphospholipid syndrome secondary to systemic lupus erythematosus. Haematologica 2000;85(1):109–10.

[157] Gong R, Liu Z, Chen Z, et al. Genetic variations in plasminogen activator inhibitor-1 gene and beta fibrinogen gene associated with glomerular microthrombosis in lupus nephritis and the gene dosage effect. Zhonghua Yi Xue Yi Chuan Xue Za Zhi 2002;19(1):1–5.

[158] Wang AY, Poon P, Lai FM, et al. Plasminogen activator inhibitor-1 gene polymorphism 4G/4G genotype and lupus nephritis in Chinese patients. Kidney Int 2001;59(4):1520–8.

[159] Tassies D, Espinosa G, Munoz-Rodriguez FJ, et al. The 4G/5G polymorphism of the type 1 plasminogen activator inhibitor gene and thrombosis in patients with antiphospholipid syndrome. Arthritis Rheum 2000;43(10):2349–58.

[160] Tolusso B, Fabris M, Gremese E, et al. Platelet GPIIb/IIIa (P1A 1/2) polymorphism in SLE: clinical and laboratory association. Ann Rheum Dis 2003;62(8):781−2.

[161] Kyogoku C, Langefeld CD, Ortmann WA, et al. Genetic association of the R620W polymophism of protein tyrosine phosphatase PTPN22 with human SLE. Am J Hum Genet 2004; 75(3):504−7.

[162] Sigurdsson S, Nordmark G, Goring HH, et al. Polymorphisms in the tyrosine kinase 2 and interferon regulatory factor 5 genes are associated with systemic lupus erythematosus. Am J Hum Genet 2005;76(3):528−37.

[163] Namjou B, Nath SK, Kilpatrick J, et al. Genome scan stratified by the presence of anti-double-stranded DNA (dsDNA) autoantibody in pedigrees multiplex for systemic lupus erythematosus (SLE) establishes linkages at 19p13.2 (SLED1) and 18q21.1 (SLED2). Genes Immun 2002;3S1:S35−41.

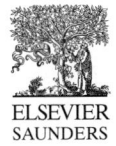

ELSEVIER
SAUNDERS

RHEUMATIC
DISEASE CLINICS
OF NORTH AMERICA

Rheum Dis Clin N Am 31 (2005) 245–254

# Review of Classification Criteria for Systemic Lupus Erythematosus

## Michelle Petri, MD, MPH

*Johns Hopkins University School of Medicine, 1830 East Monument Street,
Suite 7500, Baltimore, MD 21205, USA*

The incidence of systemic lupus erythematosus (SLE) may have tripled in the United States since the 1960s and -70s [1]. Hispanic Americans, an increasing proportion of the United States population, have SLE that is as severe as African-American SLE [2]. The survival of SLE patients has not improved since the 1980s [3]. It is imperative that SLE be recognized, referred to appropriate specialists, and treated early and effectively to prevent organ damage. Clinical trials require the inclusion of real lupus patients, if their results are to be generalizable. Disease classification criteria are an important step in this process.

### Goals of classification criteria

In SLE, the population studied affects the results obtained. The prevalence of various organ manifestations and autoantibodies differ by ethnicity. African Americans who have SLE are more likely than whites to have discoid lupus, lupus nephritis, anti-Sm, and anti-RNP. Whites who have SLE are more likely to have photosensitivity, malar rash, oral ulcers, and antiphospholipid antibodies [4]. Recent data suggest that SLE differs among nations, even beyond ethnicities. Central nervous system SLE, for example, appears to be more common in

*E-mail address:* mpetri@jhmi.edu

doi:10.1016/j.rdc.2005.01.009               *rheumatic.theclinics.com*

Sweden [5]. It is conceivable that one set of classification criteria might not be sufficient in SLE, but that subsetting by ethnicity and geographic area would be preferable. Successful classification criteria need to have high specificity and sensitivity, often best expressed as high positive predictive value.

Lupus exists not just in the systemic form, but also as chronic cutaneous lupus. Because very few (5%) of chronic cutaneous lupus patients progress to the systemic form, separate criteria for SLE and for chronic cutaneous lupus should be devised. The current American College of Rheumatology criteria for SLE include four dermatologic criteria (photosensitivity, malar rash, discoid rash, and oral ulcers) [6]. This skewing toward cutaneous lupus might lead to a bias against other organ involvement. As many as 50% of SLE patients have antiphospholipid antibodies. Four of the current American College of Rheumatology (ACR) criteria can occur in the antiphospholipid syndrome: antiphospholipid antibodies, proteinuria, seizures, and thrombocytopenia.

Systemic lupus erythematosus is a disease that evolves over time. Early in the disease course, four of the current criteria may not be present [7]. Research on stored sera of military personnel revealed that auto-antibodies are present years before any clinical symptoms of SLE [8]. This suggests that classification criteria designed to detect SLE early should emphasize the presence of specific auto-antibodies, which currently are relegated to one immunologic disorder criterion.

New knowledge should be reflected in classification criteria. In terms of SLE, entire new sets of auto-antibodies, such as anti-SR proteins [9], have been discovered, and older sets, such as antiphospholipid antibodies, are being defined further, such as beta 2 glycoprotein1-dependent anticardiolipin. New research on the interferon signature of SLE [10] may one day revolutionize diagnosis. In addition, several potential biomarkers eventually may be shown to have clinical utility [11].

Current ACR criteria were devised for classifying SLE patients for inclusion in clinical or laboratory research studies. Although often it is emphasized that they were not developed as diagnostic criteria, they often serve that purpose. This is not entirely inappropriate, given that the criteria emphasize the multi-system nature of the disease and that diagnosis (or classification) requires much more than a positive antinuclear antibody (ANA) alone.

No formal validation of the ACR classification criteria as diagnostic criteria has been performed, however. A clinical diagnosis of lupus may be bestowed in the absence of four criteria. These patients, who are thought to definitely have SLE, and, yet, do not meet classification criteria, are believed to be the most instructive group to include in the derivation of revised criteria.

Given the shortage of rheumatologists in the United States and elsewhere, it should be anticipated that classification criteria will be used by other physicians. In fact, many specialists, including dermatologists, nephrologists, and neurologists, may be the on the front line in diagnosing and treating SLE. Classification criteria need to include multiple disciplines beyond rheumatology and to be validated by these disciplines.

## Ideal classification criteria

Five rules to be met in constructing classification criteria for SLE were summarized by Fries [12]:

1. The gold standard for diagnosis (or classification) is established by highly experienced clinicians and is confirmed by: stability of the diagnosis over time and by independent review by committee members.
2. Consecutively treated patients and multiple institutions are used to minimize selection bias.
3. Control populations are chosen to represent the diagnostic problem area that will be used in selecting subjects for studies.
4. The terminology is defined with precision; a small change in definition for a criterion can make a large change in sensitivity and specificity.
5. Criteria performance is validated on a new population, because criteria always work well on the population from which they were developed.

Fries recognized that improved knowledge should lead to better disease criteria. He acknowledged the overlap of classification and diagnostic criteria, saying, "The 1982 classification has improved our diagnostic approach to SLE" [12].

## American College of Rheumatology 1982 criteria

The first classification criteria for SLE was established in 1971 and required 4 of 14 criteria [13]. In 1982, the criteria were revised to include advances in serologic testing (ANA and anti-dsDNA) and to take advantage of improved biostatistical techniques [6]. These criteria are shown in Table 1. Two items, alopecia and Raynaud's phenomenon, were removed from the 1971 criteria. The 1982 criteria have been validated [14–17].

The interpretation of some of the definitions is critical. For example, if arthritis was defined strictly as *nonerosive*, only 41% of patients filled the criteria, whereas if it was defined liberally (ie, erosions could be ruled out without the need of radiographs), 83% of patients fulfilled it.

In 1997, the Diagnostic and Therapeutic Criteria Committee of the ACR reviewed the 1982 criteria and recommended revisions to the 10th criterion of immunologic disorders [18]:

1. Delete item 10(a) (Positive LE cell preparation), and
2. Change item 10(d) to "Positive finding of antiphospholipid antibodies based on (1) an abnormal serum level of IgG or IgM anticardiolipin antibodies, (2) a positive test result for lupus anticoagulant using a standard method, or (3) a false-positive serologic test for syphilis known to be positive for at least 6 months and confirmed by *Treponema pallidum* immobilization or fluorescent treponemal antibody absorption tests."

Table 1
1982 revised systemic lupus erythematosus classification criteria

| Criterion | Definition |
| --- | --- |
| 1. Malar rash | Fixed erythema, flat or raised, over the malar eminences, tending to spare the nasolabial folds |
| 2. Discoid rash | Erythematous raised patches with adherent keratotic scaling and follicular plugging: atrophic scarring may occur in older lesions |
| 3. Photosensitivity | Skin rash as a result of unusual reaction to sunlight, by patient history or physician observation |
| 4. Oral ulcers | Oral or nasopharyngeal ulceration, usually painless, observed by a physician |
| 5. Arthritis | Nonerosive arthritis involving $\geq 2$ peripheral joints, characterized by tenderness, swelling, or effusion |
| 6. Serositis | (A) Pleuritis: convincing history of pleuritic pain or rub heard by a physician or evidence of pleural effusion<br>*or*<br>(B) Pericarditis: documented by ECG or rub or evidence of pericardial effusion |
| 7. Renal disorder | (A) Persistent proteinuria $> 0.5$ g/d or $> 3+$ if quantitation not performed<br>*or*<br>(B) Cellular casts: may be red blood cell, hemoglobin, granular, tubular, or mixed |
| 8. Neurologic disorder | (A) Seizures: in the absence of offending drugs or known metabolic derangements (eg, uremia, ketoacidosis, or electrolyte imbalance)<br>*or*<br>(B) Psychosis: in the absence of offending drugs or known metabolic derangements (eg, uremia, ketoacidosis, or electrolyte imbalance) |
| 9. Hematologic disorder | (A) Hemolytic anemia: with reticulocytosis<br>*or*<br>(B) Leukopenia: $< 4000/mm^3$ total on $\geq 2$ occasions<br>*or*<br>(C) Lymphopenia: $< 1500/mm^3$ on $\geq 2$ occasions<br>*or*<br>(D) Thrombocytopenia: $< 100,000/mm^3$ in the absence of offending drugs |
| 10. Immunologic disorder | (A) Positive LE cell preparation<br>*or*<br>(B) Anti-DNA: antibody to native DNA in abnormal titer<br>*or*<br>(C) Anti-Sm: presence of antibody to Sm nuclear antigen<br>*or*<br>(D) False positive serologic test for syphilis known to be positive for at least 6 months and confirmed by *T pallidum* immobilization or fluorescent treponemal antibody absorption test |

*(continued on next page)*

Table 1 (*continued*)

| Criterion | Definition |
| --- | --- |
| 11. Antinuclear antibody | An abnormal titer of antinuclear antibody by immunofluorescence or an equivalent assay at any point in time and in the absence of drugs known to be associated with "drug-induced lupus" syndrome |

The proposed classification is based on 11 criteria. For the purpose of identifying patients in clinical studies, a person shall be said to have systemic lupus erythematosus if any 4 or more of the 11 criteria are present, serially or simultaneously, during any interval of observation.

*From* Tan EM, Cohen AS, Fries JF, et al. The 1982 revised criteria for the classification of systemic lupus erythematosus. Arthritis Rheum 1982;25:1271–7; with permission.

These revisions were based on committee consensus, but were not subjected to any validation testing.

## Weighted criteria

It seems intuitively obvious that some criteria are more important than others (eg, lupus nephritis), and therefore, should be accorded more importance. In 1984, Clough et al applied Bayes' theorem to develop such a weighting system [19]. They assumed that various criteria occurred in individual patients independently of each other, although this is unproven. A positive (or negative) score for the presence/absence of each criterion was calculated and summed. A probability curve was constructed with the axes representing the probability of SLE versus the SLE score (Fig. 1).

In 2002, Costenbader et al revised the original Cleveland Clinic weighted criteria. The Boston Weighted criteria included antiphospholipid antibodies, renal

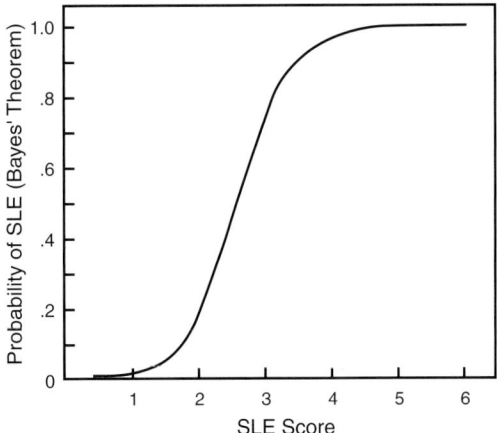

Fig. 1. Relationship of score calculated as described in text to probability of SLE as calculated from Bayes' theorem. (*From* Clough JD, Elrazak M, Calabrese LH, et al. Weighted criteria for the diagnosis of systemic lupus erythematosus. Arch Intern Med 1984;144:281–5; with permission.)

pathology, and new definitions of some criteria, such as arthritis defined as objective synovitis. For each criterion, the optimal level of sensitivity and specificity to differentiate SLE from non-SLE diagnoses was chosen. A cut-off of two points was used to identify SLE (the same cut-off used for the Cleveland Clinic Weighted Criteria) [20].

## Classification trees

Classification criteria can be presented in traditional and classification tree (recursive partitioning) formats. Using the same data set as the 1982 criteria, but with some standardization of laboratory values for ANA and complement, Edworthy et al derived several sets of classification trees [21]. The simplest tree (Fig. 2) demonstrated that just two criteria, immunologic criterion and malar rash, performed as well as the 1982 criteria set. The second classification tree (Fig. 3) contained three laboratory tests (ANA, anti-dsDNA, and complement) and three symptoms/signs (malar rash, pleurisy, and discoid rash). This second tree had a sensitivity of 97% and specificity of 95%.

## Limitations of the individual 1982 American College of Rheumatology criteria

*Cutaneous criteria*

Although all other organ systems receive only one criterion, there are four dermatologic criteria for SLE: malar rash, discoid rash, photosensitivity, and oral

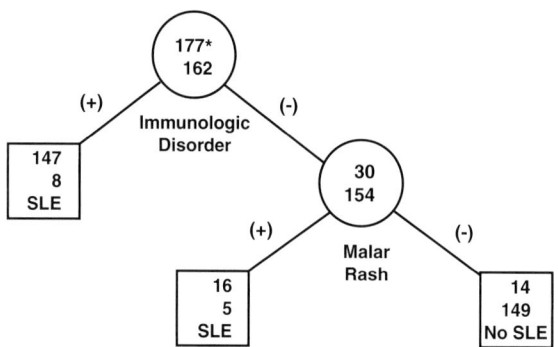

\* Upper number = SLE; Lower number = Control
Sensitivity = 92%; Specificity = 92%

Fig. 2. Classification tree for SLE. Simplest tree using 1982 criteria yielding substantial accuracy. (*From* Edworthy SM, Zatarain E, McShane DJ, et al. Analysis of the 1982 ARA lupus criteria data set by recursive partitioning methodology: new insights to the relative merit of individual criteria. J Rheumatol 1988;15:1493–8; with permission.)

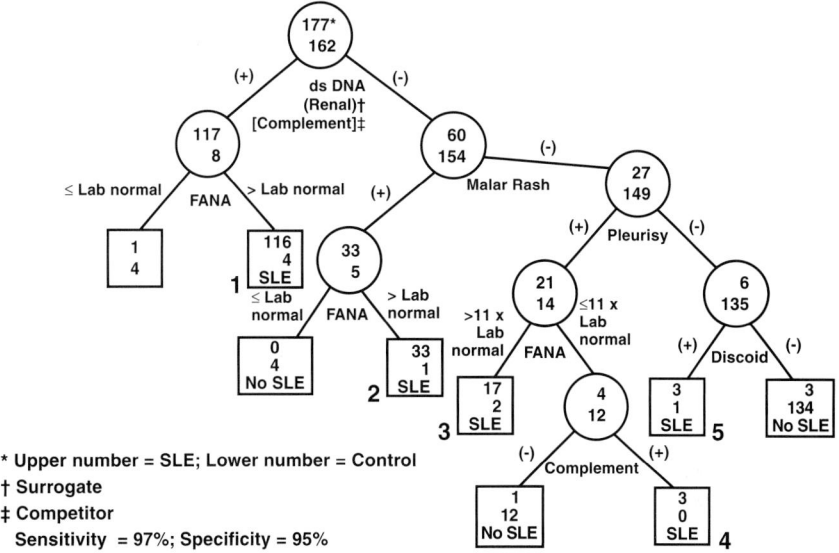

Fig. 3. Full classification tree for SLE. (*From* Edworthy SM, Zatarain E, McShane DJ, et al. Analysis of the 1982 ARA lupus criteria data set by recursive partitioning methodology: new insights to the relative merit of individual criteria. J Rheumatol 1988;15:1493–8; with permission.)

ulcers. Malar rash and photosensitivity correlate highly. They may be difficult to interpret, even if witnessed by a physician. Several other conditions, including acne rosacea, seborrheic dermatitis, actinic damage, and steroid erythema can be mistaken for a malar rash. Polymorphous light eruption, allergic reactions, and solar urticaria may be confused with lupus photosensitivity. The current criterion for oral ulcers requires that it be observed by a physician, although a history given by a reliable patient should be sufficient.

Additional criteria are needed for chronic cutaneous lupus, dermatologic lupus in the absence of systemic disease. Candidate criteria have been proposed by Werth et al [22]. They separate lupus specific from nonspecific cutaneous manifestations and emphasize the importance of biopsy confirmation.

*Arthritis*

Arthritis as a criterion is defined as nonerosive arthritis. This would require a radiograph, which rarely is done in clinical practice. Polyarthralgia, with morning stiffness, might be equally valid. Tenosynovitis and myositis are not included [23].

*Serositis*

The serositis criterion does not include a convincing history of pericarditis. This likely explains why it has only an 18% sensitivity rate [6]. Currently, peritoneal serositis [24,25] is not considered, either [26].

*Renal disorder*

The current renal criterion requires a persistent proteinuria greater than 0.5 g/d or greater than 3+. Because of the impracticality of doing 24-hour urine tests, the spot urine protein to creatinine ratio could stand in its stead [27]. The second part of the renal criterion is comprised of cellular casts. Most clinical laboratories no longer process the urinalysis properly to be able to detect casts. Active urinary sediment is more useful and should be considered. A renal biopsy showing one of the World Health Organization classes of SLE nephritis also should be sufficient [28].

*Neurologic disorder*

The ACR has developed nomenclature and case definitions for 19 potential neurologic manifestations of SLE [29]. The current neurologic criterion, however, includes only psychosis and seizure, both of which are relatively infrequent in SLE. The sensitivity, for example, of the current neurologic criterion is only 20% [6]. Unfortunately, the most common neurologic complaint in SLE, cognitive impairment, is difficult to measure, and may reflect disease damage (and, therefore, not be as useful in criteria being developed to aid in the early diagnosis of SLE). Inclusion of other neurologic manifestations, including transverse myelitis, cranial or peripheral neuropathy, mononeuritis multiplex, acute confusional state, and stroke (not caused by cardiovascular disease) would be important [30].

*Hematologic disorder*

Unlike any other organ system, the hematologic criterion requires that leukopenia and lymphopenia be present twice [31]. For lymphopenia, no clear rules exist to determine the criterion in the presence of prednisone. For leukopenia, no rules exist when the patient is taking immunosuppressive drugs. Thrombocytopenia is defined as less than $100,000/mm^3$, whereas most laboratories would define it as less than $140,000/mm^3$ to $150,000/mm^3$. Thrombocytopenia also can be associated with antiphospholipid syndrome. Operational\ rules need to be considered for these items.

*Immunologic disorder*

Not all anti-DNA assays are equally specific for SLE. ELISAs, for example, are less specific. A higher cut-off may be necessary, for example, if an ELISA is used [32]. Although hypocomplementemia was a powerful criterion in recursive partitioning, and is commonly used to support a clinical diagnosis of SLE, it was not included in the ACR criteria [33].

## Revision of the American College of Rheumatology classification criteria: role of Systemic Lupus International Collaborating Clinics

Because of the limitations of ACR classification criteria, the need to include new laboratory assays, and the need to address the omission of hypocomplementemia, the Systemic Lupus International Collaborating Clinics (SLICC) has undertaken the revision of the criteria. This process first involved defining all the potential candidate criteria by consensus. The frequency of these potential criteria then was determined in existing cohorts [5]. These potential criteria now will be tested in patients who have definite SLE by clinical diagnosis (but not necessarily by ACR criteria) and a wide range of controls (including myositis, rheumatoid arthritis, scleroderma, vasculitis, undifferentiated connective tissue disease, antiphospholipid syndrome, and fibromyalgia). A complementary exercise also will be performed by medical dermatologists to form criteria for chronic cutaneous lupus [22].

## References

[1] Uramoto KM, Michet CJJ, Thumboo J, et al. Trends in the incidence and mortality of systemic lupus erythematosus, 1950–1992. Arthritis Rheum 1999;42:46–50.

[2] Alarcon GS, Friedman AW, Straaton KV, et al. Systemic lupus erythematosus in three ethnic groups: III. A comparison of characteristics early in the natural history of the LUMINA cohort. Lupus in minority populations: nature vs nurture. Lupus 1999;8:197–209.

[3] Centers for Disease Control and Prevention. Trends in deaths from systemic lupus erythematosus—United States, 1979–1998. MMWR Morb Mortal Wkly Rep 2002;51(17): 371–4.

[4] Petri M. The effect of race on the presentation and course of SLE in the United States [abstract]. Arthritis Rheum 1997;40(Suppl 9):S162.

[5] Petri M, Urowitz M, Gladman D, et al. Frequency of current and proposed classification criteria for SLE: an international comparison study [abstract]. Arthritis Rheum 2004;50(9 Suppl):S410.

[6] Tan EM, Cohen AS, Fries JF, et al. The 1982 revised criteria for the classification of systemic lupus erythematosus. Arthritis Rheum 1982;25:1271–7.

[7] Lom-Orta H, Alarcon-Segovia D, Diaz-Jouanen E. Systemic lupus erythematosus. Differences between patients who do, and who do not, fulfill classification criteria at the time of diagnosis. J Rheumatol 1980;7(6):831–7.

[8] Arbuckle MR, McClain MT, Rubertone MV, et al. Development of auto-antibodies before the clinical onset of systemic lupus erythematosus. N Engl J Med 2003;349(16):1526–33.

[9] Neugebauer KM, Merrill JT, Wener MH, et al. SR proteins are autoantigens in patients with systemic lupus erythematosus. Importance of phosphoepitopes. Arthritis Rheum 2000;43(8): 1768–78.

[10] Baechler EC, Batliwalla FM, Karypis G, et al. Interferon-inducible gene expression signature in peripheral blood cells of patients with severe lupus. Proc Natl Acad Sci U S A 2003;100(5): 2610–5.

[11] Illei GG, Tackey E, Lapteva L, et al. Biomarkers in systemic lupus erythematosus: II. Markers of disease activity. Arthritis Rheum 2004;50(7):2048–65.

[12] Fries JF. Methodology of validation of criteria for SLE. Scand J Rheumatol 1987;14(Suppl 65): 25–30.

[13] Cohen AS, Reynolds WE, Franklin EC, et al. Preliminary criteria for the classification of systemic lupus erythematosus. Bull Rheum Dis 1971;21:643–8.

[14] Levin RE, Weinstein A, Peterson M, et al. A comparison of the sensitivity of the 1971 and 1982 American Rheumatism Association criteria for the classification of systemic lupus erythematosus. Arthritis Rheum 1984;27:530–8.

[15] Passas CM, Wong RL, Peterson M, et al. A comparison of the specificity of the 1971 and 1982 American Rheumatism Association Criteria for the classification of systemic lupus erythematosus. Arthritis Rheum 1985;28:620–3.

[16] Yokohari R, Tsunematus T. Application to the Japanese patients of the 1982 American Rheumatism Association revised criteria for the classification of systemic lupus erythematosus. Arthritis Rheum 1985;28:693–8.

[17] Davatchi F, Chams C, Akbarian M. Evaluation of the 1982 American Rheumatism Association revised criteria for the classification of systemic lupus erythematosus [letter]. Arthritis Rheum 1985;28:715.

[18] Hochberg MC. Updating the American College of Rheumatology revised criteria for the classification of systemic lupus erythematosus [letter]. Arthritis Rheum 1997;40:1725.

[19] Clough JD, Elrazak M, Calabrese LH, et al. Weighted criteria for the diagnosis of systemic lupus erythematosus. Arch Intern Med 1984;144:281–5.

[20] Costenbader KH, Karlson EW, Liang MH, et al. Defining lupus cases for clinical studies: the Boston weighted criteria for the classification of systemic lupus erythematosus. J Rheumatol 2002;29(12):2545–50.

[21] Edworthy SM, Zatarain E, McShane DJ, et al. Analysis of the 1982 ARA lupus criteria data set by recursive partitioning methodology: new insights to the relative merit of individual criteria. J Rheumatol 1988;15:1493–8.

[22] Albrecht J, Berlin JA, Braverman IM, et al. Dermatology position paper on the revision of the 1982 ACR criteria for SLE. Lupus 2004;13(11):839–49.

[23] Zoma A. Musculoskeletal involvement in SLE. Lupus 2004;13(11):851–3.

[24] Schousboe JT, Koch AE, Chang RW. Chronic lupus peritonitis with ascites? Review of the literature with a case report. Semin Arthritis Rheum 1988;18:121–6.

[25] Uzu T, Chikamori Y, Yamato M, et al. Acute lupus peritonitis during treatment of lupus nephritis: successful treatment with methylprednisolone pulse therapy. Nephron 2000;86(4):511–2.

[26] Clarke A. Proposed modification to 1982 ACR classification criteria for SLE: serositis criterion. Lupus 2004;13(11):855–6.

[27] Hartmann A, Jenssen T, Midtvedt K, et al. Protein-creatinine ratio—a simple method for proteinuria assessment in clinical practice. Tidsskr Nor Laegeforen 2002;122(22):2180–3.

[28] Dooley MA, Aranow C, Ginzler EM. Review of ACR renal criteria in SLE. Lupus 2004; 13(11):857–60.

[29] The American College of Rheumatology nomenclature and case definitions for neuropsychiatric lupus syndromes. Arthritis Rheum 1999;42:599–608.

[30] Hanly JG. ACR Classification Criteria for SLE: limitations and revisions to neuropsychiatric variables. Lupus 2004;13(11):861–4.

[31] Kao AH, Manzi S, Ramsey-Goldman R. Review of ACR hematologic criteria in SLE. Lupus 2004;13(11):865–8.

[32] Isenberg D. Anti-dsDNA antibodies—still a useful criterion for patients with systemic lupus erythematosus? Lupus 2004;13(11):881–5.

[33] Nived O, Sturfelt G. ACR classification criteria for SLE: complement components. Lupus 2004;13(11):877–9.

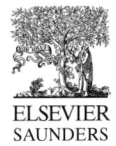

RHEUMATIC
DISEASE CLINICS
OF NORTH AMERICA

ELSEVIER
SAUNDERS

Rheum Dis Clin N Am 31 (2005) 255–272

# Antiphospholipid Syndrome in Systemic Lupus Erythematosus: Is the Whole Greater Than the Sum of Its Parts?

Carl A. Laskin, MD, Christine A. Clark, BSc,
Karen A. Spitzer, BSc

*Division of Rheumatology, Department of Medicine, University of Toronto Faculty of Medicine,
655 Bay Street, 18th Floor, Toronto, ON M5G 2K4, Canada*

Systemic lupus erythematosus (SLE) is the prototypic, non–organ-specific autoimmune disease. When coexisting with the antiphospholipid syndrome (APS), the disease can be complicated by increased hypercoagulability that may exacerbate many of the more typical features. This article compares the manifestations of SLE in the presence and absence of antiphospholipid antibodies (aPLs), the hallmark autoantibodies of APS. The authors wish to determine if individuals who have SLE with aPL present a different clinical picture or appear to be at greater risk of developing certain features compared with those who do not have aPL.

Systemic lupus erythematosus and primary APS share several features but also have some unique distinguishing characteristics. Recurrent miscarriage and thrombosis form the clinical classification criteria for APS but not SLE (Box 1) [1–3]. For many years, before APS was recognized formally as a separate syndrome, rheumatologists would classify patients who have APS as having SLE while acknowledging that such individuals would be unlikely to manifest many of the signs and symptoms of classical SLE such as arthritis, photosensitivity, leukopenia, and glomerulonephritis. Despite obvious distinctions between the

*E-mail address:* claskin@rogers.com (C.A. Laskin).

Box 1. Preliminary criteria for classification of antiphospholipid syndrome

Clinical criteria

Vascular thrombosis
Adverse pregnancy outcome

• At least one unexplained pregnancy loss beyond 10 weeks gestation
• Three or more unexplained, consecutive pregnancy losses before 10 weeks gestation
• One or more premature births of a normal neonate at or before 34 weeks' gestation because of pre-eclampsia or eclampsia, or placental insufficiency

Laboratory criteria

Moderate or high titer IgG or IgM anticardiolipin antibody measured on two or more occasions at least 6 weeks apart
Circulating anticoagulant measured on two or more occasions at least 6 weeks apart

*Data from* Wilson WA, Gharavi AE, Koike T, et al. International consensus statement on preliminary classification criteria for definite antiphospholipid syndrome. Arthritis Rheum 1999;42:1309–11.

two entities, it remains apparent that APS may, in many cases, be considered a subset of SLE.

**Primary antiphospholipid syndrome**

APS has been classified and established as a distinct clinical entity associated with thromboembolism, adverse pregnancy outcome, thrombocytopenia, Raynaud's phenomenon, and livedo reticularis in the presence of moderate or high levels of aPLs [1]. Other manifestations, most attributable to thrombotic events, have been described [4].

APLs are a family of antibodies directed against anionic, phospholipid proteins. In 1952, Conley and Hartmann first described a circulating anticoagulant associated with a hemorrhagic disorder in SLE [5]. This antibody came to be known as the lupus anticoagulant (LAC) and frequently is associated with a biologic false-positive test for syphilis (BFP). In 1963, Bowie et al [6] were the first to report that patients who have an LAC actually experienced thrombotic events rather than hemorrhage. Recurrent pregnancy loss (RPL) was noted to be associated with LAC in the mid 1970s, and in the early 1980s, many reports of recurrent thrombosis and pregnancy loss in the context of LAC were published [7,8]. Finally in 1983, Harris et al established the association of the BFP, LAC, and anticardiolipin antibodies (aCL) [9]. Since that time, a family of aPL has been described with varying reports of clinical associations. In addition to the LAC and IgG and IgM aCL, anti-β2 glycoprotein I (β2GPI) and IgA aCL are included in this family. Antibodies to other negatively charged phospholipids such as phosphatidylserine, phosphatidylinositol, phosphatidylethanolamine, and phosphatidic acid appear to be of such limited clinical significance that, outside of a research environment, there is little reason to assay for their presence. Those antibodies demonstrating the most consistent association with clinical manifestations are the IgG and IgM aCL and the LAC.

Since the early work of Harris et al [9], several workshops have established classification criteria for APS, although inconsistent laboratory methodology for the detection of aCL antibodies and the LAC remains an issue [10,11]. The major manifestations of APS are thrombosis and adverse pregnancy outcome, especially RPL. Insights into the clinical manifestations of SLE in the presence of aPL will most likely be apparent with an analysis of vascular and pregnancy-related events.

### Systemic lupus erythematosus and antiphospholipid antibodies

Anticardiolipin antibodies can be found in 2% to 5% of a normal population [11,12]. These antibodies increase in prevalence with increasing age, with IgG and IgM aCL being observed in 12% to 52% of an elderly population [13]. The frequency of the LAC is fairly well established in patients who have SLE. Approximately one-third of patients are positive [14]. In contrast, reports of aCL positivity in SLE vary considerably, from 23% to 47% [15–17]. Anti-β2GPI is found in 20% of lupus patients [17,18]. The question that arises from these data is whether aPL-positive lupus patients have an increase in thrombotic or adverse pregnancy events compared with those who do not have such antibodies. A second question, perhaps not as apparent, is whether certain vascular and pregnancy-related manifestations that have been ascribed to lupus, are seen mainly or exclusively in those who have aPL.

### Classification of syndromes with antiphospholipid antibodies

The simplistic classification system used by most physicians is that of primary and secondary APS. The former is diagnosed in patients who have clinical features consistent with those defined in the preliminary classification criteria [1].

The latter is diagnosed in those who have a specific disorder, usually a connective tissue disease, who also have thrombotic events or adverse pregnancy outcomes in the presence of apL. This classification system implies that there exists a clear distinction between APS and the connective tissue disease, but this is frequently not the case. Unfortunately, the most frequent scenario is also the most confusing: secondary APS in patients who have SLE.

Alarcon-Segovia proposed a modified classification that accepted the designations primary and secondary APS but added an intermediate group, which he named APS with lupoid features [19,20]. This group has features consistent with primary APS but fulfills fewer than four classification criteria for SLE (Fig. 1). Although this division into three subtypes of APS is not formally accepted, the concept of patients who might be experiencing a continuum of clinical manifestations helps to explain the clinical course observed in many individuals who have apL and distinguishes primary APS from SLE and illustrates the relationship of APS as a subset of SLE in many other patients.

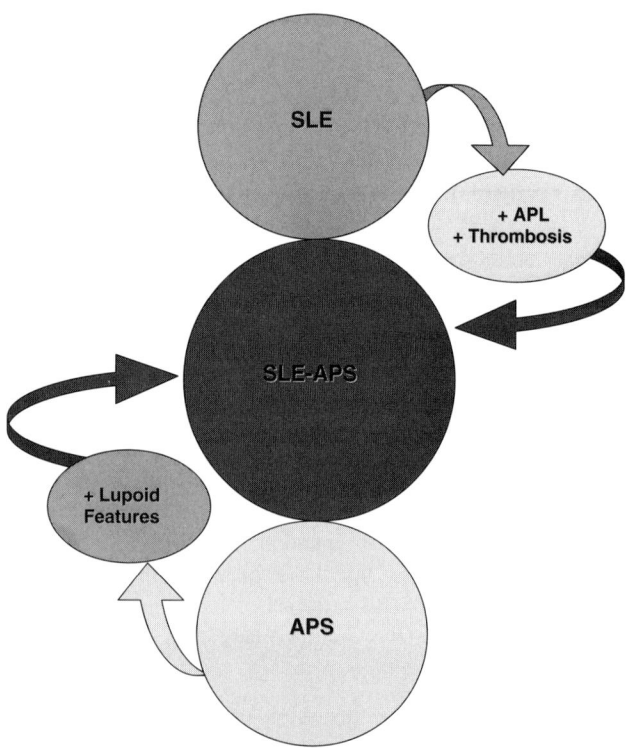

Fig. 1. The relationship of APS to SLE: APS can exist as a primary form, secondary to a connective tissue disease (usually SLE), or may be a primary form with some clinical features of SLE. The latter category can be referred to as an intermediate syndrome or APS with lupoid features.

Regardless of how these conditions are classified, one must distinguish those who have aPL from those who have aPL and clinical disease. In those who have secondary APS in association with SLE, clinical features that might be consistent with APS may not be caused by the presence of aPL. Indeed, these manifestations may be caused by some other aspect of lupus. For example, pregnancy loss may be caused by active renal disease, a flare of lupus, or even congenital heart block in the fetus (associated with anti-Ro/La antibody). Similarly, thrombosis may be caused by heavy proteinuria, which in turn leads to a hypercoagulable state independent of aPL. The question remains however, regarding the influence of the presence of aPL on SLE-specific disease manifestations and prognosis. It can be extremely difficult to tease apart clinical manifestations and attribute them to either APS or SLE when both conditions are present, and indeed, this distinction only becomes significant if therapeutic intervention differs depending upon disease attribution.

## Hypercoagulability, antiphospholipid antibodies, and systemic lupus erythematosus

The first described and hallmark manifestation in individuals who have aPL is thrombosis, either venous or arterial, regardless of vessel size. This underlying pathogenesis accounts for the major manifestations including deep venous thrombosis (DVT), stroke or other ischemic cerebral event, and pregnancy loss. It is therefore reasonable to assume that aPL may adversely affect the prognosis of patients who have SLE. Several studies have shown that there is a strong association between the presence of aPL and thromboembolism in patients who have SLE. An extensive review by Love and Santoro [15] summarized data showing that thromboembolic events occurred in 53% of 160 patients who had a LAC and in 12% of 338 patients who did not have this antibody [6,21–28]. In those who were aCL positive, 40% of 300 had thrombotic events, compared with 18% of 364 patients who were antibody negative [21,22,29–34]. Therefore the presence of aPL in the setting of SLE is associated with an increased prevalence of thromboembolism compared with patients who did not have aPL.

There appears to be an interaction between the lupus disease process and aPL that causes an increase in thrombotic events in patients who have SLE and aPL. In patients positive for aPL associated with non-SLE conditions, the frequency of thrombotic events was lower (22% of 328 patients) than that in a group of aPL-positive patients who had SLE (42% of 340 patients) [27,35–42]. A more recent study of 1519 aPL-positive patients determined that cerebrovascular thrombosis was significantly more frequent in the aPL-SLE group compared with the primary APS group [43]. These investigators also showed that venous thrombosis occurred more frequently in those who had an LAC than in those who had aCL, whereas arterial thrombosis was more frequent in the aCL-positive group compared with those who had LAC. In a study comparing lung perfusion scintigraphy in patients who had SLE, SLE with APS (SLE–APS), and primary

APS, Aung et al found 43% of those who had SLE–APS to have segmental uptake defects compared with none in the other two groups [44]. Although the groups were small, the data suggest that those lupus patients who have aPL have a significantly higher risk of pulmonary thromboembolism compared with patients who have SLE alone. Similar observations have been made regarding the incidence of stroke in patients who have SLE–APS compared with SLE alone [45,46]. Regardless of the pathogenesis of hypercoagulability in the presence of aPL, there appears to be one or more factors specific to SLE that impact significantly upon the development of thromboembolism not seen in other conditions associated with aPL.

The prognosis of lupus appears to be impacted significantly by the presence of aPL. Because thrombotic events are more common in SLE–APS, it is not surprising that the mortality in lupus is increased when aPL are present. Ruiz-Irastorza et al found cumulative survival at 15 years to be lower in patients who had APS than in those who did not have APS (65% versus 90%, $P=0.03$) [47]. A retrospective analysis determined that 8-year survival in SLE patients who did not have APS was 98%. In those who had SLE–APS, it was 75%, and in those who had primary APS 83%. The presence of APS in SLE was associated significantly with higher mortality in this study ($P=0.006$) [48]. Regression analysis of the data showed that disease activity at onset, arterial thrombosis, thrombocytopenia, valvular heart disease, capillaritis, digital necrosis, and nephritis were independent mortality risk factors. This study illustrates how the interaction between manifestations of the underlying disease and those attributable to aPL combine to adversely affect longevity in this patient population.

## Pregnancy in systemic lupus erythematosus and antiphospholipid syndrome

Insights into the clinical manifestations of SLE in the presence of aPL are most apparent upon analysis of vascular and pregnancy-related events, as adverse pregnancy outcome can be a significant problem in active SLE and APS. Indeed, pregnancy loss is one of the two clinical classification criteria of APS (see Box 1), and this issue is one that has attracted much attention among rheumatologists and obstetricians, attesting to its clinical importance.

Assessment of any woman who has a medical problem contemplating pregnancy requires an appreciation of both maternal and fetal issues. Therefore, one must address the effect of the pregnancy on the disease and the effect of the disease on the pregnancy. Ideally, a prepregnancy evaluation should be undertaken to appropriately plan the pregnancy enabling coordination of the efforts of both the rheumatologist and obstetrician. Unfortunately, unplanned pregnancies are almost the norm and require more urgent reactive rather than proactive evaluation and planning.

Pregnancy loss is the most controversial adverse outcome in both SLE and APS. The obvious questions are whether the problem in lupus is restricted to those who have apL and if the antibody exacerbates an already significant problem. APLs have been described in otherwise healthy women who have RPL, although with a frequency that is lower than might be expected. The LAC occurs in 15% of women who have RPL, while aCL might occur in 12% of a similar population [49–53]. Petri and Allbriton observed 13.1% pregnancy loss in a large lupus cohort [54]. This frequency appears to be representative when compared with other series of pregnant lupus patients [55–59]. In the presence of apL, pregnancy loss appears to be more common in women who have SLE [60–63]. Between 50% and 74% of lupus patients who have a history of RPL have an LAC, and up to 36% have aCL [60,61].

In the presence of apL, pregnancy loss can occur at any stage of pregnancy, although the classic description is that of late pregnancy loss. Both early and late pregnancy loss in lupus can be attributed to factors other than apL, including active disease and an exacerbation of underlying renal disease. It is always problematic to assess the etiology of very early pregnancy loss, and even more difficult to determine the role of apL in early pregnancy loss in lupus. The case becomes clearer if a patient who has SLE and apL has a history of RPL even when her disease is under good control.

Later pregnancy losses may be assessed more readily for etiology. APLs have been associated with the development of placental thrombosis leading to placental insufficiency and intrauterine growth restriction (IUGR) culminating in fetal demise [63]. In the context of active lupus, the etiologic evidence for late pregnancy loss is far more subjective if placental pathology is either unavailable or inconclusive. The exception to this might be active renal disease with heavy proteinuria, which can precipitate pre-eclampsia. This in turn can lead to placental insufficiency with resultant IUGR, which occurs with increased frequency in lupus pregnancies with or without fetal demise. In this case, hypercoagulability is the common feature that could lead to a similar clinico–pathologic picture as APS. Therefore, although pregnancy loss may occur in SLE, the presence of apL appears to place the pregnancy at greater risk. Unfortunately, data have yet to support intervention in pregnant women who have or do not have lupus when apL is present if there is no previous history of pregnancy loss.

Pregnancy loss in SLE, regardless of apL status, must be evaluated methodically. It would be wrong to make the a priori assumption that a loss is caused by either underlying disease or apL. Any woman who has recurrent or late pregnancy loss should be investigated for anatomic, hormonal, or genetic abnormalities that might account for the losses, and it is essential that patients who have lupus be assessed using the same thorough protocol. Furthermore, if placental pathology is available and consistent with ischemic pregnancy loss even if apL are negative, other thrombophilias such as protein C or S deficiency, factor V Leiden mutation, prothrombin gene mutation, antithrombin III deficiency, or hyperhomocysteinemia should be considered. The latter abnormality however, may be quite uncommon, because homocysteine levels are reduced by folic acid, a vitamin commonly taken by any woman contemplating a pregnancy.

Preterm birth (no later than 37 weeks' gestation) is common in SLE (40.5% of live births) [64,65] and can be related to disease activity, pre-eclampsia, placental insufficiency, or possibly premature rupture of the membranes [66,67]. In addition, preterm delivery also may be a reflection of advanced perinatal care where the obstetrician intervenes owing to threatened fetal demise [68]. Corticosteroids also have been associated with premature birth, but usually the neonate is appropriate size for gestational age [53]. Some authors also have suggested that the development of pre-eclampsia may be caused by the use of high doses of corticosteroids for disease control [69]. It is quite possible, however, that the steroids have little direct impact on the onset of pre-eclampsia and are actually an epiphenomenon in the etiology of pre-eclampsia. Rather, an exacerbation of disease activity or a flare of renal disease with heavy proteinuria may be the underlying problem, which is likely the reason for the institution of the high doses of corticosteroids. APLs have been associated with an increased frequency of pre-eclampsia, which could result in placental insufficiency, so the presence of aPL may be an additive factor in the high frequency of premature births commonly seen in women who have SLE.

Maternal complications are described in pregnant women with SLE. Although one would expect an increase in disease flares owing to the hyperestrogenic environment, the results of several studies are quite conflicting [64,66,70–77]. Among the medical complications are hypertension, diabetes mellitus, pre-eclampsia, and thrombosis [69,78]. Although these are more common in lupus, they may not be caused by disease activity. The higher risk of thrombosis is described in lupus pregnancies [78]. Even in uncomplicated pregnancies in healthy women, the third trimester, the immediate postpartum period, and after a cesarean section are characterized by hypercoagulability, and there is a greater risk associated with hypercoagulability in those who have SLE, which is increased further when aPL are present.

A particular problem arises when the woman who has SLE requires contraception. The easiest and most effective choice would be estrogen-containing oral contraceptive pills (OCP). Because lupus is a disease often exacerbated by a hyperestrogenic state, the use of OCP remains controversial owing to the risk of inducing a flare of the disease. If the patient is also positive for aPL, then OCP likely should be avoided. In this latter case, OCP may not only exacerbate the underlying disease (ie, SLE) but also place the woman at greater risk of thrombosis. Indeed, the presence of aPL should be considered at least a relative contraindication to the use of estrogen-containing OCP [79].

Women who have SLE or SLE–APS do not have any decrease in fertility. Although there is some debate regarding subfertility and an association with aPL, there is no good evidence to support that contention. There are however, two scenarios that may affect fertility adversely. The first is increased disease activity that could interfere with ovulation. The second issue is drug therapy. Cyclophosphamide may compromise ovarian function and potentially lead to ovarian failure.

It is possible for women who have SLE with or without APS to have infertility, as could any woman who does not have these conditions. Treatment for the lupus patient may be problematic, however, owing to the hyperestrogenicity resulting from ovulation induction or superovulation therapy using exogenous follicle stimulating hormone (FSH). As with OCP, a hyperestrogenic environment may lead to exacerbation of SLE. There are cases of documented flares, but these have been mild [80]. Providing the disease is under good control, FSH therapy can be used with appropriate monitoring by the rheumatologist. The presence of aPL however, complicates the situation. Again, elevated estrogen levels may increase the tendency to thrombosis. Although there have been no large studies attesting to the safety of such therapy in women who have aPL, ovulation induction could be undertaken cautiously if there is no history of prior thrombosis, but the patient and all physicians involved should be counseled regarding potential risks.

## Renal disease

The involvement of the kidney in SLE is known and described. Renal involvement has been part of the classification criteria of SLE from the outset [2,3]. With the exception of membranous disease, the renal lesions are inflammatory, targeting the glomerulus. Most patients who have SLE have some degree of renal disease, but it is not always clinically detectable without the benefit of immunofluorescence or electronmicroscopic evaluation of a kidney biopsy [81]. In the case of APS, renal involvement is not observed commonly. When present, the pathology is characterized by a thrombotic microangiopathy with thrombosis involving arterial and arteriolar lesions resulting in cortical ischemic atrophy [82,83]. The clinical manifestations of APS vascular nephropathy are characterized by hypertension, acute or chronic renal insufficiency, and low-grade proteinuria [84].

Daugas et al [84] retrospectively studied 114 patients who had SLE for renal disease in the presence or absence of aCL or LAC. The results revealed that APS nephropathy occurred in 32% of patients who had SLE in addition to lupus nephritis. The APS lesions were associated with LAC but not with aCL. Renal lesions occurred when there was evidence of extra-renal arterial thromboses and pregnancy loss but were not associated with venous thromboses. Most significantly, APS renal involvement appeared to be independent of the lupus-associated nephritis, and resulted in hypertension, renal insufficiency, and interstitial fibrosis. It is therefore likely that APS nephropathy contributes to increased morbidity and a poorer prognosis in this target lupus population because of its superimposition on lupus nephritis.

Renal transplantation in patients who have SLE appears to have a similar prognosis as transplantation in other conditions. The caveat to this reported observation, however, is the poorer prognosis seen in patients who have aPL [85–87]. Patients who have SLE–APS suffer an increased number of thromboembolic events posttransplant. There is a significant frequency of thrombotic microangiopathy recurring in the graft and a higher incidence of thrombosis of the renal graft vein compared with lupus patients who do not have aPL.

## Neurologic manifestations

Central nervous system (CNS) lupus is difficult to diagnose and manage. The manifestations have been variously reported as seizures, psychosis, stroke, transient ischemic attacks (TIA), chorea, cognitive dysfunction, and headaches. The pathology has been difficult to define, as it may be entirely normal. There is no gold standard test to diagnose CNS lupus, and physicians must rely on their clinical judgment. The most common neurologic manifestations of APS are stroke and TIA caused by arterial obstruction [88]. Although neuropsychiatric disorders have been linked to aPL, the association is tenuous. Neurologic involvement however, appears to be greater in those lupus patients who have aPL [15]. A review of the literature demonstrated neurologic disorders in 38% of LAC-positive patients compared with 21% in SLE patients lacking LAC. Similarly, 49% of lupus patients who had aCL had neurologic manifestations compared with 12% in aCL-negative lupus patients [15]. These data strongly suggest that CNS disease is more common in SLE–APS than in SLE without APS. Furthermore, as expected, aPL are associated more strongly with vascular neurologic events such as stroke, retinal artery occlusion, or amaurosis fugax. A recent multicenter study demonstrated a significant association of epilepsy with aPL positivity that appears to be secondary to CNS vascular disease [89].

## Cardiac involvement

In 1924, Libman and Sacks described a verrucous endocarditis affecting the heart valves in patients who had SLE [90]. The lesions can be found in 30% to 50% of autopsy or echocardiographic studies but are not often of clinical significance during life. The valvular disease is usually mild and rarely leads to compromise of cardiac function. In APS, the valvular abnormalities are essentially identical to those seen in SLE. There are no data indicating that patients who have SLE–APS have a higher incidence of valvular disease compared with SLE alone, but Vianna et al [91] did find a higher incidence of valvular disease in patients who had SLE–APS compared with patients who had APS alone. These investigators did find, however, that 41% of SLE–APS patients who had valvular disease had significant mitral regurgitation, which was far in excess of that seen in SLE without aPL [92]. The more severe involvement in aPL-positive patients may be caused by a direct effect of aPL damaging the endocardium. Therefore, aPL appears to enhance the pathogenic mechanism operational in lupus as it affects cardiac valves. Moreover, there is an additional risk in the presence of both aPL and endocardial vegetations, which results in a higher frequency of embolic neurologic events [93,94].

## Atherosclerosis in systemic lupus erythematosus and antiphospholipid syndrome

In 1976, Urowitz et al published a landmark paper documenting a bimodal mortality pattern in SLE [95]. Early deaths were caused by infection and renal disease, whereas later mortality was caused by atherosclerotic vascular disease. Recent studies observed that lupus patients have a 50-fold higher risk of developing cardiovascular disease and stroke beyond the conventional risk factors [96]. In the general population, aCL may be an independent risk factor for atherosclerotic vascular disease as evidenced by a 15% prevalence of aCL in middle-aged patients who had documented peripheral vascular disease [97]. In primary APS, IgG aCL was identified as an independent predictor of intima media thickness, a marker of atherosclerotic vascular disease [98]. Although lipid profile abnormalities have been described extensively in SLE, this is not the case in primary APS [99–101]. Alves and Ames contrasted the close association of dyslipidemia with atherosclerotic disease in SLE with the relative lack of such an abnormality in primary APS. They did, however, find a subgroup of patients who had primary APS lacking any lipid abnormality but having high titers of aCL, thereby implying a direct effect of aCL promoting atherosclerosis. Furthermore, these authors demonstrated an inhibitory effect of anti-β2GPI antibodies on the naturally occurring antioxidant paraoxonase [102]. Therefore in primary APS, atherosclerotic vascular disease appears to be promoted by aCL. Further evidence is provided that aPL may be an additive risk for atherosclerosis in SLE that is not accounted for by the traditional risk factors [103,104].

## Other disease manifestations in systemic lupus erythematosus and antiphospholipid syndrome

Several other manifestations exist in SLE and APS that characterize each of these conditions. Thrombocytopenia is described in both disorders. It is frequently milder in APS than in SLE. There is no evidence to suggest that this cytopenia is more frequent in SLE–APS than in SLE alone. Similarly, Coombs-positive hemolytic anemia is described in APS and SLE. It is, however, more characteristic of lupus, and if occurring in primary APS, it may be an indicator of the evolution of APS into SLE.

The skin is a target in both conditions. Although livedo reticularis has been purported to be one of the hallmarks of APS, it appears to occur with equal frequency in SLE without aPL. Similarly, leg ulcers, digital gangrene, necrotizing purpura, and nailfold infarcts appear to be as common in SLE as in APS [105,106].

Catastrophic APS is a rare condition of small vessel vasculopathy affecting multiple organ systems associated with a high mortality [107]. It must be distinguished from thrombotic thrombocytopenic purpura and disseminated intravascular coagulation [108]. The distinguishing marker however, is aCL or

LAC positivity. This condition can occur in primary APS or SLE–APS where the presence of aPL renders patients who have SLE at risk for this often fatal complication.

### Antiphospholipid syndrome and evolving systemic lupus erythematosus

The intermediate classification of APS with lupoid features proposed by Alarcon-Segovia [19] suggests that APS in some patients may be the first manifestation of SLE. Just as rheumatologists initially thought of APS as a subset of SLE, perhaps it may exist as evolving SLE. In a cohort of 165 patients who had APS followed over a median period of 78 months, Mujic et al [109] reported 3 of 80 patients who had primary APS developing features of SLE. Although one patient evolved into SLE after 4 years, the other two did not show features of lupus until 10 years after the diagnosis of primary APS. Similarly, a case report of a woman who had primary APS was diagnosed with SLE 15 years later [110]. In another case report of APS evolving into SLE 12 years after the first manifestations of APS, Derksen et al [111] suggest that a strongly positive antinuclear antibody in a patient who has primary APS may be the marker for later development of SLE. Carbone et al [112] reported that 3 (9%) of 33 patients who had a history of RPL and aPL developed features of SLE over a 6-year follow-up. The authors' group [113] found 3 of 32 women who had the same history of RPL also evolved into SLE or SLE–APS after a mean follow-up period of 12 years. Although some immunogenetic studies have been undertaken to determine if a particular haplotype is associated with APS occurring with SLE, the findings are rather preliminary. Despite the limited evidence, it is apparent that the evolution of APS into definite SLE does occur and may do so after many years.

### Summary

SLE is the prototypical, autoimmune disease characterized by immune-mediated inflammation in multiple organ systems. Although many of the auto-antibodies found in this condition appear to be merely markers of the presence of the disease or indicators of disease activity, some are definitely pathogenic. Morbidity and mortality in lupus are caused by the severity of the inflammation and the specific organ system involved. In addition, drug therapy often has significant impact on morbidity.

APS is an autoimmune disease characterized less by inflammation but more by hypercoagulability and thrombotic events. The disorder was initially described as a subset of SLE, but it is now known to exist as a separate entity in what is described as primary APS. Morbidity and mortality in this condition are caused by thrombosis and are dependent upon the organs affected. In addition, the impact of the disease on prognosis also may be determined by the type of vascular involvement, with venous usually being of less concern than arterial. Therapy plays less of a role in morbidity than in SLE. The combination of SLE and APS appears to be of greater concern than either entity alone. APS complicates SLE by adding a vaso–occlusive factor to the inflammatory component that adversely affects the prognosis of those who have lupus and aPL. The discovery of aPL in SLE and the diagnosis of the thrombotic complications associated with the APS aspect of the combined disorder, however, have significant implications therapeutically. Rather than instituting a regimen of corticosteroids and immunosuppressive agents with all of their attendant adverse effects, anticoagulation may be a safer and more appropriate therapeutic option. It is therefore incumbent upon the physician to clearly define the entity and evaluate the patient based upon a complete knowledge of the underlying disease processes.

## References

[1] Wilson WA, Gharavi AE, Koike T, et al. International consensus statement on preliminary classification criteria for definite antiphospholipid syndrome. Arthritis Rheum 1999;42: 1309–11.

[2] Tan EM, Cohen AS, Fries JF, et al. The 1982 revised criteria for the classification of systemic lupus erythematosus. Arthritis Rheum 1982;25:1271–7.

[3] Hochberg MC. Updating the American College of Rheumatology revised criteria for the classification of systemic lupus erythematosus. Arthritis Rheum 1997;40:1725.

[4] Cervera R, Piette J-C, Font J, et al. Anti-phospholipid syndrome. Clinical and immunologic manifestations of disease expression in a cohort of 1000 patients. Arthritis Rheum 2002;46: 1019–27.

[5] Connley CL, Hartmann RC. Hemorrhagic disorder caused by circulating anticoagulant in patients with disseminated lupus erythematosus. J Clin Invest 1952;31:621–2.

[6] Bowie EJ, Thompson JH, Pascuzzi CA, et al. Thrombosis in systemic lupus erythematosus despite circulating anticoagulants. J Lab Clin Med 1963;62:416–30.

[7] Nilsson IM, Astedt B, Hedner V, Berezin D. Intrauterine death and circulating anticoagulant (anti-thromboplastin). Acta Med Scand 1975;197:153–9.

[8] Carreras LO, Defreyn G, Machin SJ, et al. Arterial thrombosis, intrauterine death and lupus anticoagulant: detection of immunoglobulin interfering with prostacyclin formation. Lancet 1981;1:244–6.

[9] Harris EN, Gharavi AE, Boey ML, et al. Anticardiolipin antibodies: detection by radioimmunoassay and association with thrombosis in systemic lupus erythematosus. Lancet 1983;2:1211–4.

[10] Lockshin MD, Sammaritano LS, Schwartzman SS. Validation of the Sapporo criteria for antiphospholipid antibody syndrome. Arthritis Rheum 2000;43:440–3.

[11] Fields RA, Toubbeh H, Searles RP, et al. The prevalence of anticardiolipin antibodies in a healthy elderly population and its association with antinuclear antibodies. J Rheumatol 1989; 16:623–5.

[12] Vila P, Hernandez MC, Lopez-Fernandez MF, et al. Prevalence, follow-up and clinical significance of the anticardiolipin antibodies in normal subjects. Thromb Haemost 1994;72: 209–13.

[13] Manoussakis MN, Tzioufas AG, Silis MP, et al. High prevalence of anticardiolipin and other autoantibodies in a healthy elderly population. Clin Exp Immunol 1987;69:557–65.

[14] McNeil HP, Chesternam CN, Krilis SA. Immunology and clinical importance of antiphospholipid antibodies. Adv Immunol 1991;49:193–280.

[15] Love PE, Santoro SA. Antiphospholipid antibodies: anticardiolipin and the lupus anticoagulant in systemic lupus erythematosus (SLE) and non-SLE disorders. Ann Intern Med 1990; 112:682–98.

[16] Abu-Shakra M, Gladman D, Urowitz MB, et al. Anticardiolipin antibodies in systemic lupus erythematosus: clinical and laboratory correlations. Am J Med 1995;99:624–8.

[17] Sebastiani GD, Galeazzi M, Tincani A, et al. Anticardiolipin and anti-beta2GPI antibodies in a large series of European patients with systemic lupus erythematosus: prevalence and clinical associations. Scand J Rheumatol 1999;28:344–51.

[18] Bruce IN, Clark-Soloninka CA, Spitzer KA, et al. Prevalence of antibodies to B2-glycoprotein I in systemic lupus erythematosus and their association with antiphospholipid antibody syndrome criteria: a single centre study and literature review. J Rheumatol 2000;27:2833–7.

[19] Aracon-Segovia D, Cabral AR. The concept and classification of antiphospholipid/cofactor syndromes. Lupus 1996;5:364–7.

[20] Webe M, Hayem G, De Bandt M, et al. Classification of an intermediate group of patients with antiphospholipid syndrome and lupus-like disease: primary or secondary antiphospholipid syndrome? J Rheumatol 1999;26:2131–6.

[21] Derksen RH, Hasselaar P, Blizijl L, et al. Coagulation screen is more specific than the anticardiolipin antibody ELISA in defining a thrombotic subset of lupus patients. Ann Rheum Dis 1988;47:364–71.

[22] Petri M, Rheinschmidt M, Whiting-O'Keefe Q, et al. the frequency of lupus anticoagulant in systemic lupus erythematosus. A study of sixty consecutive patients by activated partial thromboplastin time, Russell viper venom time, and anticardiolipin antibody. Ann Intern Med 1987;106:523–31.

[23] Angles-Cano E, Sultan Y, Clauvel JP. Predisposing factors to thrombosis in systemic lupus erythematosus. J Lab Clin Med 1979;94:312–23.

[24] Boey ML, Colaco CB, Gharavi AE, et al. Thrombosis in systemic lupus erythematosus: striking association with the presence of circulating lupus anticoagulant. BMJ 1983;287:1021–3.

[25] Colaco CB, Elkon KB. The lupus anticoagulant. A disease marker in antinuclear antibody negative lupus that is cross-reactive with autoantibodies to double-stranded DNA. Arthritis Rheum 1985;28:67–74.

[26] Pauzner R, Rosner E, Many A. Circulating anticoagulant in systemic lupus erythematosus: clinical manifestations. Acta Haematol (Basel) 1986;76:90–4.

[27] Derksen RH, Bouma BN, Kater L. The prevalence and clinical associations of the lupus anticoagulant in systemic lupus erythematosus. Scand J Rheumatol 1987;16:185–92.

[28] Averbuch M, Koifman B, Levo Y. Lupus anticoagulant, thrombosis and thrombocytopenia in systemic lupus erythematosus. Am J Med Sci 1987;293:2–5.

[29] Tincani A, Meroni PL, Brucato A, et al. Anti-phospholipid and anti-mitochondrial type M5 antibodies in systemic lupus erythematosus. Clin Exp Rheumatol 1985;3:321–6.

[30] Meyer O, Piette JC, Bourgeois P, et al. Antiphospholipid antibodies: a disease marker in 25 patients with antinuclear antibody negative systemic lupus erythematosus (SLE). Comparison with a group of 91 patients with antinuclear antibody positive SLE. J Rheumatol 1987;14: 502–6.

[31] Fort JG, Cowchock FS, Abruzzo JL, et al. Anticardiolipin antibodies in patients with rheumatic diseases. Arthritis Rheum 1987;30:752–60.

[32] Manoussakis MN, Gharavi AE, Drosos AA, et al. Anticardiolipin antibodies in unselected autoimmune rheumatic disease patients. Clin Immunol Immunopathol 1987;44:297–307.

[33] Kalunian KC, Peter JB, Middlekauff HR, et al. Clinical significance of a single test for anti-cardiolipin antibodies in patients with systemic lupus erythematosus. Am J Med 1988;85: 602–8.

[34] Harris EN, Chan JK, Asherson RA, et al. Thrombosis, recurrent fetal loss, and thrombocytopenia. Predictive value of the anticardiolipin test. Arch Intern Med 1986;146:2153–6.

[35] Mannucci PM, Canciani MT, Mari D, et al. The varied sensitivity of partial thromboplastin and prothrombin time reagents in the demonstration of the lupus-like anticoagulant. Scand J Haematol 1979;22:423–34.

[36] Gastineau DA, Kazmier FJ, Nichols WL, et al. Lupus anticoagulant: an analysis of the clinical and laboratory features of 219 cases. Am J Hematol 1985;19:265–75.

[37] Jude B, Goudemand J, Dolle I, et al. Lupus anticoagulant: a clinical and laboratory study of 100 cases. Clin Lab Haematol 1988;10:41–51.

[38] Triplett DA, Brandt JT, Musgrave KA, et al. The relationship between lupus anticoagulants and antibodies to phospholipid. JAMA 1988;259:550–4.

[39] Mueh JR, Herbst KD, Rapaport SI. Thrombosis in patients with the lupus anticoagulant. Ann Intern Med 1980;92:156–9.

[40] Elias M, Eldor A. Thromboembolism in patients with the "lupus"-type circulating anticoagulant. Arch Intern Med 1984;144:510–5.

[41] Carreras LO, Vermylen JG. Lupus" anticoagulant and thrombosis–possible role of inhibition of prostacyclin formation. Thromb Haemost 1982;38:38–40.

[42] Waddell CC, Brown JA. The lupus anticoagulant in 14 male patients. JAMA 1982;248:2493–5.

[43] Soltesz P, Veres K, Lakos G, et al. Evaluation of clinical and laboratory features of antiphospholipid syndrome: a retrospective study of 637 patients. Lupus 2003;12:302–7.

[44] Aung W, Murata Y, Ishida R, et al. Comparison of lung perfusion scintigraphic findings in pulmonary thromboembolism in systemic lupus erythematosus, SLE plus antiphospholipid syndrome, and primary antiphospholipid syndrome. Nucl Med Commun 2000;21:299–304.

[45] Chaves CJ. Stroke in patients with systemic lupus erythematosus and antiphospholipid antibody syndrome. Curr Treat Options Cardiovasc Med 2004;6:223–9.

[46] Kitagawa Y, Gotoh F, Koto A, et al. Stroke in systemic lupus erythematosus. Stroke 1990;21: 1533–9.

[47] Ruiz-Irastorza G, Egurbide MV, Ugalde J, et al. High impact of antiphospholipid syndrome on irreversible organ damage and survival of patients with systemic lupus erythematosus. Arch Intern Med 2004;164:77–82.

[48] Reshetniak TM, Alekberova ZS, Kotel'nikova GP, et al. [Survival and prognostic factors of death risk in antiphospholipid syndrome: results of 8-year follow-up]. Ter Arkh 2003;75(5): 46–51 [in Russian].

[49] Edelman P, Rouquette AM, Verdy E, et al. Autoimmunity, fetal losses, lupus anticoagulant: beginning of systemic lupus erythematosus or new autoimmune entity with gynaeco-obstetrical expression? Hum Reprod 1986;1:295–7.

[50] Cowchock S, Smith JB, Gocial B. Antibodies to phospholipids and nuclear antigens in patients with repeated abortions. Am J Obstet Gynecol 1986;155:1002–10.

[51] Howard MA, Firkin BG, Healy DL, et al. Lupus anticoagulant in women with multiple spontaneous miscarriage. Am J Hematol 1987;26:175–8.

[52] Petri M, Golbus M, Anderson R, Whiting-O"Keefe Q, Corash L, Hellmann D. Antinuclear antibody, lupus anticoagulant, and anti-cardiolipin antibody in women with idiopathic habitual abortion. A controlled, prospective study of forty-four women. Arthritis Rheum 1987;30: 601–6.

[53] Laskin CA, Bombardier C, Hannah ME, et al. Prednisone and aspirin in women with autoantibodies and unexplained recurrent fetal loss. N Engl J Med 1997;337:148–53.

[54] Petri M, Allbritton J. Fetal outcome of lupus pregnancy: a retrospective case-control study of the Hopkins Lupus Cohort. J Rheumatol 1993;20:650–6.

[55] Engelbert HJ, Derue GM, Loizou S, et al. Pregnancy and lupus: prognostic indicators and response to treatment. Q J Med 1988;66:125–36.

[56] Hanly JG, Gladman DD, Rose TH, et al. Lupus pregnancy: a prospective study of placental changes. Arthritis Rheum 1988;31:358–66.

[57] Lockshin MD, Druzin ML, Goei S, et al. Antibody to cardiolipin as a predictor of fetal distress or death in pregnancy patients with systemic lupus erythematosus. N Engl J Med 1985;313: 152–6.

[58] Lockshin MD, Qamar T, Druzin ML, et al. Antibody to cardiolipin, lupus anticoagulant, and fetal death. J Rheumatol 1987;14:259–62.

[59] Koskela P, Vaarala O, Makitalo R, et al. Significance of false positive syphilis reactions

and anticardiolipin antibodies in a nationwide series of pregnant women. J Rheumatol 1988;15: 70–3.

[60] Derue GJ, Englert JH, Harris EN, et al. Fetal loss in systemic lupus: association with anticardiolipin antibodies. J Obstet Gynaecol 1985;5:207–9.

[61] Clauvel JP, Tchobroutsky C, Danon F, et al. Spontaneous recurrent fetal wastage and autoimmune abnormalities: a study of fourteen cases. Clin Immunol Immunopathol 1986;39: 523–30.

[62] Lockshin MD, Druzin ML, Qamar MA. Prednisone does not prevent recurrent fetal death in women with antiphospholipid antibody. Am J Obstet Gynecol 1989;169:439–43.

[63] Rahman P, Gladman DD, Urowitz MB. Clinical predictors of fetal outcome in systemic lupus erythematosus. J Rheumatol 1998;25:1526–30.

[64] Johns KR, Morand EF, Littlejohn GO. Pregnancy outcome in systemic lupus erythematosus (SLE): a review of 54 cases. Aust N Z J Med 1998;28:18–22.

[65] Kleinman D, Katz VL, Kuller JA. Perinatal outcomes in women with systemic lupus erythematosus. J Perinatol 1998;18:178–82.

[66] Aggarawal N, Sawhney H, Vasishta K, et al. Pregnancy in patients with systemic lupus erythematosus. Aust N Z J Obstet Gynaecol 1999;39:28–30.

[67] Johnson MJ, Petri M, Witter FR, et al. Evaluation of preterm delivery in a systemic lupus erythematosus pregnancy clinic. Obstet Gynecol 1995;86:396–9.

[68] Clark CA, Spitzer KA, Nadler JN, et al. Preterm deliveries in women with systemic lupus erythematosus. J Rheumatol 2003;30:2127–32.

[69] Petri M. Hopkins Lupus Pregnancy Center: 1987 to 1996. Rheum Dis Clin North Am 1997;23: 1–14.

[70] Lockshin MD, Reinitz E, Druzin ML, et al. Lupus pregnancy. I. Case-control prospective study demonstrating absence of lupus exacerbation during or after pregnancy. Am J Med 1984;77: 893–8.

[71] Meehan RT, Dorsey JK. Pregnancy among patients with systemic lupus erythematosus receiving immunosuppressive therapy. J Rheumatol 1987;14:252–8.

[72] Petri M, Howard D, Repke J. Frequency of lupus flare in pregnancy: the Hopkins Lupus pregnancy Center experience. Arthritis Rheum 1991;34:1538–45.

[73] Urowitz MB, Gladman DD, Farewell VT, et al. Lupus and pregnancy studies. Arthritis Rheum 1993;36:1392–7.

[74] Ruiz-Irastorza G, Lima F, Alves J, et al. Increased rate of lupus flare during pregnancy and the puerperium: a prospective study of 78 pregnancies. Br J Rheumatol 1996;35:133–8.

[75] Le Huong Î, Wechsler B, Vauthier-Brouzes D, et al. Outcome of planned pregnancies in systemic lupus erythematosus: a prospective study on 62 pregnancies. Br J Rheumatol 1997;36: 772–7.

[76] Carmona F, Font J, Cervera R, et al. Obstetrical outcome of pregnancy in patients with systemic lupus erythematosus. A study of 60 cases. Eur J Obstet Gynecol Reprod Biol 1999;83: 137–42.

[77] Georgiou PE, Politi EN, Katsimbrei P, et al. Outcome of lupus pregnancy: a controlled study. Rheumatology (Oxford) 2000;39:1014–9.

[78] Yasmeen S, Wilkins EE, Field NT, et al. Pregnancy outcomes in women with systemic lupus erythematosus. J Matern Fetal Med 2001;10:91–6.

[79] Lakasing L, Khamashta M. Contraceptive practices in women with systemic lupus erythematosus and/or antiphospholipid syndrome: what advice should we be giving? J Fam Plann Reprod Health Care 2001;27:7–12.

[80] Huong du LT, Wechsler B, Vauthier-Brouzes D, et al. Importance of planning ovulation induction therapy in systemic lupus erythematosus and antiphospholipid syndrome: a single center retrospective study of 21 cases and 114 cycles. Semin Arthritis Rheum 2002;32:174–88.

[81] Golbus J, McCune WJ. Lupus nephritis. Classification, prognosis, immunopathogenesis and treatment. Rheum Dis Clin North Am 1994;20:213–42.

[82] Nochy D, Daugas E, Droz D, et al. The intrarenal vascular lesions associated with primary antiphospholipid syndrome. J Am Soc Nephrol 1999;10:507–18.

[83] Kincaid-Smith P, Nicholls K. Renal thrombotic microvascular disease associated with lupus anticoagulant. Nephron 1990;54:285–8.

[84] Daugas E, Nochy D, Huong du LT, et al. Antiphospholipid syndrome nephropathy in systemic lupus erythematosus. J Am Soc Nephrol 2002;13:42–52.

[85] McIntyre JA, Wagenknecht DR. Antiphospholipid antibodies – risk assessments for solid organ, bone marrow and tissue transplantation. Rheum Dis Clin North Am 2001;27:611–31.

[86] Radhakrishnan J, Williams GS, Appel GB, et al. Renal transplantation in anticardiolipin antibody-positive lupus erythematosus patients. Am J Kidney Dis 1994;23:286–9.

[87] Amigo MC, Khamashta MA. Antiphospholipid (Hughes) syndrome in systemic lupus erythematosus. Rheum Dis Clin N Am 2000;331–48.

[88] Brey RL. Differential diagnosis of central nervous system manifestations of the antiphospholipid antibody syndrome. J Autoimmun 2000;15:133–8.

[89] Shoenfeld Y, Lev S, Blatt I, et al. Features associated with epilepsy in the antiphospholipid syndrome. J Rheumatol 2004;31:1344–8.

[90] Libman E, Sacks B. A hitherto undescribed form of valvular and mural endocarditis. Arch Intern Med 1924;33:701–7.

[91] Vianna JL, Khamashta MA, Ordi-Ros J, et al. Comparison of the primary and secondary antiphospholipid syndrome: A European multicentre study of 114 patients. Am J Med 1994;96: 3–9.

[92] Khamashta MA, Cervera R, Asherson RA, et al. Association of antibodies against phospholipids with heart valve disease in systemic lupus erythematosus. Lancet 1990;335:1541–4.

[93] Hojnik M, George J, Ziporen I, et al. Heart involvement (Libman-Sacks endocarditis) in the antiphospholipid syndrome. Circulation 1996;93:1579–87.

[94] Morelli S, Bernardo ML, Viganego F, et al. Left-sided heart valve abnormalities and risk of ischemic cerebrovascular accidents in patients with systemic lupus erythematosus. Lupus 2003;12:805–12.

[95] Urowitz MB, Bookman AA, Koehler BF, et al. The bimodal mortality pattern of systemic lupus erythematosus. Am J Med 1976;60:221–5.

[96] Manzi S, Meilahn EN, Rairie JE, et al. Age-specific incidence rates of myocardial infarction and angina in women with systemic lupus erythematosus: comparison with the Framingham Study. Am J Epidemiol 1997;14:408–15.

[97] Glueck CJ, Lang JE, Tracy T, et al. Evidence that anticardiolipin antibodies are independent risk factors for atherosclerotic vascular disease. Am J Cardiol 1999;83:1490–4.

[98] Ames PR, Margarita A, Delgado Alves J, et al. Anticardiolipin antibody titre and plasma homocysteine level independently predict intima media thickness of carotid arteries in subjects with idiopathic antiphospholipid antibodies. Lupus 2002;11:208–14.

[99] Lahita RG, Rivkin E, Cavanagh I, et al. Low levels of total cholesterol, high-density lipoprotein, and apolipoprotein A1 in association with anticardiolipin antibodies in patients with systemic lupus erythematosus. Arthritis Rheum 1993;36:1566–74.

[100] Delgado AJ, Ames PRJ, Donohue S, et al. Antibodies towards high density lipoprotein and beta-2-glycoprotein–I are inversely correlated with paraoxonase activity in systemic lupus erythematosus (SLE) and primary antiphospholipid antibody syndrome (PAPS). Arthritis Rheum 2002;46:2686–94.

[101] Ames PR, Tommasino C, Alves J, et al. Antioxidant susceptibility of pathogenic pathways in subjects with antiphospholipid antibodies: a pilot study. Lupus 2000;9:688–95.

[102] Alves JD, Ames PR. Atherosclerosis, oxidative stress and auto-antibodies in systemic lupus erythematosus and primary antiphospholipid syndrome. Immunobiology 2003;207:23–8.

[103] Jara LJ, Medina G, Vera-Lastra O, et al. Atherosclerosis and antiphospholipid syndrome. Clin Rev Allergy Immunol 2003;25:79–88.

[104] Vlachoyiannopoulos PG, Kanellopoulos PG, Ioannidis JP, et al. Atherosclerosis in premenopausal women with antiphospholipid syndrome and systemic lupus erythematosus: a controlled study. Rheumatology (Oxford) 2003;42:645–51.

[105] Gibson GE, Su WP, Pittelkow MR. Antiphospholipid syndrome and the skin. J Am Acad Dermatol 1997;36:970–82.

[106] Naldi L, Locati F, Marchesi L, et al. Cutaneous manifestations associated with antiphospholipid antibodies in patients with suspected primary antiphospholipid syndrome: a case-control study. Ann Rheum Dis 1993;52:219–22.

[107] Asherson RA, Cervera R, Piette JC, et al. Catastrophic antiphospholipid syndrome. Clinical and laboratory features of 50 patients. Medicine (Baltimore) 1998;77:195–207.

[108] Asherson RA, Cervera R, de Groot PG, et al. Catastrophic Antiphospholipid Syndrome Registry Project Group. Catastrophic antiphospholipid syndrome: international consensus statement on classification criteria and treatment guidelines. Lupus 2003;12:530–4.

[109] Muljic F, Cuadrado MJ, Lloyd M, et al. Primary antiphospholipid syndrome evolving into systemic lupus erythematosus. J Rheumatol 1995;22:1589–92.

[110] Al Attia HM. Progression of primary APS (Hughes syndrome) into serological SLE: case report. Rheumatol Int 2001;20:79–80.

[111] Derksen RH, Gmelig-Meijling FH, de Groot PG. Primary antiphospholipid syndrome evolving into systemic lupus erythematosus. Lupus 1996;5:77–80.

[112] Carbone J, Orera M, Rodriguez-Mahou M, et al. Immunological abnormalities in primary APS evolving into SLE: 6 years follow-up in women with repeated pregnancy loss. Lupus 1999; 8:274–8.

[113] Clark CA, Spitzer KA, Goldberg AS, et al. A. Long-term follow-up of women with autoantibodies and recurrent pregnancy loss (RPL) [abstract]. Arthritis Rheum 2002;6(Suppl):S45.

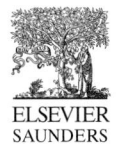
ELSEVIER
SAUNDERS

RHEUMATIC
DISEASE CLINICS
OF NORTH AMERICA

Rheum Dis Clin N Am 31 (2005) 273–298

# Neuropsychiatric Lupus

## John G. Hanly, MD, MRCPI, FRCPC

*Division of Rheumatology, Arthritis Center of Nova Scotia,
Queen Elizabeth II Health Sciences Centre, Dalhousie University, 1341 Summer Street, 2nd Floor,
Halifax, NS B3H 4K4, Canada*

Potential involvement of the nervous system by systemic lupus erythematosus (SLE) has been recognized ever since the multisystem nature of the disease first was appreciated. Clinical features include both neurologic (N) and psychiatric (P) manifestations, which may involve both the central and peripheral nervous systems. Although there have been significant advances in understanding of some aspects of neuropsychiatric (NP) SLE in recent years, nervous system disease continues to pose diagnostic, therapeutic, and scientific challenges for physicians and researchers alike. This article summarizes current thinking on this aspect of lupus with an emphasis on recent developments.

## Classification of neuropsychiatric systemic lupus erythematosus

It generally is accepted that the NP manifestations of SLE include a much broader spectrum of disease than the two features included in the current American College of Rheumatology (ACR) classification criteria [1,2], namely seizures and psychosis. Central nervous system (CNS) involvement predominates over peripheral nervous system disease and may take the form of diffuse disease (eg, psychosis and depression) or focal disease (eg, stroke and transverse myelitis) depending upon the anatomic location of pathology. Over time, several classifications have been developed for NP-SLE [3–5], none of which has received universal acceptance.

A deficiency in many of the classifications of NP-SLE has been the lack of definitions of individual manifestations and lack of standardization for inves-

Supported by a grant from the Canadian Institutes of Health Research.
*E-mail address:* john.hanly@cdha.nshealth.ca

tigation and diagnosis. In 1999, the ACR research committee produced a standard nomenclature and set of case definitions for NP-SLE [6]. Using a consensus approach and drawing on a pool of experts from several subspecialties including rheumatology, neurology, immunology, psychiatry, and neuropsychology, 19 NP syndromes (Box 1) were defined, and diagnostic criteria were developed [6]. For each NP syndrome, potential etiologies other than SLE were identified for either exclusion, or recognition as an association, acknowledging that in some clinical presentations it is not possible to be definitive about attribution. The issue of the identification of other potential causes for NP events in SLE patients is critical and was not addressed adequately in previous studies of NP-SLE.

---

**Box 1. Neuropsychiatric syndromes in systemic lupus erythematosus as defined by the American College of Rheumatology nomenclature**

*Central nervous system*

    Aseptic meningitis
    Cerebrovascular disease
    Demyelinating syndrome
    Headache
    Movement disorder
    Myelopathy
    Seizure disorders
    Acute confusional state
    Anxiety disorder
    Cognitive dysfunction
    Mood disorder
    Psychosis

*Peripheral nervous system*

    Guillain-Barré syndrome
    Autonomic neuropathy
    Mononeuropathy
    Myasthenia gravis
    Cranial neuropathy
    Plexopathy
    Polyneuropathy

*Adapted from* The American College of Rheumatology nomenclature and case definitions for neuropsychiatric lupus syndromes. Arthritis Rheum 1999;42(4):599–608.

Guidelines for reporting standards also were developed by the ACR research committee, and specific diagnostic tests were recommended for each syndrome. The result of this initiative was an important advance and addressed many of the deficiencies that had hampered previous attempts to classify NP-SLE.

## Epidemiology

The ACR nomenclature and case definitions for NP-SLE have been validated in a cross-sectional, population-based study by Ainiala et al [7]. Forty-six SLE patients were compared with 46 individuals randomly selected from the Finnish population register and matched by age, gender, education, and municipality of residence. Study procedures performed on both SLE and control subjects included a complete clinical assessment, neurologic examination, and a battery of neuropsychologic tests. At least one NP manifestation was identified in 91% of the 46 Finnish patients compared with 54% of controls. This provided an odds ratio of 9.5 (95% confidence interval (CI) 2.21 to 40.8) for the occurrence of an NP event and specificity of 46%. In view of the high prevalence of NP disease in both SLE and controls, the authors suggested several modifications to how the criteria should be used. Thus, by excluding headache, anxiety, mild depression, mild cognitive impairment, and polyneuropathy without electrophysiologic confirmation, the prevalence of NP disease fell from 91% to 46% in SLE patients and from 54% to 7% in controls. This provided an odds ratio of 7.0 (95% CI 2.09 to 23.47) and specificity of 93%.

In addition to the study of Ainiala et al, at least four other groups [8–11] have used the ACR nomenclature to classify their SLE cohorts for NP-SLE manifestations (Table 1). The overall prevalence of NP disease in these patient populations has varied between 37% and 95%. The most common 4 of the 19 NP syndromes in each of these five SLE cohorts are summarized in Table 2. Most of the other NP syndromes were infrequent, with a prevalence of less than 1% in most cases (Table 3). Of interest, the range in the prevalence of NP-SLE in these studies was as wide as that reported before the introduction of the ACR nomenclature. In previous studies, NP disease was reported in 14% to 75% of SLE patients [12–14].

The attribution of individual NP events to SLE or to an alternative etiology remains a challenge. In the absence of a diagnostic gold standard for most of the NP-SLE syndromes, attribution is determined on the basis of exclusion using the best available clinical, laboratory, and imaging data. The ACR nomenclature [6] provide a basis for addressing this issue in a systematic manner, because for each NP syndrome there is a comprehensive list of exclusions and associations, the presence of which may indicate an alternative etiology. Using this approach and taking into consideration the temporal relationship between the NP event and the diagnosis of SLE, a recent study has determined that up to 41% of all NP events in SLE patients may be attributed to factors other than lupus [9].

Table 1
Prevalence of neuropsychiatric systemic lupus erythematosus as defined by the American College of Rheumatology nomenclature in five individual studies

| Characteristics | Study | | | | |
| --- | --- | --- | --- | --- | --- |
| | Ainiala et al, 2001 [7] (Tampere, Finland) | Brey et al, 2002 [8] (San Antonio, TX) | Sanna et al, 2003 [10] (London, UK, & Cagliari, Italy) | Hanly et al, 2004 [9] (Halifax, Canada) | Sibbitt Jr et al, 2002 [11] (Albuquerque, NM)[a] |
| No. of patients | 46 | 128 | 323 | 111 | 75 |
| Disease duration (mean ± SD years) | 14 ± 8 | 8 | 11 ± 8 | 10 ± 1 | 7 ± 8 |
| NP-SLE (%) | 91 | 80 | 57 | 37 | 95 |

[a] Pediatric population.
*Adapted from* The American College of Rheumatology nomenclature and case definitions for neuropsychiatric lupus syndromes. Arthritis Rheum 1999;42(4):599–608.

Table 2
The four most common manifestations of neuropsychiatric systemic lupus erythematosus defined by the American College of Rheumatology nomenclature in five individual studies

| Criteria | Study | | | | |
|---|---|---|---|---|---|
| | Ainiala et al, 2001 [7] (%)[a] | Brey et al, 2002 [8] (%)[b] | Sanna et al, 2003 [10] (%) | Hanly et al, 2004 [9] (%) | Sibbitt et al, 2002 [11] (%)[b] |
| Cognitive dysfunction | 80 | 69 | — | — | 55 |
| Headache | 54 | 57 | 24 | 28 | 72 |
| Mood disorder | — | 40 | — | 14 | 57 |
| Cerebrovascular disease | 15 | — | 18 | 5 | — |
| Seizures | — | — | 8 | 6 | 51 |
| Polyneuropathy | 28 | — | — | — | — |
| Anxiety | — | 24 | — | — | — |
| Psychosis | — | — | 8 | — | — |

[a] Formal neuropsychologic assessments done on all patients.
[b] Pediatric population.
*Adapted from* Hanly JG. ACR Classification Criteria for SLE; Limitations and Revisions to Neuropsychiatric Variables. Lupus 2004;13:861–4.

The results of these clinical studies serve to reinforce previous conclusions on NP-SLE and introduce new concepts. Despite the improved definitions for individual NP syndromes, there continues to be substantial variability in the overall prevalence of NP disease between different populations. Whether this represents inherent differences between study cohorts or a bias in data acquisition remains to be determined. None of the individual NP manifestations are unique to lupus, and indeed some occur with considerable frequency in the general population. Thus, the inclusion of control groups is critical to determine whether the

Table 3
The least common manifestations (< 1%) neuropsychiatric systemic lupus erythematosus defined by the American College of Rheumatology nomenclature in five individual studies

| Manifestation | Study | | | | |
|---|---|---|---|---|---|
| | Ainiala et al, 2001 [7] | Brey et al, 2002 [8] | Sanna et al, 2003 [10] | Hanly et al, 2004 [9] | Sibbitt et al, 2002 [11] |
| Movement disorder | + | + | — | + | — |
| Demyelinating syndrome | + | + | + | — | — |
| Myelopathy | + | + | — | + | + |
| Myasthenia gravis | + | + | — | + | + |
| Guillain-Barré syndrome | + | + | + | + | + |
| Autonomic disorder | + | + | + | + | + |
| Plexopathy | + | + | + | + | + |
| Aseptic meningitis | — | + | + | + | + |

*Adapted from* Hanly JG. ACR Classification Criteria for SLE; Limitations and Revisions to Neuropsychiatric Variables. Lupus 2004;13:861–4.

prevalence of NP disease in SLE patients is in excess of that found in the normal population and in other chronic disease groups. Because many of the NP syndromes are quite rare (less than 1%), multicenter efforts will be required to assemble sufficient numbers of patients for study. Attribution of NP disease in individual patients remains a challenge, particularly in the absence of a diagnostic gold standard. Nevertheless, current evidence suggests that non-SLE factors likely contribute to a substantial proportion of NP disease in SLE patients, particularly the softer NP manifestations such as headache, anxiety, and some mood disorders. Future studies will need to define which of the many NP manifestations have the greatest clinical impact.

## Etiology of neuropsychiatric systemic lupus erythematosus

Given the plethora of NP manifestations reported in SLE patients, it is unlikely that there is a single pathogenic mechanism. NP events in SLE may be caused by a primary manifestation of the disease, secondary complications of the disease or therapy such as hypertension or infection, or a coincidental problem unrelated to lupus (Fig. 1). Primary manifestations of NP-SLE likely reflect a mixture of

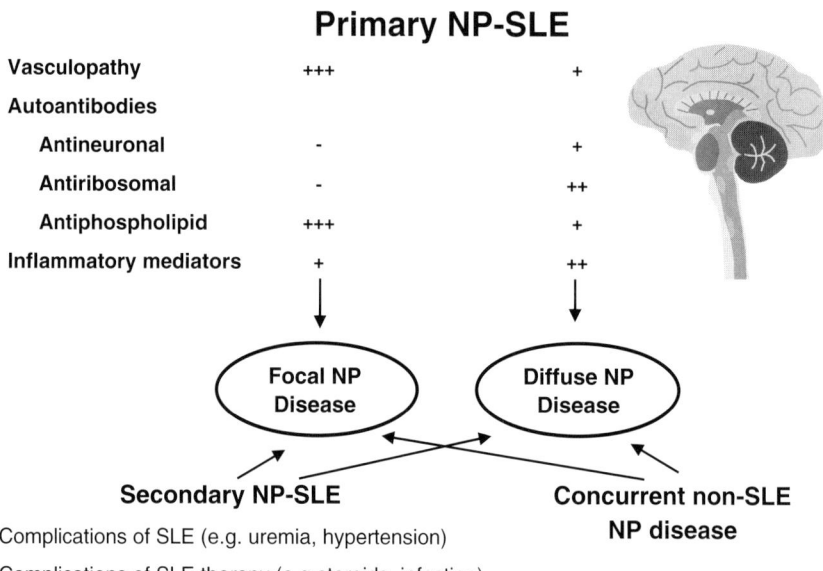

Fig. 1. Factors contributing to the pathogenesis of neuropsychiatric (NP) disease in systemic lupus erythematosus (SLE). (*Adapted from* Hanly JG. Neuropsychiatric lupus. Curr Rheumatol Rep 2001; 3:205–12; with permission.)

---

**Box 2. Pathogenesis of neuropsychiatric systemic lupus erythematosus**

*Vascular abnormalities*

Noninflammatory vasculopathy
Vasculitis
Thrombosis

*Autoantibodies*

Antineuronal antibodies
Antiribosomal P antibodies
Antiphospholipid antibodies

*Inflammatory mediators*

IL-2, -6, -8, and -10
Interferon-α
Tumor necrosis factor–α
Matrix metalloproteinase (MMP)–9

*Adapted from* Hanly JG. Neuropsychiatric lupus. Curr Rheumatol Rep 2001;3:205–12; with permission.

---

pathogenic mechanisms that include vascular abnormalities, autoantibodies, and the local production of inflammatory mediators (see Fig. 1 and Box 2).

*Vasculopathy*

Evidence in support of vascular abnormalities in NP-SLE may be found in neuropathologic studies [15–18]. A bland, noninflammatory vasculopathy involving small vessels was the predominant finding in these studies. In contrast, inflammatory disease of small or large vessels was rare. Brain microinfarcts occurred in association with, and were attributed to the microangiopathy [16]. Although instructive, there are significant limitations to using brain pathology as a means of advancing understanding of NP-SLE. First, patients who come to autopsy, which has been the most frequent source of brain tissue, represent a subset of patients with the most severe disease. Second, there is frequently a temporal disconnect between the NP event and tissue sampling. Third, this approach is restricted to the detection of structural abnormalities. Finally, confounding factors such as infection, hypertension, or corticosteroids may modify the original pathology that occurs as a consequence of the disease. The solution to these problems may come from advances in imaging technology that can act as a surrogate for brain biopsy.

*Autoantibodies*

A humoral immune response directed against several families of autoantigens on neurons, ribosomes, and phospholipid-associated proteins has been implicated to a varying extent in the pathogenesis of NP-SLE. The data from human studies implicating antineuronal antibodies is largely circumstantial. This includes the temporal relationship between clinical events and serologic findings [19], the presence of autoantibodies in the cerebrospinal fluid (CSF) [20], and, to a very limited extent, their identification in neuronal tissues from patients succumbing to the disease [21]. The presence of autoantibodies in the CSF of SLE patients is likely because of passive transfer from the circulation through a permeabilized blood–brain barrier [22,23], and, independently, to direct intrathecal production [19,22]. More direct evidence for the pathogenic potential of antineuronal antibodies is derived from animal studies in which the intracranial injection of autoantibodies reactive with neuronal tissues has been shown to induce memory deficits, seizures, and neuropathologic changes [24–26]. Considerable effort has gone into identifying the fine specificity of this family of autoantibodies. For example, Hanson et al [27] described reactivity to a 50-kd neuronal membrane protein in SLE patients. These autoantibodies bound to the surface of cultured rat neuroblastoma cells, and on Western blotting identified a protein of comparable size in human fetal brain and bovine adult brain. Although there was a significant association between these autoantibodies and NP-SLE, this was not restricted to any particular clinical subset of NP disease. Autoantibodies to gangliosides, which are a family of acid glycolipids predominantly located on neuronal and myelin membranes in the central and peripheral nervous system, have been studied extensively in SLE and in neurologic disorders such as multiple sclerosis. Although present in serum [19,28,29] and CSF [30] of SLE patients, there has not been a consistent association with NP manifestations of the disease.

Most recently, attention has been focused on anti-NR2 glutamate receptor antibodies as a potentially novel system that could explain some of the complexities of NP-SLE. The NMDA (N-methyl-D-aspartate) receptors NR2a and NR2b bind the neurotransmitter glutamate and are present on neurons throughout the forebrain [31–33]. The hippocampus, which is the anatomical structure closely linked to learning and memory, has the highest density of brain NMDA receptors [32]. In addition to their putative role in learning and memory [34], these receptors display altered expression in major psychoses [35], and if engaged by receptor antagonists, they cause hallucinations and paranoia [36]. A recent study [37] has shown that a subset of anti-DNA antibodies, derived from both murine models of SLE and from four human subjects with the disease, cross-react with a pentapeptide consensus sequence that is present in the extracellular, ligand binding domain of NR2 receptors. Moreover, these antibodies induced apoptotic cell death of neurons in vitro and in vivo and were present in the CSF of one SLE patient with progressive cognitive decline. Thus, in contrast to the previously described antineuronal antibodies in SLE, the anti-NR2 glutamate receptor antibodies appear to have a functional consequence leading to neuronal injury in a manner similar to that seen in excitatory amino acid toxicity [38]. In this model, excessive stimulation of the receptor is followed by increased entry of calcium into the cell and subsequent cell death. Although of interest in elucidating a novel pathway for neuronal injury in SLE, these findings are preliminary, largely derived from animal studies, and require confirmation in human subjects with NP-SLE.

Antiribosomal (anti-P) antibodies first were described in SLE patients in 1985 and are quite specific for SLE, with a prevalence of 13% to 20% depending upon the ethnic group [39,40]. In 1987, these autoantibodies were linked to NP-SLE, in particular psychosis [41]. Subsequent work has either supported, refuted, or extended this initial observation to include depression [39,40,42,43]. Potential explanations for the differences is study outcomes include different diagnostic criteria for psychiatric disease, variance in the temporal relationship between clinical events and serologic testing, and differences in assay technique, particularly antigen preparation and purity. One of the largest studies [42] examined 394 SLE patients, 63 (16%) of whom had anti-P antibodies. There was a significant association with psychosis and depression, with odds ratios between 4 and 10. Because of the low prevalence of clinical events, however, the positive predictive value was only 13% and 16% for psychosis and depression, respectively. This has important implications for the application of this serologic test in decision-making for individual patients. In contrast, a more recent study of 149 patients [43], 12% of whom had anti-P antibodies, did not find an association with any of the NP syndromes as defined by the ACR nomenclature [6].

Additional observations on anti-P antibodies are of interest and may provide insight into their pathogenic mechanisms. Koren et al [44] have reported an association between anti-P and antineuronal antibodies, and furthermore, demonstrated that anti-P antibodies bind a 38-kd surface protein on human neuroblastoma cells. In a study of 87 SLE patients, Isshi et al [45] found a significant elevation in circulating anti-P antibodies in 34 patients who had lupus psychosis, but there was no increase in the level of serum antineuronal antibodies. In contrast, examination of the CSF from the same patients revealed a significant elevation in antineuronal antibodies but not in anti-P antibody levels. These data suggest potential interaction between these two families of autoantibodies in the pathogenesis of NP-SLE.

Autoimmune antiphospholipid antibodies, which are directed against phospholipid-binding proteins such as $\beta_2$-glycoprotein I and prothrombin [46], are associated with predominately focal manifestations of NP-SLE. The most common neurologic disorders are those of vascular origin such as transient cerebral ischemia or stroke, but other associations include seizures, chorea, transverse myelitis, and cognitive dysfunction [47]. In a review of over 1000 SLE patients, Love and Santoro reported neuropsychiatric manifestations in 38% of patients who had lupus anticoagulant compared with 21% of patients who did not have these antiphospholipid antibodies [48]. The favored pathogenic mechanism for this subset of autoantibodies in NP-SLE is thrombosis within vessels of different caliber and subsequent cerebral ischemia. A procoagulant state may be induced through acquired resistance to protein C and protein S, platelet aggregation, and direct activation of endothelial cells [46]. However, the intrathecal production of antiphospholipid antibodies in NP-SLE patients [22], their association with diffuse cognitive impairment [49,50], and in vitro evidence indicating modulation of neuronal cell function [51] raise the possibility of an alternative pathogenic mechanism.

*Inflammatory mediators*

The potential role of proinflammatory cytokines in neuropsychiatric lupus has received increasing attention in recent years. Studies in Japan were the first to report an association between enhanced intracranial production of interleukin (IL)-6 with seizures [52] and interferon-$\alpha$ with lupus psychosis [53]. Subsequent studies have provided further evidence for the intrathecal production of IL-6 [54–57] and have identified other potential candidate cytokines such as IL-10 [57,58], IL-2 [59], IL-8 [56] and tumor necrosis factor–$\alpha$ [57]. Potential sources for the intrathecal production of these cytokines include neuronal [53,55] and glial cells [53]. The stimulus for, and regulation of this enhanced cytokine response remain to be determined. Although potentially an epiphenomenon, it also may be a consequence of cell activation mediated by autoantibodies within the intrathecal space. Measuring CSF cytokine levels unselectively in patients who had any manifestation of NP-SLE, however, is unlikely to be of diagnostic value [60].

Other potentially important inflammatory mediators are MMPs, a family of endoperoxidases that can degrade extracellular matrix components [61]. MMP-9 is a gelatinase and is secreted by a variety of cells in the vessel wall, including macrophages, T lymphocytes, and endothelial and smooth muscle cells [62]. Implicated in the pathogenesis of plaque rupture [63], elevated levels also have been associated with other conditions, including multiple sclerosis [64], Guillain-Barré syndrome [65], rheumatoid arthritis [66], and SLE [67]. A recent study [68] examined the association between circulating levels of MMP-9 and NP-SLE. Although there was no difference in the levels of MMP-9 between SLE patients and healthy population controls, elevated levels of MMP-9 were associated with NP-SLE, and in particular with cognitive impairment. There was a positive correlation between circulating MMP-9 levels and both T1 and T2 lesions on brain MRI. It is also of interest that increased expression of MMP-9 is found in the disrupted blood–brain barrier following cerebral ischemia and may facilitate lymphocyte migration into and possibly through the arterial wall [69].

## Specific neuropsychiatric manifestations

As with other organ involvement in SLE, nervous system disease may occur at any time in the disease course. Nevertheless, it is of interest that NP-SLE frequently presents early in the disease course, either before or following the diagnosis of lupus [70,71]. NP events in patients who have active multiorgan disease from lupus is well recognized [16], and when it occurs, it provides support for the notion that lupus is the most likely cause of the NP manifestation. NP-SLE, however, may also occur in the setting of globally quiescent lupus [72]. In the following comments on specific NP manifestation, the prevalence of individual manifestations is derived from studies using the 1999 ACR definitions for NP-SLE [6].

*Cognitive function*

Cognitive dysfunction, assessed using neuropsychologic assessment techniques, has been reported in up to 80% of SLE patients [7], although most studies have found prevalence between 17% and 66% [12,73]. These tests evaluate the functional integrity of the CNS through systematic assessment of performance on specific tasks. The tests are administered and scored in a standardized manner and assess multiple areas of cognitive function, including simple and complex attention, memory, visual–spatial processing, language, reasoning, psychomotor speed, and executive functions. Results can be expressed in relation to normative data or in terms of the estimated premorbid level of function or competence. As most SLE patients who have cognitive impairment have relatively mild deficits, the careful selection and assessment of cognitive performance in control groups is of critical importance to define expected levels of function in healthy individuals and those with other chronic diseases. Although cognitive impairment may be viewed as a distinct subset of NP-SLE, it also can serve as a surrogate of overall brain health in SLE patients, which may be affected by several factors including other NP syndromes.

The range in prevalence of cognitive impairment in SLE [12,73] is most likely because of differences in selection of patients for study and lack of uniform definitions for cognitive impairment. There is no specific or unique pattern of cognitive impairment in SLE, and many individual patients have subclinical deficits. For example, a review of 14 cross-sectional studies of cognitive function in SLE revealed subclinical cognitive impairment in 11% to 54% of patients [73]. This latter observation raises several clinical questions. For example, what is the evolution of these cognitive deficits over time, and does their detection predict the subsequent development of other more profound clinically overt forms of NP disease?

The outcome of cognitive impairment in SLE patients has been examined in several studies. For example, in a 5-year prospective study of 70 SLE patients using a standardized panel of neuropsychologic tests [74], the prevalence of overall cognitive impairment in SLE patients fell from 21% to 13% over the period of study. Five patterns of cognitive performance were observed over the 5-year period. Eighty-three percent of patients were either never impaired or had resolution of cognitive impairment without specific therapeutic interventions. An additional 13% of patients demonstrated an emerging or fluctuating pattern of impairment, and only 4% (two patients) showed persisting deficits that were stable over time. Similar benign changes in cognitive performance over time have been reported by Waterloo et al [75] in 28 patients over 5 years, by Hay et al [76] in a 2-year prospective study, and by Carlomagno et al [77].

Predictors of cognitive decline over time also have been examined. In a study by Hanly et al [74], when patients who were cognitively impaired at the initial assessment were compared with those who were not impaired, the differences between groups in tests of recent memory and delayed free recall decreased over 5 years. A similar result was reported by Waterloo et al [75]. Patients who had clinically overt NP-SLE at any time in their disease course, however, had a statistically significant decline in memory performance over 5 years when compared with patients who did not have a history of clinically overt NP-SLE [74]. These results suggest that the occurrence of clinically overt NP events, rather than the identification of isolated subclinical cognitive impairment, is a more reliable predictor of deterioration in selective aspects of memory function over time.

The association between cognitive function and anticardiolipin (aCL) anti-bodies has been examined in several cross-sectional and prospective studies. In work completed at the author's center, 51 SLE patients were divided into those who were persistently aCL antibody positive or negative on the basis of up to seven antibody determinations over a 5-year period [49]. The relative change in performance on individual neuropsychologic tests then was compared between patients who were antibody positive and negative. Those who were persistently IgG aCL antibody positive demonstrated a greater reduction in psychomotor speed compared with those who were antibody negative. In contrast, patients who were persistently IgA aCL antibody positive had significantly poorer perfor-mance in conceptual reasoning and executive ability. Similar results have been reported by Menon et al in a 2-year prospective study of 45 SLE patients [50]. These data suggest that IgG and IgA aCL may be responsible for long-term subtle deterioration in cognitive function in SLE patients.

*Headache*

The association between SLE and headache is controversial. The reported prevalence of headache has varied widely between 24% and 72% [7–11], but the prevalence of headache in the general population is also high, with up to 40% of individuals reporting a severe headache at least once per year [78]. Two of the most recent studies [79,80], which were methodologically more robust than earlier work, found no increase in the prevalence of headache in SLE. Fur-thermore, there is only one study [81] reporting an association between head-ache and other clinical features of active lupus. Thus, although headache may be a component of active SLE in individual patients, particularly in patients who have active systemic disease, it is more likely that most headaches in SLE patients are unrelated to SLE [82].

*Psychosis, mood disorders, and anxiety*

Psychosis is reported in up to 8% of SLE patients [7–11,83], and it is characterized by either the presence of delusions (false belief despite evidence to the contrary) or hallucinations (perceptual experiences occurring in the absence of external stimuli). The latter are most frequently auditory. Psychosis is a rare but dramatic manifestation of NP-SLE, and when present it must be distinguished form other causes, including drug abuse, schizophrenia, and depression. Depression and anxiety are common symptoms in lupus patients and occur in 24% to 57% of patients [7–11,43]. As there are no features of these syndromes that are unique to SLE patients, however, there is often uncertainty about the etiology and attribution in individual cases. The association between psychosis, depression, and anti-P antibodies in SLE is supported by some but not all studies [39,41–43].

*Cerebrovascular disease*

The many forms of cerebrovascular disease are reported in 5% to 18% of SLE patients [7–11] and are likely multifactorial in etiology. Accelerated atherosclerosis is recognized in SLE, particularly in relation to coronary heart disease, where there is a 5 to 10 times higher rate of events compared with control populations [83]. This also contributes to the increased rate of cerebrovascular events in SLE. An additional etiologic factor is the prothrombotic state as a consequence of antiphospholipid antibodies [46], which provides a rationale for therapeutic intervention with anticoagulants in selected cases.

*Seizures*

Generalized and focal seizures are reported in 6% to 51% [7–11] of patients and may occur either in the setting of active generalized multisystem lupus or as isolated neurologic events. Their occurrence frequently is associated with the presence of antiphospholipid antibodies [10], which are associated with microangiopathy, arterial thrombosis, and subsequent cerebral infarction.

*Demyelination, transverse myelopathy, and chorea*

These are rare manifestations of nervous system disease in SLE and occur no more frequently than in 1% to 3% of patients [7–11,14]. Clinical and neuroimaging evidence of demyelination has been described and may be indistinguishable from multiple sclerosis [84]. This may represent a concordance or overlap of two autoimmune conditions. Transverse myelopathy [85] and chorea

[86] present acutely and frequently are associated with antiphospholipid antibodies [85,86]. Although an arterial thrombotic event is a likely mechanism for transverse myelopathy, the cause of chorea is less clear, and there has been speculation that it may be a consequence of a direct interaction of antiphospholipid antibodies with neuronal structures in the basal ganglia [87].

*Neuropathy*

A sensorimotor neuropathy has been reported in up to 28% [7–11] of SLE patients and frequently occurs independently of other disease characteristics [88]. The abnormalities are persistent, but in one study, 67% of patients had no change in their neuropathy over a 7-year period [88]. A controlled immunohistologic study of skin biopsies in SLE patients has demonstrated involvement of small nerve fibers [89].

## Clinical impact and prognosis of neuropsychiatric systemic lupus erythematosus

The clinical impact of NP events in SLE has been determined by examining the association with several clinical indicators including quality of life. In a recent study [9], NP events were associated with significantly lower scores on most subscales of the SF-36, a generic self-report measure of quality of life, and with higher fatigue scores. These associations were present regardless of the attribution of the NP event to SLE or an alternative etiology, but they did not occur in patients who have a history of renal disease. Jonsen et al [70] also reported a higher frequency of disability in SLE patients who have NP disease compared with patients who do not have NP events and the general population. Collectively, these data indicate that NP events in SLE patients, regardless of their etiology and attribution, have a negative impact on quality of life.

Although the overall clinical impact of NP-SLE may be detrimental, it is likely that individual NP manifestations differ in their prognostic implications. For example, the subtle cognitive deficits detected by formal neuropsychologic testing have not been associated with a negative impact on quality of life, at least as determined by self-report questionnaires [74,90]. In another study [91] 70% of patients who have cognitive difficulties were able to maintain their work capacity, and 86% had no change in their social functioning.

Relatively few studies have examined the course of NP-SLE over time. Karassa et al [92] examined the prognosis of NP disease in 32 patients who had been hospitalized for NP-SLE and followed for 2 years. The outcome was generally favorable, with either substantial improvement (69%) or stabilization (19%) accounting for most cases. A high number of prior NP events and the occurrence of the antiphospholipid syndrome were predictors of an unfavorable clinical outcome at 2 years. There is no consensus in the literature on the association between NP-SLE and mortality. Some studies report increased mortality

[93–97] in SLE patients who have NP disease, and others report no such association [71,98–100]. One cause of mortality in SLE is suicide, which has been reported in association with NP manifestations in a recent study involving a small number of patients [101].

## Diagnostic imaging and neuropsychiatric systemic lupus erythematosus

When considering neuroimaging in NP-SLE it is helpful to incorporate an assessment of brain structure and brain function. Although CT scanning is the preferred technique for the diagnosis of acute intracranial hemorrhage, it largely has been replaced by MRI for detecting other abnormalities because of its increased sensitivity [102]. Abnormalities on MRI scanning may be found in 19% [103] to 70% [104] of SLE patients. $T_2$-weighted MRI images identify pathologic processes that cause edema and is more sensitive than $T_1$-weighted images for detecting abnormalities in NP-SLE patients. Applying the technique of fluid-attenuating inversion recovery (FLAIR), to dampen the CSF signal and highlight areas of edema, further enhances the utility of $T_2$-weighted images [84,105]. Focal neurologic disease is associated with predominately fixed lesions in the preventricular and subcortical white matter usually in the territory of a major cerebral blood vessel [106]. These multiple white matter lesions are quite nonspecific, however, and more commonly are attributed to hypertension, disease duration, and age-related small vessel disease than to the presence of NP-SLE [107–109]. If the lesions are larger, occur in the corpus collosum, and are seen on $T_1$-weighted images, then the diagnosis of multiple sclerosis has to be considered [84]. Diffuse NP clinical presentations are associated with transient subcortical white matter lesions and patchy hyperintensities in the gray matter that usually are not confined to the territories of major cerebral blood flow [106]. Other abnormalities detected on MRI scanning in SLE patients include cerebral infarction, venous sinus thrombosis, and increased signal in the spinal cord accompanying the clinical presentation of myelopathy [84]. MRI also provides quantitative volumetric analysis of brain atrophy.

The most objective neuroimaging study of brain function is positron emission tomography (PET) scanning, but practical considerations limit its applicability [4]. Single photon emission computed tomography (SPECT) scanning often is regarded as the poor man's PET [110]. This provides semiquantitative analysis of regional cerebral blood flow and metabolism. It is exquisitely sensitive, and in studies of SLE patients [111–115], SPECT imaging has identified diffuse and focal deficits that may be fixed or reversible. The findings are not specific for SLE [111], however, and do not always correlate with clinical NP manifestations [116]. The interpretation of what these imaging abnormalities indicate is not always clear. The most common explanation is that they reflect a primary or secondary reduction in blood flow. In the brain, however, there is sometimes disassociation between metabolism and blood flow. Changes in blood flow and metabolism can occur in sites distant from those of the pathologic lesion, a phenomenon known as diaschisis. A study [117] of concurrent SPECT and PET imaging in 25 SLE patients, 13 of whom had a history of NP-SLE, indicated the superiority of PET scanning. Furthermore, the abnormalities in glucose metabolism detected by PET scanning are reversible with the institution of anti-inflammatory and immunosuppressive therapies [118,119] but may also progress to structural changes within the brain as detected by subsequent MRI [118].

The application of several technologies to MRI scanning has provided additional opportunities to assess brain metabolism and function. Magnetic resonance angiography (MRA) permits a nonevasive visualization of cerebral blood flow, although it is probably not optimal for visualization of flow in small caliber vessels, which are the ones primarily involved in NP-SLE. Magnetic resonance spectroscopy (MRS) allows the identification and quantification of brain metabolites, thereby providing indirect evidence of cellular changes [102]. Thus, the amount of N-acetyl (NA) compounds, which reflect the quantity and integrity of neuronal cells, is reduced in lupus brains. Studies of SLE patients have found an association between reduced NA brain levels with neurocognitive dysfunction [120] and independently with elevated IgG antiphospholipid antibodies [121]. Brain lactate levels also are elevated, indicating ischemia and inflammation, while choline compounds are increased, reflecting damaged cell membranes and myelin destruction.

Magnetization transfer imaging (MTI) is particularly suited to the detection and quantification of diffuse brain damage. This technique quantifies the exchange of protons between water within a macromolecule such as myelin and protons in free water. Either the loss of myelin or the accumulation of edema will alter the transfer, which is expressed as the magnetization transfer ratio (MTR) [122]. Studies have revealed a lower MTR in patients who have NP-SLE and multiple sclerosis, while there was no difference between healthy controls and SLE patients who did not have NP disease [104,123,124]. The findings in SLE patients correlated with the results of cognitive assessment and psychiatric functioning [125]. As both MRS and MTI identified abnormalities in SLE patients who have normal MRI scans, these techniques provide a means for detecting and quantifying brain injury in NP-SLE patients that is not apparent with other imaging modalities. Diffusion weighted imaging (DWI) is highly effective for detecting hyperacute brain injury, in particular acute ischemia following stroke when the diffusion of water is highly restricted because of the acute shift of fluid into the intracellular compartment and cytotoxic edema [84,122]. Such abnormalities are not seen in multiple sclerosis. In a study of 20 SLE patients by Moritani et al [126], DWI abnormalities were detected in four cases. Functional MRI measures cerebral blood flow and neuronal activity by measuring oxygenation status of hemoglobin, and studies of SLE patients using this technique are awaited with interest. Although none of these techniques identify abnormalities that are unique to NP-SLE patients it will be of considerable interest to examine their clinical significance and evolution over time and to determine the potential for reversibility.

## Biologic markers of nervous system damage

Nonspecific abnormalities may be found in the CSF of 33% of patients who have NP disease [127]. They include pleocytosis and elevated protein levels. A recent study [128] indicated more specific markers of cellular damage. Thus, elevated levels of CSF neurofilament triplet protein (NFL), which reflects neuronal and in particular axonal damage, were increased in SLE patients who have NP-SLE compared with SLE patients who do not have NP disease and healthy controls. The sensitivity was 74% and specificity 65%. Likewise, the level of CSF glial fibrillary acidic protein (GFAP), which indicates astrogliosis or scarring, was increased in the same patient population, with a sensitivity of 48% and specificity of 87%. Moreover, the levels of both NFL and GFAP were associated with abnormalities on MRI scanning and were reduced following the successful treatment of several NP manifestations with cyclophosphamide. Although elevated levels of NFL and GFAP are not restricted to SLE, these data indicate a potentially objective, biologic indicator of nervous system disease in lupus patients.

## Diagnosis and management of neuropsychiatric systemic lupus erythematosus

The first step in the management of a patient with SLE who presents with a NP event is to determine whether the event can be convincingly attributed to SLE, a complication of the disease or its therapy, or whether it reflects a coincidental disease process. This is achieved largely by a process of exclusion, given the absence of a diagnostic gold standard for most of the NP manifestations that occur in SLE. Thus, the correct diagnosis is derived from a careful analysis of the clinical, laboratory, and imaging data on a case-by-case basis. The spectrum of diagnostic tests available is listed in Box 3, and these may be used to a varying extent depending upon the clinical circumstances. Examination of the CSF should be considered primarily to exclude infection. Analysis of CSF autoanti-bodies, cytokines, and biomarkers of neurologic damage is still in the research arena. In considering autoantibodies, those that are most likely to provide the greatest diagnostic yield are antiphospholipid antibodies. The value of measuring anti-P antibodies remains uncertain given the conflicting results to date, while the role of anti-NR2 antibodies in NP-SLE is unknown. Neuroimaging should include a modality to assess brain structure and another to assess brain function. Neuropsychologic testing only should be done to address specific concerns about cognitive ability, as the detection of isolated subclinical deficits appears to have little clinical significance.

Management will need to be tailored according to the individual patient's needs (Box 4), and there remains a paucity of controlled studies to guide treatment decisions. Once a diagnosis of NP-SLE is established, the first step is to

---

**Box 3. Investigations in the assessment of systemic lupus erythematosus patients for neuropsychiatric disease**

*Cerebrospinal fluid*
- Exclude infection
- Autoantibodies (?)
- Cytokines (?)

*Autoantibodies*
- Antiphospholipid
- Antineuronal (?)
- Antiribosomal P (?)

*Neuroimaging*
- Brain structure (CT, MRI)
- Brain function (PET, SPECT, MRI, MRA, MRS, MTI, DWI, FMRI)

*Neuropsychologic assessment*

*Abbreviations:* DWI, diffusion weighted imaging; FMRI, functional MRI; MRA, magnetic resonance angiography; MRS, magnetic resonance spectroscopy; MTI, magnetization transverse imaging; PET, positron emission tomography; SPECT, single photon emission computed tomography.

*Adapted from* Hanly JG. Neuropsychiatric lupus. Curr Rheumatol Rep 2001;3:205–12; with permission.

---

identify and treat potential aggravating factors such as hypertension, infection, and metabolic abnormalities. Symptomatic therapy with, for example, anticonvulsants, antidepressants, and antipsychotic medications, should be considered if appropriate. Immunosuppressive therapy with high-dose corticosteroids, cyclophosphamide, and azathioprine has been used to treat many NP-SLE manifestations. With the exception of one study [129], there are no placebo-controlled studies examining the benefit of oral or intravenous corticosteroids [130,131] in NP lupus. Similarly, pulse intravenous cyclophosphamide therapy [132–140], akin to that which has been used in the treatment of lupus nephritis, has been reported to be beneficial in NP-SLE, although no controlled studies have been performed. A recent open-label study of 13 patients who had lupus psychosis reported a favorable outcome in all patients treated with oral cyclophosphamide for 6 months followed by maintenance therapy with azathioprine [141]. In virtually all of these studies, immunosuppressive therapy has been used in conjunction with corticosteroids in addition to symptomatic therapies, such as antipsychotic medications. More targeted immunosuppressive therapies, for example B lymphocyte depletion with anti-CD20 used alone or in com-

---

**Box 4. Management of neuropsychiatric events in patients who have systemic lupus erythematosus**

*Establish diagnosis of NP-SLE*
*Identify aggravating factors*
  • Hypertension
  • Infection
  • Metabolic abnormalities
*Symptomatic therapy*
  • Anticonvulsants
  • Psychotropics
  • Anxiolytics
*Immunosuppression*
  • Corticosteroids
  • Azathioprine,
  • Cyclophosphamide
  • B-lymphocyte depletion
*Anticoagulation*
  • Heparin
  • Warfarin

*Adapted from* Hanly JG. Neuropsychiatric lupus. Curr Rheumatol Rep 2001;3:205–12; with permission.

---

bination with cyclophosphamide [142,143], are promising but require further study. Anticoagulation is indicated strongly for focal disease when antiphospholipid antibodies are implicated, and such therapy usually will be lifelong [47, 144,145].

There are several opportunities for novel or improved therapies in the future. The optimal management of intracranial thrombosis should become clearer following the completion of controlled studies of anticoagulation therapy in patients who have primary antiphospholipid antibody syndrome, although studies to date have yielded conflicting results [144,145]. Depending on the outcome of studies of thrombolytic therapy in patients who have degenerative vascular disease, there also may be a role for such therapy in SLE. Novel therapies in development for Alzheimer's disease and vascular dementias also may hold some promise for selected SLE patients who have major cognitive dysfunction. If the role of cytokines in the pathogenesis of specific subsets of NP-SLE is confirmed, then consideration should be given to anticytokine therapies. Finally, studies of non-pharmacologic therapies also should be considered, as exemplified by a recent placebo-controlled trial of a theory-based psychoeducational intervention that reported positive outcomes at 6 and 12 months of follow-up [146].

## Summary

Nervous system disease in SLE patients spans a wide spectrum of neurologic and psychiatric features that may be attributed to a primary manifestation of SLE, complications of the disease or its therapy, or a coincidental disease process. The ACR nomenclature and case definitions have provided a basis for the classification of NP disease and provide the standard for categorizing patients in clinical studies of NP-SLE. Despite this advance, there continues to be considerable variability in the prevalence of NP disease reported in different cohorts of SLE patients, and the rarity of many of the NP syndromes emphasizes the need for multicenter studies. The etiology of primary NP disease is multifactorial and includes vascular injury of intracranial vessels, autoantibodies to neuronal antigens, ribosomes and phospholipid-associated proteins, and the intracranial generation of cytokines and possibly other inflammatory mediators. In the absence of a diagnostic gold standard for most of the NP-SLE syndromes, many investigations are employed to support the clinical diagnosis and determine the severity of NP disease. The advancement in technology employing MRI holds particular promise in this regard. Treatment remains largely empiric in the absence of controlled studies and draws upon the experience in the management of other serious organ involvement such as lupus nephritis. Current strategies include the use of immunosuppressive therapies, appropriate symptomatic interventions, and the treatment of non-SLE factors when identified.

## References

[1] Tan EM, et al. The 1982 revised criteria for the classification of systemic lupus erythematosus. Arthritis Rheum 1982;25(11):1271–7.

[2] Hochberg MC. Updating the American College of Rheumatology revised criteria for the classification of systemic lupus erythematosus. Arthritis Rheum 1997;40(9):1725.

[3] West SG. Neuropsychiatric lupus. Rheum Dis Clin North Am 1994;20(1):129–58.

[4] Hanly JG. Evaluation of patients with CNS involvement in SLE. Baillieres Clin Rheumatol 1998;12(3):415–31.

[5] How A, et al. Antineuronal antibodies in neuropsychiatric systemic lupus erythematosus. Arthritis Rheum 1985;28(7):789–95.

[6] The American College of Rheumatology nomenclature and case definitions for neuropsychiatric lupus syndromes. Arthritis Rheum 1999;42(4):599–608.

[7] Ainiala H, et al. Validity of the new American College of Rheumatology criteria for neuropsychiatric lupus syndromes: a population-based evaluation. Arthritis Rheum 2001;45(5): 419–23.

[8] Brey RL, et al. Neuropsychiatric syndromes in lupus: prevalence using standardized definitions. Neurology 2002;58(8):1214–20.

[9] Hanly JG, McCurdy G, Fougere L, et al. Neuropsychiatric disease in systemic lupus erythematosus (SLE): attribution and clinical significance. J Rheumatol 2004;31:2156–62.

[10] Sanna G, et al. Neuropsychiatric manifestations in systemic lupus erythematosus: prevalence and association with antiphospholipid antibodies. J Rheumatol 2003;30(5):985–92.

[11] Sibbitt Jr WL, et al. The incidence and prevalence of neuropsychiatric syndromes in pediatric onset systemic lupus erythematosus. J Rheumatol 2002;29(7):1536–42.

[12] Hanly JG, Liang MH. Cognitive disorders in systemic lupus erythematosus. Epidemiologic and clinical issues. Ann N Y Acad Sci 1997;823:60–8.

[13] McCune WJ, Golbus J. Neuropsychiatric lupus. Rheum Dis Clin North Am 1988;14(1):149–67.

[14] Jennekens FG, Kater L. The central nervous system in systemic lupus erythematosus. Part 1. Clinical syndromes: a literature investigation. Rheumatology (Oxford) 2002;41(6):605–18.

[15] Johnson RT, Richardson EP. The neurological manifestations of systemic lupus erythematosus. Medicine (Baltimore) 1968;47(4):337–69.

[16] Hanly JG, Walsh NM, Sangalang V. Brain pathology in systemic lupus erythematosus. J Rheumatol 1992;19(5):732–41.

[17] Devinsky O, Petito CK, Alonso DR. Clinical and neuropathological findings in systemic lupus erythematosus: the role of vasculitis, heart emboli, and thrombotic thrombocytopenic purpura. Ann Neurol 1988;23(4):380–4.

[18] Ellis SG, Verity MA. Central nervous system involvement in systemic lupus erythematosus: a review of neuropathologic findings in 57 cases, 1955–1977. Semin Arthritis Rheum 1979; 8(3):212–21.

[19] Weiner SM, Klein R, Berg PA. A longitudinal study of autoantibodies against central nervous system tissue and gangliosides in connective tissue diseases. Rheumatol Int 2000;19(3):83–8.

[20] Bluestein HG, Williams GW, Steinberg AD. Cerebrospinal fluid antibodies to neuronal cells: association with neuropsychiatric manifestations of systemic lupus erythematosus. Am J Med 1981;70(2):240–6.

[21] Zvaifler NJ, Bluestein HG. The pathogenesis of central nervous system manifestations of systemic lupus erythematosus. Arthritis Rheum 1982;25(7):862–6.

[22] Martinez-Cordero E, Rivera Garcia BE, Aguilar Leon DE. Anticardiolipin antibodies in serum and cerebrospinal fluid from patients with systemic lupus erythematosus. J Investig Allergol Clin Immunol 1997;7(6):596–601.

[23] Abbott NJ, Mendonca LL, Dolman DE. The blood–brain barrier in systemic lupus erythematosus. Lupus 2003;12(12):908–15.

[24] Karpiak SE, Graf L, Rapport MM. Antiserum to brain gangliosides produces recurrent epileptiform activity. Science 1976;194(4266):735–7.

[25] Kobiler D, Fuchs S, Samuel D. The effect of antisynaptosomal plasma membrane antibodies on memory. Brain Res 1976;115(1):129–38.

[26] Gaburo NJ, Timo-Iaria C, Bueno C, et al. "In vivo" effects of anti-ribosomal P protein antibodies injections into lateral of the rat brain. Arthritis Rheum 1995;38(9):S297.

[27] Hanson VG, et al. Systemic lupus erythematosus patients with central nervous system involvement show autoantibodies to a 50-kD neuronal membrane protein. J Exp Med 1992; 176(2):565–73.

[28] Galeazzi M, et al. Antiganglioside antibodies in a large cohort of European patients with systemic lupus erythematosus: clinical, serological, and HLA class II gene associations. European Concerted Action on the Immunogenetics of SLE. J Rheumatol 2000;27(1):135–41.

[29] Martinez X, et al. Antibodies against gangliosides in patients with SLE and neurological manifestations. Lupus 1992;1(5):299–302.

[30] Pereira RM, et al. Antiganglioside antibodies in patients with neuropsychiatric systemic lupus erythematosus. Lupus 1992;1(3):175–9.

[31] Prins JM, de Glas-Vos JW. Cerebral disseminated lupus erythematosus; brain-racking for patient and physician. Ned Tijdschr Geneeskd 1990;134(46):2252–6.

[32] Ozawa S, Kamiya H, Tsuzuki K. Glutamate receptors in the mammalian central nervous system. Prog Neurobiol 1998;54(5):581–618.

[33] Scherzer CR, et al. Expression of N-methyl-D-aspartate receptor subunit mRNAs in the human brain: hippocampus and cortex. J Comp Neurol 1998;390(1):75–90.

[34] Morris RG, et al. Selective impairment of learning and blockade of long-term potentiation by an N-methyl-D-aspartate receptor antagonist, AP5. Nature 1986;319(6056):774–6.

[35] Akbarian S, et al. Selective alterations in gene expression for NMDA receptor subunits in prefrontal cortex of schizophrenics. J Neurosci 1996;16(1):19–30.

[36] Jentsch JD, Roth RH. The neuropsychopharmacology of phencyclidine: from NMDA receptor hypofunction to the dopamine hypothesis of schizophrenia. Neuropsychopharmacology 1999; 20(3):201–25.

[37] DeGiorgio LA, et al. A subset of lupus anti-DNA antibodies cross-reacts with the NR2 glutamate receptor in systemic lupus erythematosus. Nat Med 2001;7(11):1189–93.

[38] Lipton SA, Rosenberg PA. Excitatory amino acids as a final common pathway for neurologic disorders. N Engl J Med 1994;330(9):613–22.

[39] Teh LS, Isenberg DA. Antiribosomal P protein antibodies in systemic lupus erythematosus. A reappraisal. Arthritis Rheum 1994;37(3):307–15.

[40] Tzioufas AG, et al. The clinical relevance of antibodies to ribosomal-P common epitope in two targeted systemic lupus erythematosus populations: a large cohort of consecutive patients and patients with active central nervous system disease. Ann Rheum Dis 2000;59(2):99–104.

[41] Bonfa E, et al. Association between lupus psychosis and anti-ribosomal P protein antibodies. N Engl J Med 1987;317(5):265–71.

[42] Arnett FC, et al. Ribosomal P autoantibodies in systemic lupus erythematosus. Frequencies in different ethnic groups and clinical and immunogenetic associations. Arthritis Rheum 1996; 39(11):1833–9.

[43] Gerli R, et al. Clinical and serological associations of ribosomal P autoantibodies in systemic lupus erythematosus: prospective evaluation in a large cohort of Italian patients. Rheumatology (Oxford) 2002;41(12):1357–66.

[44] Koren E, et al. Autoantibodies to the ribosomal P proteins react with a plasma membrane-related target on human cells. J Clin Invest 1992;89(4):1236–41.

[45] Isshi K, Hirohata S. Differential roles of the anti-ribosomal P antibody and antineuronal antibody in the pathogenesis of central nervous system involvement in systemic lupus erythematosus. Arthritis Rheum 1998;41(10):1819–27.

[46] Hanly JG. Antiphospholipid syndrome: an overview. CMAJ 2003;168(13):1675–82.

[47] Sanna G, et al. Central nervous system involvement in the antiphospholipid (Hughes) syndrome. Rheumatology (Oxford) 2003;42(2):200–13.

[48] Love PE, Santoro SA. Antiphospholipid antibodies: anticardiolipin and the lupus anticoagulant in systemic lupus erythematosus (SLE) and in non-SLE disorders. Prevalence and clinical significance. Ann Intern Med 1990;112(9):682–98.

[49] Hanly JG, et al. A prospective analysis of cognitive function and anticardiolipin antibodies in systemic lupus erythematosus. Arthritis Rheum 1999;42(4):728–34.

[50] Menon S, et al. A longitudinal study of anticardiolipin antibody levels and cognitive functioning in systemic lupus erythematosus. Arthritis Rheum 1999;42(4):735–41.

[51] Chapman J, et al. Antiphospholipid antibodies permeabilize and depolarize brain synaptoneurosomes. Lupus 1999;8(2):127–33.

[52] Hirohata S, Miyamoto T. Elevated levels of interleukin-6 in cerebrospinal fluid from patients with systemic lupus erythematosus and central nervous system involvement. Arthritis Rheum 1990;33(5):644–9.

[53] Shiozawa S, et al. Interferon-alpha in lupus psychosis. Arthritis Rheum 1992;35(4):417–22.

[54] Jara LJ, et al. Prolactin and interleukin-6 in neuropsychiatric lupus erythematosus. Clin Rheumatol 1998;17(2):110–4.

[55] Hirohata S, Hayakawa K. Enhanced interleukin-6 messenger RNA expression by neuronal cells in a patient with neuropsychiatric systemic lupus erythematosus. Arthritis Rheum 1999;42(12): 2729–30.

[56] Trysberg E, Carlsten H, Tarkowski A. Intrathecal cytokines in systemic lupus erythematosus with central nervous system involvement. Lupus 2000;9(7):498–503.

[57] Dellalibera-Joviliano R, et al. Kinins and cytokines in plasma and cerebrospinal fluid of patients with neuropsychiatric lupus. J Rheumatol 2003;30(3):485–92.

[58] Rood MJ, et al. Neuropsychiatric systemic lupus erythematosus is associated with imbalance in interleukin 10 promoter haplotypes [see comments]. Ann Rheum Dis 1999;58(2):85–9.

[59] Gilad R, et al. Cerebrospinal fluid soluble interleukin-2 receptor in cerebral lupus. Br J Rheumatol 1997;36(2):190–3.

[60] Jonsen A, et al. The heterogeneity of neuropsychiatric systemic lupus erythematosus is reflected in lack of association with cerebrospinal fluid cytokine profiles. Lupus 2003;12(11): 846–50.

[61] Lijnen HR. Plasmin and matrix metalloproteinases in vascular remodeling. Thromb Haemost 2001;86(1):324–33.

[62] Kalela A, et al. Serum matrix metalloproteinase-9 concentration in angiographically assessed coronary artery disease. Scand J Clin Lab Invest 2002;62(5):337–42.

[63] Ross R. Atherosclerosis–an inflammatory disease. N Engl J Med 1999;340(2):115–26.

[64] Lee MA, et al. Serum gelatinase B, TIMP-1 and TIMP-2 levels in multiple sclerosis. A longitudinal clinical and MRI study. Brain 1999;122:191–7.

[65] Creange A, et al. Matrix metalloproteinase-9 is increased and correlates with severity in Guillain-Barre syndrome. Neurology 1999;53(8):1683–91.

[66] Ahrens D, et al. Expression of matrix metalloproteinase 9 (96-kd gelatinase B) in human rheumatoid arthritis. Arthritis Rheum 1996;39(9):1576–87.

[67] Faber-Elmann A, et al. Activity of matrix metalloproteinase-9 is elevated in sera of patients with systemic lupus erythematosus. Clin Exp Immunol 2002;127(2):393–8.

[68] Ainiala H, et al. Increased serum matrix metalloproteinase 9 levels in systemic lupus erythematosus patients with neuropsychiatric manifestations and brain magnetic resonance imaging abnormalities. Arthritis Rheum 2004;50(3):858–65.

[69] Montaner J, et al. Matrix metalloproteinase-9 pretreatment level predicts intracranial hemorrhagic complications after thrombolysis in human stroke. Circulation 2003;107(4):598–603.

[70] Jonsen A, et al. Outcome of neuropsychiatric systemic lupus erythematosus within a defined Swedish population: increased morbidity but low mortality. Rheumatology (Oxford) 2002; 41(11):1308–12.

[71] Sibley JT, et al. The incidence and prognosis of central nervous system disease in systemic lupus erythematosus. J Rheumatol 1992;19(1):47–52.

[72] Hermosillo-Romo D, Brey RL. Diagnosis and management of patients with neuropsychiatric systemic lupus erythematosus (NPSLE). Best Practice and Research Clinical Rheumatology 2002;16(2):229–44.

[73] Denburg SD, Denburg JA. Cognitive dysfunction and antiphospholipid antibodies in systemic lupus erythematosus. Lupus 2003;12(12):883–90.

[74] Hanly JG, Cassell K, Fisk JD. Cognitive function in systemic lupus erythematosus: results of a 5-year prospective study. Arthritis Rheum 1997;40(8):1542–3.

[75] Waterloo K, et al. Neuropsychological function in systemic lupus erythematosus: a five-year longitudinal study. Rheumatology (Oxford) 2002;41(4):411–5.

[76] Hay EM, et al. A prospective study of psychiatric disorder and cognitive function in systemic lupus erythematosus. Ann Rheum Dis 1994;53(5):298–303.

[77] Carlomagno S, et al. Cognitive impairment in systemic lupus erythematosus: a follow-up study. J Neurol 2000;247(4):273–9.

[78] Raskin N. Headache. In: Fauci BE, Isselbacher KJ, editors. Harrison's principles of internal medicine. New York: McGraw Hill; 1998. p. 68–72.

[79] Sfikakis PP, et al. Headache in systemic lupus erythematosus: a controlled study. Br J Rheumatol 1998;37(3):300–3.

[80] Fernandez-Nebro A, et al. Chronic or recurrent headache in patients with systemic lupus erythematosus: a case control study. Lupus 1999;8(2):151–6.

[81] Amit M, et al. Headache in systemic lupus erythematosus and its relation to other disease manifestations. Clin Exp Rheumatol 1999;17(4):467–70.

[82] Mitsikostas DD, Sfikakis PP, Goadsby PJ. A meta-analysis for headache in systemic lupus erythematosus: the evidence and the myth. Brain 2004;127:1200–29.

[82] Bodani M, Kopelman MD. A psychiatric perspective on the therapy of psychosis in systemic lupus erythematosus. Lupus 2003;12(12):947–9.

[83] Wajed J, et al. Prevention of cardiovascular disease in systemic lupus erythematosus–proposed guidelines for risk factor management. Rheumatology (Oxford) 2004;43(1):7–12.

[84] Graham JW, Jan W. MRI and the brain in systemic lupus erythematosus. Lupus 2003;12(12): 891–6.

[85] Kovacs B, et al. Transverse myelopathy in systemic lupus erythematosus: an analysis of 14 cases and review of the literature. Ann Rheum Dis 2000;59(2):120–4.

[86] Cervera R, et al. Chorea in the antiphospholipid syndrome. Clinical, radiologic, and immunologic characteristics of 50 patients from our clinics and the recent literature. Medicine (Baltimore) 1997;76(3):203–12.

[87] Katzav A, Chapman J, Shoenfeld Y. CNS dysfunction in the antiphospholipid syndrome. Lupus 2003;12(12):903–7.

[88] Omdal R, et al. Peripheral neuropathy in systemic lupus erythematosus–a longitudinal study. Acta Neurol Scand 2001;103(6):386–91.

[89] Omdal R, et al. Small nerve fiber involvement in systemic lupus erythematosus: a controlled study. Arthritis Rheum 2002;46(5):1228–32.

[90] Hanly JG, et al. Clinical course of cognitive dysfunction in systemic lupus erythematosus. J Rheumatol 1994;21(10):1825–31.

[91] Ginsburg KS, et al. A controlled study of the prevalence of cognitive dysfunction in randomly selected patients with systemic lupus erythematosus. Arthritis Rheum 1992;35(7):776–82.

[92] Karassa FB, et al. Predictors of clinical outcome and radiologic progression in patients with neuropsychiatric manifestations of systemic lupus erythematosus. Am J Med 2000;109(8): 628–34.

[93] Estes D, Christian CL. The natural history of systemic lupus erythematosus by prospective analysis. Medicine (Baltimore) 1971;50(2):85–95.

[94] Feng PH, Cheah PS, Lee YK. Mortality in systemic lupus erythematosus: a 10-year review. BMJ 1973;4(895):772–4.

[95] Cheatum DE, et al. Renal histology and clinical course of systemic lupus erythematosus. A prospective study. Arthritis Rheum 1973;16(5):670–6.

[96] Lee P, et al. Systemic lupus erythematosus. A review of 110 cases with reference to nephritis, the nervous system, infections, aseptic necrosis and prognosis. Q J Med 1977;46(181): 1–32.

[97] Ginzler EM, et al. A multicenter study of outcome in systemic lupus erythematosus. I. Entry variables as predictors of prognosis. Arthritis Rheum 1982;25(6):601–11.

[98] Sergent JS, et al. Central nervous system disease in systemic lupus erythematosus. Therapy and prognosis. Am J Med 1975;58(5):644–54.

[99] Feinglass EJ, et al. Neuropsychiatric manifestations of systemic lupus erythematosus: diagnosis, clinical spectrum, and relationship to other features of the disease. Medicine (Baltimore) 1976;55(4):323–39.

[100] Kovacs JA, Urowitz MB, Gladman DD. Dilemmas in neuropsychiatric lupus. Rheum Dis Clin North Am 1993;19(4):795–814.

[101] Karassa FB, Magliano M, Isenberg DA. Suicide attempts in patients with systemic lupus erythematosus. Ann Rheum Dis 2003;62(1):58–60.

[102] Sibbitt Jr WL, Sibbitt RR, Brooks WM. Neuroimaging in neuropsychiatric systemic lupus erythematosus [see comments]. Arthritis Rheum 1999;42(10):2026–38.

[103] McCune WJ, et al. Identification of brain lesions in neuropsychiatric systemic lupus erythematosus by magnetic resonance scanning. Arthritis Rheum 1988;31(2):159–66.

[104] Rovaris M, et al. Brain involvement in systemic immune mediated diseases: magnetic resonance and magnetisation transfer imaging study. J Neurol Neurosurg Psychiatry 2000;68(2): 170–7.

[105] Sibbitt Jr WL, et al. Fluid Attenuated Inversion Recovery (FLAIR) imaging in neuropsychiatric systemic lupus erythematosus. J Rheumatol 2003;30(9):1983–9.

[106] Bell CL, et al. Magnetic resonance imaging of central nervous system lesions in patients with lupus erythematosus. Correlation with clinical remission and antineurofilament and anticardiolipin antibody titers [see comments]. Arthritis Rheum 1991;34(4):432–41.

[107] Gonzalez-Crespo MR, et al. Magnetic resonance imaging of the brain in systemic lupus erythematosus. Br J Rheumatol 1995;34(11):1055–60.

[108] Stimmler MM, Coletti PM, Quismorio Jr FP. Magnetic resonance imaging of the brain in neuropsychiatric systemic lupus erythematosus. Semin Arthritis Rheum 1993;22(5):335–49.

[109] Cauli A, et al. Abnormalities of magnetic resonance imaging of the central nervous system in patients with systemic lupus erythematosus correlate with disease severity. Clin Rheumatol 1994;13(4):615–8.

[110] Hanly JG. Single photon emission computed tomography scanning in neuropsychiatric systemic lupus erythematosus [editorial; comment]. J Rheumatol 1998;25(3):401–3.

[111] Nossent JC, et al. Single-photon-emission computed tomography of the brain in the evaluation of cerebral lupus. Arthritis Rheum 1991;34(11):1397–403.

[112] Oku K, et al. Cerebral imaging by magnetic resonance imaging and single photon emission computed tomography in systemic lupus erythematosus with central nervous system involvement. Rheumatology (Oxford) 2003;42(6):773–7.

[113] Rubbert A, et al. Single-photon-emission computed tomography analysis of cerebral blood flow in the evaluation of central nervous system involvement in patients with systemic lupus erythematosus [see comments]. Arthritis Rheum 1993;36(9):1253–62.

[114] Rogers MP, et al. I-123 iofetamine SPECT scan in systemic lupus erythematosus patients with cognitive and other minor neuropsychiatric symptoms: a pilot study. Lupus 1992;1(4):215–9.

[115] Kovacs JA, et al. The use of single photon emission computerized tomography in neuropsychiatric SLE: a pilot study [see comments]. J Rheumatol 1995;22(7):1247–53.

[116] Waterloo K, et al. Neuropsychological dysfunction in systemic lupus erythematosus is not associated with changes in cerebral blood flow. J Neurol 2001;248(7):595–602.

[117] Kao CH, et al. The role of FDG-PET, HMPAO-SPET and MRI in the detection of brain involvement in patients with systemic lupus erythematosus. Eur J Nucl Med 1999;26(2): 129–34.

[118] Weiner SM, et al. Alterations of cerebral glucose metabolism indicate progress to severe morphological brain lesions in neuropsychiatric systemic lupus erythematosus. Lupus 2000; 9(5):386–9.

[119] Otte A, et al. Neuropsychiatric systemic lupus erythematosus before and after immunosuppressive treatment: a FDG PET study. Lupus 1998;7(1):57–9.

[120] Brooks WM, et al. Relationship between neurometabolite derangement and neurocognitive dysfunction in systemic lupus erythematosus. J Rheumatol 1999;26(1):81–5.

[121] Sabet A, et al. Neurometabolite markers of cerebral injury in the antiphospholipid antibody syndrome of systemic lupus erythematosus. Stroke 1998;29(11):2254–60.

[122] Peterson PL, et al. Quantitative magnetic resonance imaging in neuropsychiatric systemic lupus erythematosus. Lupus 2003;12(12):897–902.

[123] Bosma GP, et al. Evidence of central nervous system damage in patients with neuropsychiatric systemic lupus erythematosus, demonstrated by magnetization transfer imaging. Arthritis Rheum 2000;43(1):48–54.

[124] Bosma GP, et al. Detection of cerebral involvement in patients with active neuropsychiatric systemic lupus erythematosus by the use of volumetric magnetization transfer imaging. Arthritis Rheum 2000;43(11):2428–36.

[125] Bosma GP, et al. Association of global brain damage and clinical functioning in neuropsychiatric systemic lupus erythematosus. Arthritis Rheum 2002;46(10):2665–72.

[126] Moritani T, et al. Diffusion-weighted echo-planar MR imaging of CNS involvement in systemic lupus erythematosus. Acad Radiol 2001;8(8):741–53.

[127] Small P, et al. Central nervous system involvement in SLE. Diagnostic profile and clinical features. Arthritis Rheum 1977;20(3):869–78.

[128] Trysberg E, et al. Neuronal and astrocytic damage in systemic lupus erythematosus patients with central nervous system involvement. Arthritis Rheum 2003;48(10):2881–7.

[129] Denburg SD, Carbotte RM, Denburg JA. Corticosteroids and neuropsychological functioning in patients with systemic lupus erythematosus. Arthritis Rheum 1994;37(9):1311–20.

[130] Barile L, Lavalle C. Transverse myelitis in systemic lupus erythematosus–the effect of IV pulse methylprednisolone and cyclophosphamide. J Rheumatol 1992;19(3):370–2.

[131] Eyanson S, et al. Methylprednisolone pulse therapy for nonrenal lupus erythematosus. Ann Rheum Dis 1980;39(4):377–80.

[132] Trevisani VF, et al. Cyclophosphamide versus methylprednisolone for the treatment of neuropsychiatric involvement in systemic lupus erythematosus (Cochrane review). Cochrane Database Syst Rev 2000:3;CD00265.

[133] Baca V, et al. Favorable response to intravenous methylprednisolone and cyclophosphamide in children with severe neuropsychiatric lupus. J Rheumatol 1999;26(2):432–9.

[134] Leung FK, Fortin PR. Intravenous cyclophosphamide and high dose corticosteroids improve MRI lesions in demyelinating syndrome in systemic lupus erythematosus. J Rheumatol 2003; 30(8):1871–3.

[135] Boumpas DT, et al. Pulse cyclophosphamide for severe neuropsychiatric lupus. Q J Med 1991; 81(296):975–84.

[136] Neuwelt CM, et al. Role of intravenous cyclophosphamide in the treatment of severe neuropsychiatric systemic lupus erythematosus. Am J Med 1995;98(1):32–41.

[137] Ramos PC, et al. Pulse cyclophosphamide in the treatment of neuropsychiatric systemic lupus erythematosus. Clin Exp Rheumatol 1996;14(3):295–9.

[138] Mok CC, et al. Acute transverse myelopathy in systemic lupus erythematosus: clinical presentation, treatment, and outcome. J Rheumatol 1998;25(3):467–73.

[139] Galindo-Rodriguez G, et al. Cyclophosphamide pulse therapy in optic neuritis due to systemic lupus erythematosus: an open trial. Am J Med 1999;106(1):65–9.

[140] McCune WJ, et al. Clinical and immunologic effects of monthly administration of intravenous cyclophosphamide in severe systemic lupus erythematosus. N Engl J Med 1988; 318(22):1423–31.

[141] Mok CC, Lau CS, Wong RW. Treatment of lupus psychosis with oral cyclophosphamide followed by azathioprine maintenance: an open-label study. Am J Med 2003;115(1):59–62.

[142] Gorman C, Leandro M, Isenberg D. Does B cell depletion have a role to play in the treatment of systemic lupus erythematosus? Lupus 2004;13(5):312–6.

[143] Saito K, et al. Successful treatment with anti-CD20 monoclonal antibody (rituximab) of life-threatening refractory systemic lupus erythematosus with renal and central nervous system involvement. Lupus 2003;12(10):798–800.

[144] Crowther MA, et al. A comparison of two intensities of warfarin for the prevention of recurrent thrombosis in patients with the antiphospholipid antibody syndrome. N Engl J Med 2003;349(12):1133–8.

[145] Khamashta MA, et al. The management of thrombosis in the antiphospholipid-antibody syndrome [see comments]. N Engl J Med 1995;332(15):993–7.

[146] Karlson EW, et al. A randomized clinical trial of a psychoeducational intervention to improve outcomes in systemic lupus erythematosus. Arthritis Rheum 2004;50(6):1832–41.

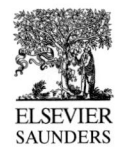

ELSEVIER
SAUNDERS

RHEUMATIC
DISEASE CLINICS
OF NORTH AMERICA

Rheum Dis Clin N Am 31 (2005) 299–313

# Neonatal Lupus: Basic Research and Clinical Perspectives

## Jill P. Buyon, MD[a,b],*, Robert M. Clancy, PhD[a,b]

[a]Division of Rheumatology, Department of Medicine, New York University School of Medicine, New York, NY, USA
[b]Department of Rheumatic Diseases and Molecular Medicine, Hospital for Joint Diseases, 301 East 17th Street, Room 1608, New York, NY 10003, USA

The study of neonatal lupus (NL) exemplifies not only translational research, which inherently draws upon clinical observations and explores them in the laboratory, but also integrational research, which attempts to fit critical clinical and basic observations together, even those seemingly at odds.

Congenital heart block (CHB), absent structural abnormalities and detected in the second trimester, almost universally is associated with maternal auto-antibodies reactive with the intracellular soluble ribonucleoproteins 48 kD SSB/La, 52 kD SSA/Ro, or 60 kD SSA/Ro [1,2]. An erythematous skin rash with a predilection for the scalp and periorbital region, most often apparent in the first 8 weeks after birth, also is linked strongly to these maternal antibodies and to antibodies against U1 RNP [2,3]. Permanent cardiac and transient cutaneous diseases are the most common manifestation of NL, initially named because of the resemblance of the skin rash to subacute cutaneous lupus erythematosus (SCLE). Less often, abnormalities of the liver or blood affect newborns exposed in utero to maternal anti-SSA/Ro-SSB/La antibodies [4–7]. Fetal and neonatal injuries are presumed to result from the transplacental passage of IgG anti-Ro/La antibodies from the mother into the fetal circulation [8]. Fetal/neonatal disease is independent of maternal disease; mothers may have systemic lupus erythematosus (SLE), Sjögren's syndrome (SS), or other autoimmune symptoms, or be

This work has been supported in part by National Institutes of Health Grant AR42455 and contract AR4-2220 (Research Registry for Neonatal Lupus).

* Corresponding author. Department of Rheumatic Diseases and Molecular Medicine, Hospital for Joint Diseases, 301 East 17th Street, Room 1608, New York, NY 10003.

*E-mail address:* jill.buyon@nyumc.org (J.P. Buyon).

Table 1
Outcome of 94 pregnancies immediately subsequent to the birth of a child who has congenital heart block

| Outcome | N | (%) |
|---|---|---|
| Healthy | 67 | 71 |
| Manifestations of NL | | |
|    CHB only | 15 | 16 |
|    CHB + rash | 3 | 3 |
|    Rash only | 7 | 7 |
| Fetal demise | 1 | 1 |
| Neonatal death (heart valve dysfunction and heart failure) | 1 | 1 |

*Data from* the Research Registry for Neonatal Lupus; September 15, 2004.

entirely asymptomatic [9]. The fetal heart appears to be uniquely vulnerable, because complete block only has been reported in a single mother [10], despite mothers' exposure to identical circulating levels of the autoantibodies. CHB carries a significant mortality (15%–30%, primarily fetal and neonatal) and morbidity (67% of surviving affected children require permanent pacing before adulthood) [9]. The recurrence rate of CHB in subsequent pregnancies is approximately 19% [11] (Table 1), or at least ninefold greater than the risk for CHB in a primigravida with the candidate antibodies [10]. Extensive work from several laboratories has resulted in the molecular characterization of the maternal autoantibody responses and the cloning of genes expressing the cognate antigens whose structural features suggest a role in transcriptional regulation. Anecdotal cases support the use of dexamethasone for the treatment of in utero effusions, hydrops, and incomplete block, but prospective evaluation of dexamethasone or other prophylactic therapy for the at-risk pregnancy remains to be reported.

## Proposed mechanisms of injury

*In vitro apoptosis, opsonization, and fibrosis*

Bridging the gap from identification of the target antigens recognized by the maternal autoantibodies to the mechanism by which these antibodies result in tissue damage and overt clinical disease represents a major challenge. The necessity of anti-SSA/Ro-SSB/La antibodies is supported by their presence in more than 85% of mothers whose fetuses are identified with conduction abnormalities in a structurally normal heart [1,2]. When Brucato et al [10] prospectively evaluated 118 pregnancies in 100 patients who had anti-SSA/Ro antibodies, however, the frequency of CHB in a fetus was only 1.7%. Gladman [12] reported no cases of CHB in 100 live births to 96 women who had anti-SSA/Ro or -SSB/La antibodies and no history of a previous child who had NL. This low frequency suggests that a fetal factor or the in utero environment likely amplifies the effects of the antibody, which may be necessary but insufficient to cause fibrotic replacement of the atrioventricular (AV) node and in some cases a cardiomyopathy. Notably, one mother in the series reported by Brucato et al [10], who gave birth to two healthy children, developed complete heart block herself, raising the possibility that her heart had acquired fetal factors. Clearly, this is a unique situation and one that needs to be studied further, because it likely will contribute important clues to pathogenesis.

To account for the accessibility of the normally sequestered intracellular target antigens and the vulnerability of the fetal heart, apoptosis has been the focus of attention in two laboratories. Tran et al [13,14] recently identified physiologic apoptosis, translocation of SSB/La, and binding of anti-SSB/La antibodies in the developing murine heart. These in vivo observations are supported by the findings of Clancy et al [15]. In vitro, human fetal cardiocytes rendered apoptotic by culturing on plates coated with poly-2-(hydroxymethacrylate) (pHEMA) are bound by anti-SSA/Ro-SSB/La antibodies.

Physiologic apoptosis results in translocation of the intracellular SSA/Ro-SSB/La antigens to the cell surface [16], leading to binding by cognate maternal antibodies (opsonization), which triggers an inflammatory response by macrophages [17]. In vitro studies employing cardiac myocytes and fibroblasts separately isolated and cultured from human fetal hearts provide evidence for a pathologic link between antibodies and injury [15]. Cocultured macrophages have been demonstrated to phagocytose opsonized apoptotic cardiocytes and secrete inflammatory cytokines such as tumor necrosis factor α (TNF-α) [17] and tumor growth factor β (TGF-β) [18]. Other investigators also have demonstrated that phagocytosis of opsonized apoptotic cells is proinflammatory [19–21], as exemplified by the observation that ingestion of apoptotic cells bound by anti-cardiolipin antibodies results in the release of macrophage TNF-α [21].

A potential role for TGF-β in fibrosis of the AV node was supported by additional experiments. Human fetal cardiac fibroblasts exposed to supernatants obtained from macrophages incubated with opsonized apoptotic cardiocytes markedly increased expression of the myofibroblast marker, smooth muscle actin (SMAc), associated with scarring. This effect was blocked by anti–TGF-βantibodies [15].

*In vitro congenital heart block model*

Immunohistology of the heart from a term male infant (diagnosed with AV block at 24 weeks of gestation and dying shortly after birth) supported macrophage crosstalk despite the 2-month lag time from detection to death [15]. The ventricular tissue revealed microcalcification in which a predominant SMAc[+] infiltrate could be observed readily. Macrophages also were seen in areas of scar tissue. Notably, the fibrosis was not bland but involved an infiltrate of activated myofibroblasts months after the initial insult. Recently, this heart and two others from fetuses who had CHB (20- and 22-week fetal deaths) were examined for myofibroblasts, which were found in all specimens, supporting the persistence of the myofibroblast phenotype, because this collection encompassed a spectrum of disease severity and timing of death relative to clinical detection [22]. Fig. 1 illustrates the presence of myofibroblasts and macrophages in a 23-week fetal CHB heart, and their absence in tissue from a normal abortus, previously unpublished.

To evaluate the extent of fibrosis, cardiac sections were stained with picro-sirius for detection of collagen. In both the 20- and 22-week CHB hearts, there was extensive fibrosis in the inferior portion of the atrial wall where the AV node is likely to reside. Collagen deposition was absent in the septal tissue of a normal (fetal age-matched) control heart. In the 20- and 22-week CHB hearts, TGF-β immunoreactivity was seen in the conduction tissue. In several sections, intense TGF-β staining was present in the extracellular fibrous matrix between SMAc⁺ myofibroblasts concentrated in the adjacent subendocardium and infiltrating CD68⁺ macrophages. Double labeling revealed colocalization of TGF-β in the cytoplasm of macrophages, including multinucleate giant cells. No fibrosis or TGF-β immunostaining was seen in conduction tissue or ventricles of control hearts from 22- or 23-week abortuses [22].

*Genetic considerations in the proposed pathogenesis of congenital heart block*

It is clear that maternal antibodies are not sufficient to directly cause cardiac scarring and that additional maternal and fetal factors such as genetics are likely to convert predisposition to clinical expression. At present, no model of inheritance for CHB is known, making this a complex genetic problem. As noted previously, CHB occurs in 19% of siblings born subsequent to a CHB-affected infant [11], a rate 3000 times higher than the population prevalence (1/20,000), implying a strong genetic effect. Driven by the proposed pathologic cascade

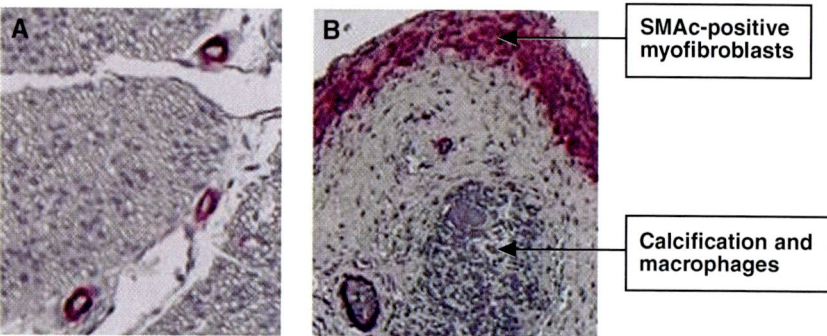

Fig. 1. Histologic evidence of myofibroblasts in cardiac conduction tissue from a fetus that died of CHB at 23 weeks' gestation. Shown are low magnification images of longitudinal sections through the septa of a 23-week CHB-heart (*B*) and a normal heart of similar gestational age (*A*) stained with antismooth muscle actin (SMAc) and alkaline phosphatase conjugated antimouse IgG (red). SMAc⁺ cells line the blood vessels of the affected and normal fetal heart as expected. Myofibroblasts (*upper arrow*) were adjacent to an area of fibrosis and in proximity to an area of calcification and macrophages (*lower arrow*).

supported by in vitro and in vivo data, the authors have begun an initial analysis of TGF-β and TNFα polymorphisms.

The human gene encoding TGF-β is on chromosome 19q13 and is highly polymorphic. Awad et al [23] identified five polymorphisms in the *TGF-β* gene: two in the promoter region at positions −800 and −509, one at position +72 in a nontranslated region, and two in the signal sequence at positions +869 and +915. The polymorphisms at positions +869 and +915, which change codon 10 (T→C, leucine→proline) and codon 25 (G→C, arginine→proline) are associated with interindividual variation in the levels of TGF-β production. This has clinical relevance because several animal and human studies have shown that high TGF-β producers develop significantly more lung fibrosis in response to a number of inflammatory triggers such as radiation [24], chemotherapy [25], and lung transplantation [26]. The Pro$^{25}$ allele is associated with lower TGF-β synthesis in vitro and in vivo, whereas the Arg$^{25}$ allele is associated with allograft fibrosis in transbronchial biopsies when compared with controls and with nonallograft fibrosis [27]. It has been reported that lung allograft recipients who have the Leu$^{10}$ allele produced the highest amounts of TGF-β [23], and chronic rejection after lung transplant is linked with high levels of TGF-β [27]. In parallel with the authors' hypothesis that high levels of TGF-β permit the development of CHB because of enhancement of extracellular matrix and increased fibrosis, patients who have cystic fibrosis and develop rapid deterioration in lung function have an increased frequency of the Leu$^{10}$ homozygosity [28].

Codons 10 and 25 of the *TGF-β* gene were evaluated in 88 children (40 who had CHB, 17 who had rashes, and 31 unaffected siblings) and 74 mothers from the Research Registry for Neonatal Lupus (RRNL) [29]. The TGF-β polymorphism Leu$^{10}$ (associated with increased fibrosis) was significantly higher in CHB children (genotypic frequency 60%, allelic frequency 78%) than unaffected offspring (genotypic frequency 29%, $P$=0.016; allelic frequency 56%, $P$=0.011) and controls, while there were no significant differences between controls and other NL groups. For the TGF-β polymorphism, Arg$^{25}$, there were no significant differences between NL groups and controls.

*Genetic considerations in the proposed pathogenesis of neonatal lupus rash*

Neonatal lupus rash, as noted previously, resembles SCLE and is often photosensitive. There is evidence that the release of TNF-α by ultraviolet light-exposed keratinocytes contributes to the lesions of SCLE in individuals who have the haplotype −308A TNF-α/DRB1*03 [30,31]. The gene encoding TNF-α is highly polymorphic, and a substitution of G→A at position −308 (TNF2) in the promoter region has been associated with increased production of this cytokine [32]. The common (wild-type) allele, −308G (TNF1), has a frequency of approximately 80% in whites and 92% in African Americans [33]. The link between anti-SSA/Ro antibodies, photosensitivity, and TNF-α promoter polymorphisms extends to HLA class II molecules. In Whites, there is a strong linkage disequilibrium between the −308A allele and HLA-DRB1*03 [34]. The presence of DRB1*03 is also common in individuals who synthesize anti-SSA/Ro and SSB/La antibodies.

DNA was isolated from 92 children (22 who had rashes, 31 unaffected siblings, and 39 who had CHB) and 79 mothers from the RRNL for genotyping of the TNF-$\alpha$ −308-promoter region and HLA-DRB1 [35]. There was a significantly higher −308A carrier frequency in children who have rash compared with healthy controls (64% versus 23%; $P$ = 0.002). The DRB1 distribution for DRB1*03 was significantly higher in children who have rash compared with controls (64% versus 17%; $P$ = 0.014). The carrier frequency of DRB1*03 was also significantly higher than controls for children who have CHB (54%) and for mothers (73%) but not unaffected children (39%). Although the carrier frequency was higher in children who have rash compared with children who do not have rash, the difference did not reach statistical significance.

In the children with rash, the prevalence of the −308A allele paralleled the prevalence of DRB1*03. When individual subjects were tabulated by the presence or absence of −308A and DRB1*03, the two alleles together were significantly greater in the children who have rash, children who have CHB, and mothers, compared with population controls. In contrast, unaffected children were not significantly different from controls. For children who have rash, the association between the −308A allele and DRB1*03 occurred in all but one case (7%) ($P$ = 0.012 versus control). For children who have CHB and unaffected children, however, the presence of −308A in the absence of DRB1*03 was 25% and 38%, respectively, which did not differ significantly from controls.

### Clinical observations and considerations

*Classification and progression of heart block*

Again, the issue of complete versus incomplete heart block warrants clarification. It is recognized that heart block might progress through various stages. Therefore, cases have been assigned loosely as CCHB (congenital complete heart block) when in fact the rhythm was second-degree block. It is anticipated that, as echocardiograms are done more frequently during pregnancies of mothers who have anti-SSA/Ro-SSB/La antibodies, this point will be clarified. Presently, CHB is used best to describe congenital heart block, which can be first-, second- or third-degree.

To ascertain the spectrum of arrhythmias associated with maternal anti-SSA/Ro-SSB/La antibodies, Askanase et al [36] reviewed records of all children enrolled in the RRNL. Of 187 children who have CHB whose mothers had anti-Ro/La antibodies, nine had a prolonged PR interval on EKG at birth, four of whom progressed to more advanced AV block. A child whose younger sibling had third-degree block was diagnosed with first-degree block at age 10 years at the time of surgery for a broken wrist. Two children diagnosed in utero who had second-degree block were treated with dexamethasone and reverted to normal sinus rhythm by birth, but ultimately progressed to third-degree block. Four children had second-degree block at birth: of these, two progressed to third-degree block. These data have important research and clinical implications. Perhaps many fetuses sustain mild inflammation, but resolution is variable, as suggested by the presence of incomplete AV block. Because subsequent progression of less-advanced degrees of block can occur, an EKG should be performed on all infants born to mothers with anti-Ro/La antibodies.

The Toronto registry group retrospectively analyzed the single-center outcome of children who had isolated CHB presenting from 1965 to 1998, up to age 20 years [37]. Cases were diagnosed from fetal life through childhood. There were a total of 102 cases, divided in three groups. Fetal presentation in 29 cases had a 43% mortality rate. Neonatal presentation in 33 cases had a 6% mortality rate. There were no deaths in the 40 cases presenting in childhood, but 19 out of 20 tested had negative maternal antibody levels. Risk factors for death were a fetal diagnosis, the presence of hydrops, gestational age under 33 weeks, or the development of endocardial fibroelastosis (EFE) with ejection fraction no more than 40%. Three neonates who had been diagnosed before birth were treated with corticosteroids. Most of the cases (88%–89%) were paced by age 20. Late cardiomyopathy occurred in 5% of patients overall, but in the antibody-positive cases, late cardiomyopathy occurred in 11% of patients. There was progression noted also in the degree of heart block over time. Pacemaker insertions were associated with complications in 25% of cases, and there was a frequent need for pacemaker revisions.

The Toronto group also retrospectively reviewed the clinical history, echocardiography, and pathology of fetuses and children from five medical centers who had EFE associated with CHB and were born to mothers positive for anti-SSA/Ro or anti-SSB/La antibodies [38]. Thirteen patients were identified: six who had a prenatal and 7 a postnatal diagnosis. Severe ventricular dysfunction was seen in all fetal and postnatal cases. Four fetal and three postnatal cases had EFE at initial presentation. Two fetal and four postnatal cases, however, developed EFE 6 to 12 weeks and 7 months to 5 years from CHB diagnosis, respectively, even despite ventricular pacing in six postnatal cases. Eleven patients (85%) either died (N = 9) or underwent cardiac transplantation (N = 2) secondary to the EFE. Pathologic assessment of the explanted heart, available in 10 cases, revealed moderate-to-severe EFE in seven cases and mild EFE in three cases, predominantly involving the left ventricle. Immunohistochemistry in four cases (including three fetuses) demonstrated deposition of IgG in four, IgM in three, and T-cell infiltrates in three cases, suggesting an immune response by the affected fetus or child. The important conclusion from this study was that EFE occurs despite adequate ventricular pacing and is associated with significant mortality, whether developing in fetal or postnatal life.

This same group of investigators also described a unique clinical series of three cases of isolated EFE (one fetus, two infants, all female) with antibody-positive mothers in the absence of CHB [39]. Two died and one received a heart transplant. Histologic evaluation revealed EFE with diffuse IgG deposition

and T-cell infiltration but no detectable apoptosis. This latter observation remains unexplained.

*Management of the at-risk pregnancy and of congenital heart block detected in*
*utero*

The clinical approach to cardiac manifestations of NL includes obstetric and
rheumatologic management of the fetus who has a normal heart rate but at risk
of developing CHB and the fetus identified with heart block.

All pregnant women who have anti-SSA/Ro-SSB/La antibodies should have
serial fetal echocardiography done by an experienced pediatric cardiologist
weekly from 16 to 26 weeks, and every other week until about 34 weeks. Until
recently, the in utero detection of first-degree block was not technically feasible.
Now, however, the EKG equivalent of the PR interval can be measured by
echocardiography [40]. Using the gated-pulsed Doppler technique, time intervals
from the onset of the mitral A wave (atrial systole) to the onset of the aortic
pulsed Doppler tracing (ventricular systole) within the same left ventricular
cardiac cycle may be measured. This time interval represents the mechanical PR
interval. Its validity was confirmed by neonatal electrocardiographic correlation
to the pulsed Doppler mechanical PR interval [41]. The normal mechanical PR
interval in the fetus is $0.12 \pm 0.02$ seconds (95% confidence intervals 0.10–0.14).

A prospective National Institutes of Health (NIH)-supported multicenter study,
PR Interval and Dexamethasone Evaluation (PRIDE) in CHB is underway to
examine the mechanical PR interval weekly in pregnant woman who has anti-
SSA/Ro or -SSB/La antibodies. One of the goals of this trial is to identify the
prevalence of first-degree block and to determine whether it is a marker for more
advanced destruction of the conducting system. Such information will provide
the optimal opportunity for reversibility.

It also is recommended strongly that all neonates born to mothers who
have anti-SSA/Ro-SSB/La antibodies have an EKG at birth to detect first-
degree block.

The initiation of dexamethasone or plasmapheresis as a preventative measure
has been considered. With regard to prophylactic therapy of the high-risk mother
(documentation of high titer anti-SSA/Ro and SSB/La antibodies, anti-48kD
SSB/La and 52kD SSA/Ro on immunoblot, and a previous child who had NL),
administration of prednisone, dexamethasone, or plasmapheresis is not yet jus-
tified. Maternal prednisone (at least in low and moderate doses) early in pregnancy does not prevent the development of CHB [42]. This might be anticipated,
because prednisone given to the mother is not active in the fetus [43], and levels
of anti-SSA/Ro and anti-SSB/La antibodies remain relatively constant during
steroid therapy.

Kaaja and Julkunen [44] recently reported their experience using intravenous immunoglobulin (IVIG) and corticosteroids in highest-risk mothers (those
who have anti-SSA/Ro antibodies and a previous child who had CHB).

Conclusions are limited by the small number of treated patients (N = 8) and the absence of a control group. The one mother who did have a second CHB baby received only IVIG and no corticosteroids. Effectiveness of treatment is difficult to assess in this study. To formally evaluate the efficacy of treatment, a randomized placebo-controlled trial would need to be conducted and probably only include mothers who had a previous CHB child. An example of a power analysis is a follows: if one accepts a clinically meaningful outcome as a reduction of the recurrence rate of CHB from 19% to 10%, 261 mothers will be needed in each group; from 19% to 5%, 97 mothers would be needed ($\alpha$ = 80%).

The mechanism of potential efficacy is unknown, but effective decrease of circulating antibody in the fetus might involve idiotype/anti-idiotype regulation, a decrease in placental transport, or perhaps induction of surface expression of the inhibitory Fc receptor, $Fc\gamma RIIB$, on macrophages [45]. Precedent for decrease of anti-Ro/La transport has been provided by a murine model [13,14]. Modulation of inhibitory signaling could be a potent therapeutic strategy for attenuating autoantibody-triggered inflammatory diseases.

The rationale for treatment of identified heart block and prevention of potential heart block is to diminish a generalized inflammatory insult and reduce or eliminate maternal autoantibodies. Accordingly, several intrauterine therapeutic regimens have been tried, including dexamethasone, which is not metabolized by the placenta and is available to the fetus in an active form. In the largest retrospective study published to date, it was observed that fluorinated glucocorticoids ameliorated incomplete AV block and hydropic changes in autoimmune-associated congenital heart block but did not reverse established third-degree block [46]. Maternal risks of dexamethasone are similar to any glucocorticoid and include infection, osteoporosis, osteonecrosis, diabetes, hypertension, and preeclampsia. Fetal risks include oligohydramnios, intrauterine growth retardation, and adrenal suppression. Intervention with glucocorticoids might decrease acute inflammation but not necessarily prevent subsequent fibrosis. A second goal of the PRIDE Trial is to assess the efficacy of maternal oral dexamethasone (4 mg/d) in reversing or preventing the progression of AV block newly detected in utero. Under the PRIDE protocol, if third-degree block has remained present with no improvement through 6 weeks of dexamethasone therapy, the drug is tapered and discontinued. Continued use of dexamethasone is warranted in such a case only if hydropic changes are present.

Available data support serial cardiac monitoring of all fetuses who have any bradyarrhythmias detected in utero and of neonates who have incomplete blocks at birth whose mothers are known previously or currently identified to have anti-SSA/Ro-SSB/La antibodies. Fetal echocardiogram is essential to diagnose and follow the course of disease, and may suggest the presence of an associated myocarditis by the finding of decreased contractility in addition to the secondary changes associated with myocarditis such as an increase of cardiac size, pericardial effusions, and tricuspid regurgitation. The obstetric management should be guided by the degree of cardiac failure noted on the ultrasound images. The in utero environment is preferred as long as possible because of the low-resistance circulatory pathways, thereby affording minimal work to maintain cardiac output.

A case report in which ritodrine was given intravenously to the mother to increase the heart rate of a 28-week fetus who had CHB and a ventricular rate of 54 beats per minute serves as a reminder that nonimmunosuppressive approaches may have a role in therapy. Sympathomimetics can increase fetal heart rate transiently, although they do not restore coordination of AV conduction on which the heart is dependent for adequate filling [47].

Current treatment recommendations for CHB diagnosed in utero are summarized in Fig. 2. Fig. 3 provides an overview of the translational approach to prevention and therapy, including current and investigational strategies.

### Transient manifestations of neonatal lupus: skin, liver, and blood

Neonatal lupus skin lesions generally become manifest several weeks into postnatal life; less commonly the rash is present at birth. Ultraviolet light exposure may be an initiating factor and can exacerbate an existing rash [2,48]. Cutaneous activity, inclusive of erythema and the continued appearance of new

| SITUATION | $\rightarrow$ | TREATMENT |
|---|---|---|
| *Degree of block at presentation:* | | |
| • 3rd ° (>2 wk from detection) | $\rightarrow$ | Evaluation by serial echos; no therapy. |
| • 3rd ° (<2 wk from detection) | $\rightarrow$ | 4 mg p.o. dexamethasome daily for 6 wk. If improvement to 2nd ° or better, continue until delivery. |
| • Alternating 2nd ° / 3rd °<br><br>• 2nd °<br><br>• Prolonged mechanical PR interval (1st °) | $\rightarrow$ | 4 mg dex to delivery, unless progression to 3rd ° for 6 wk. |
| Block associated with signs of myocarditis, CHF and/or hydropic changes | $\rightarrow$ | 4 mg dex until improvement. |
| Severely hydropic fetus | $\rightarrow$ | 4 mg dex plus apheresis to rapidly remove maternal antibodies. |

Fig. 2. Currently recommended therapeutic approach to CHB diagnosed in utero. Given the risks to mother and fetus of maternal oral dexamethasone, and the irreversibility (to date) of established third-degree heart block, the use of dexamethasone is recommended only in the scenarios outlined here. When discontinuation is indicated, the dosage must be tapered. CHF, congestive heart failure.

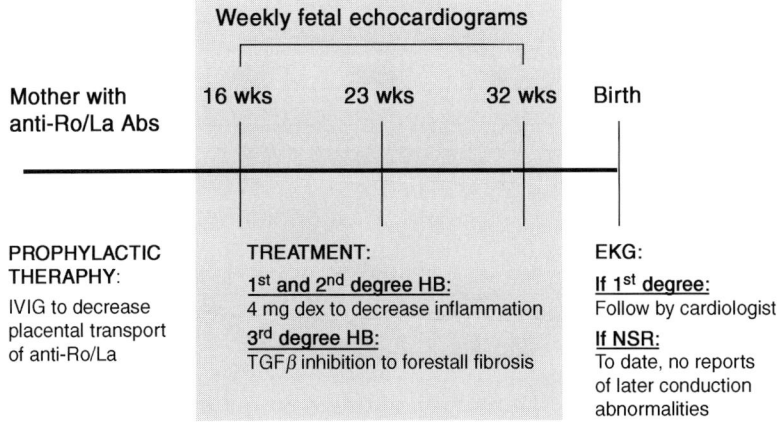

Fig. 3. Translational approach to CHB. Monitoring and treatment options for pregnancy and birth in women with anti-Ro/La antibodies, including currently recommended practice and promising approaches under investigation. Current recommendations include: weekly echocardiograms between 16 and 32 weeks of gestation, treatment with 4 mg dexamethasone to the mother (as detailed in Fig. 2), and an EKG at birth (any conduction abnormality at birth should be followed by a cardiologist, but no later conduction abnormalities have been reported to date in an infant with normal sinus rhythm at birth). Treatment of the mother with intravenous immune globulin (IVIG) to reduce transplacental transport of anti-Ro/La antibodies is being evaluated. Recent laboratory findings point to inhibition of TGF-β production as a promising therapeutic target to forestall fibrosis in the fetus with third-degree block in utero.

lesions, is generally present for several weeks, with resolution by 6 to 8 months of age coincident with the clearance of maternal autoantibodies from the baby's circulation. The rash frequently involves the face and scalp, with a characteristic predilection for the upper eyelids, but it may be present in other locations and in some instances covers virtually the entire body. Lesions are superficial inflammatory plaques resembling subacute cutaneous lupus erythematosus of the adult, typically annular or elliptical with erythema and scaling. Hypopigmentation is frequent and may be a prominent feature. It may persist into the second year of life. The more characteristic lesions of adult discoid lupus such as follicular plugging, dermal atrophy, and scarring generally are not observed in the neonatal skin rash. A recent assessment of NL rash (absent heart disease) in 57 infants in the RRNL found no significant difference with regard to residual sequelae (hypopigmentation, telengectasias, pitting, scarring, and atrophy) between untreated infants and those treated with topical corticosteroids.

It is most important for the clinician to consider the outcomes of pregnancies subsequent to the birth of a child who has NL rash. Among RRNL mothers, 25% of such pregnancies resulted in a child who had CHB (Table 2).

To extend the information base on the hepatobiliary manifestations of NL, Lee et al [6] evaluated records from 219 children enrolled in the RRNL. Nineteen (9%) had probable or possible hepatobiliary disease, 16 of whom also had cardiac or cutaneous manifestations of NL. Three clinical variants of hepatobiliary

Table 2
Outcome of 36 pregnancies immediately subsequent to the birth of a child who has cutaneous
manifestations of neonatal lupus

| Outcome | N | (%) |
|---|---|---|
| Healthy | 13 | 36 |
| Manifestations of NL | | |
|   CHB only | 3 | 8 |
|   CHB + rash | 6 | 17 |
|   Rash only | 14 | 39 |
| Fetal demise | 0 | 0 |

*Data from* the Research Registry for Neonatal Lupus; September 15, 2004.

disease were observed: (1) severe liver failure present during gestation or in the neonatal period, often with the phenotype of neonatal iron storage disease; (2) conjugated hyperbilirubinemia with mild or no elevations of aminotransferases, occurring in the first few weeks of life; and (3) mild elevations of aminotransferases occurring at approximately 2 to 3 months of life. The prognosis for the children in the last two categories was excellent.

Thrombocytopenia has been observed together with other manifestations of NL [5], but may in some cases result from antiplatelet rather than anti-SSA/Ro-SSB/La antibodies targeting the surface of fetal cells. Kanagasegar et al [7] recently reported an infant who had neutropenia and mildly abnormal liver functions, but no cardiac or cutaneous manifestations of NL, born to a mother who had anti-SSA/Ro-SSB/La antibodies. The child's neutropenia improved as maternal antibody was metabolized. Sera from this child and mother, and sera from two RRNL mothers who gave birth to infants who had CHB and neutropenia, were shown to bind the cell surface of intact neutrophils [7]. Binding to neutrophils then was inhibited (more than 80%) by incubating the sera with 60kD Ro antigen, suggesting that anti-60kD SSA/Ro is involved directly in the pathogenesis of neutropenia.

*Breast feeding*

Finally, some comment on breast feeding is warranted, because this is so often a concern among physicians and their patients. To first determine whether human breast milk contains anti-Ro/La antibodies, breast milk was obtained from nine antibody-positive mothers and evaluated by ELISA and immunoblot [49]. All mothers had anti-Ro/La antibodies of IgG and IgA isotypes in their breast milk. These results paralleled those obtained from the respective sera, with lower titers measured in the milk.

A questionnaire was sent to all mothers in the RRNL (by definition, all mothers have anti-Ro/La antibodies and a child who has NL) to ascertain precise details of their breast-feeding history for their affected and unaffected children. Based on a questionnaire returned by 129 of 237 mothers, of 77 children who had NL rash, 45 were breast-fed, compared with 60 of 117 unaffected siblings ($P$ = not significant). There were insufficient numbers of patients who had cardiomyopathies to ascertain the influence of breast feeding on this serious complication.

## Summary

Currently, the presence of anti-SSA/Ro antibodies in a primigravid woman predicts a risk of about 2% for CHB in an offspring. This suggests the contribution of fetal factors. In considering the pathogenesis of CHB, unresolved challenges remain. The antigen system is considered by definition to be associated with RNA and not normally expressed on cell surface membranes, and the maternal heart is not affected. Apoptosis may explain, in part, accessibility of antigen to maternal antibody and developmental vulnerability. Fetal factors are being sought, with the focus on those that promote fibrosis. Postnatal development of cardiomyopathy continues to be reported and carries a poor prognosis. Incorporation of the mechanical PR interval in serial fetal echocardiographic assessments of mothers who have anti-SSA/Ro-SSB/La antibodies may provide a window of opportunity for treatment. Because postnatal progression of less-advanced degrees of block can occur, an EKG should be performed on all infants born to mothers who have the candidate antibodies. With the establishment of two large research registries, one in the United States and the other in Canada, significant advances in the management of high-risk pregnancies and assessment of long-term outcomes of mothers and children should be made.

## References

[1] Buyon JP. Neonatal lupus syndrome. In: Lahita RG, editor. Systemic lupus erythematosus. 4th edition. San Diego (CA): Elsevier Academic Press; 2004. p. 449–50.

[2] Lee LA. Neonatal lupus erythematosus. J Invest Dermatol 1993;100:9s–13s.

[3] Solomon BA, Laude TA, Shalita AR. Neonatal lupus erythematosus: discordant disease expression of $U_1$RNP-positive antibodies in fraternal twins — is this a subset of neonatal lupus erythematosus or a new distinct syndrome? J Am Acad Dermatol 1995;32:858–62.

[4] Laxer RM, Roberts EA, Gross KR, et al. Liver disease in neonatal lupus erythematosus. J Pediatr 1990;116:238–42.

[5] Watson R, Kang JE, May M, et al. Thrombocytopenia in the neonatal lupus syndrome. Arch Dermatol 1988;124:560–3.

[6] Lee LA, Sokol RJ, Buyon JP. Hepatobiliary disease in neonatal lupus erythematosus: prevalence and clinical characteristics in cases enrolled in a national registry. Pediatrics 2002;109:e11.

[7] Kanagasegar S, Cimaz R, Kurien BT, et al. Neonatal lupus manifests as isolated neutropenia and mildly abnormal liver functions. J Rheumatol 2002;29:187–91.

[8] Story CM, Mikulska JE, Simister NE. A major histocompatibility complex class I-like Fc receptor cloned from human placenta: possible role in transfer of immunoglobulin G from mother to the fetus. J Exp Med 1994;180:2377–81.

[9] Buyon JP, Hiebert R, Copel J, et al. Autoimmune-associated congenital heart block: Mortality, morbidity, and recurrence rates obtained from a national neonatal lupus registry. J Am Coll Cardiol 1998;31:1658–66.

[10] Brucato A, Frassi M, Franceschini F, et al. Risk of congenital heart block in newborns of mothers with anti-Ro/SSA antibodies detected by counterimmunoelectrophoresis. Arthritis Rheum 2001;44:1832–5.

[11] Solomon DG, Rupel A, Buyon JP. Birth order and recurrence rate in autoantibody-associated congenital heart block: implications for pathogenesis and family counseling. Lupus 2003;12: 646–7.

[12] Gladman G, Silverman ED, Yuk-Law, et al. Fetal echocardiographic screening of pregnancies of mothers with anti-Ro and/or anti-La antibodies. Am J Perinatol 2002;19:73–80.

[13] Tran HB, Ohlsson M, Beroukas D, et al. Subcellular redistribution of La(SS-B) autoantigen during physiologic apoptosis in the fetal mouse heart and conduction system: a clue to the pathogenesis of congenital heart block. Arthritis Rheum 2002;46:202–8.

[14] Tran HB, Macardle PJ, Hiscock J, et al. Anti-La (SS-B) antibodies transported across the placenta bind apoptotic cells in fetal organs targeted in neonatal lupus. Arthritis Rheum 2002;46: 1572–9.

[15] Clancy RM, Askanase AD, Kapur RP, et al. Transdifferentiation of cardiac fibroblasts, a fetal factor in anti-SSA/Ro-SSB/La antibody-mediated congenital heart block. J Immunol 2002;169: 2156–63.

[16] Miranda ME, Tseng CE, Rashbaum W, et al. Accessibility of SSA/Ro and SSB/La antigens to maternal autoantibodies in apoptotic human fetal cardiac myocytes. J Immunol 1998;161: 5061–9.

[17] Miranda-Carus ME, Askanase AD, Clancy RM, et al. Anti-SSA/Ro and -SSB/La autoantibodies bind the surface of apoptotic fetal cardiocytes and promote secretion of tumor necrosis factor alpha by macrophages. J Immunol 2000;165:5345–51.

[18] Clancy RM, Buyon JP. Clearance of apoptotic cells: TGF-beta in the balance between inflammation and fibrosis. J Leukoc Biol 2003;74:959–60.

[19] Fadok VA, Bratton DA, Konowal A, et al. Macrophages that have ingested apoptotic cells in vitro inhibit proinflammatory cytokine production through autocrine/paracrine mechanisms involving TGF-β, PGE2 and PAF. J Clin Invest 1998;101:890–8.

[20] Brown JR, Goldblatt D, Buddle J, et al. Diminished production of anti-inflammatory mediators during neutrophil apoptosis and macrophage phagocytosis in chronic granulomatous disease (CGD). J Leukoc Biol 2003;73:591–9.

[21] Manfredi AA, Rovere P, Galati G, et al. Apoptotic cell clearance in systemic lupus erythematosus. I. Opsonization by antiphospholipid antibodies. Arthritis Rheum 1998;41:205–14.

[22] Clancy RM, Kapur RP, Molad Y, et al. Immunohistologic evidence supports apoptosis, IgG deposition and novel macrophage/fibroblast crosstalk in the pathologic cascade leading to congenital heart block. Arthritis Rheum 2004;50:173–82.

[23] Awad MR, El-Gamel A, Hasleton P, et al. Genotypic variation in the transforming growth factor-beta1 gene: association with transforming growth factor-beta1 production, fibrotic lung disease, and graft fibrosis after lung transplantation. Transplantation 1998;66:1014–20.

[24] Franko AJ, Sharplin J, Ghahary A, et al. Immunohistochemical localization of transforming growth factor beta and tumor necrosis factor alpha in the lungs of fibrosis-prone and non-fibrosing mice during the latent period and early phase after irradiation. Radiat Res 1997;147: 245–56.

[25] Phan SH, Kunkel SL. Lung cytokine production in bleomycin-induced pulmonary fibrosis. Exp Lung Res 1992;18:29–43.

[26] Nakamura Y, Tate L, Ertl RF, et al. Bronchial epithelial cells regulate fibroblast proliferation. Am J Physiol 1995;269:L377–87.

[27] El-Gamel A, Awad MR, Hasleton PS, et al. Transforming growth factor-beta (TGF-beta1) genotype and lung allograft fibrosis. J Heart Lung Transplant 1999;18:517–23.

[28] Arkwright PD, Laurie S, Super M, et al. TGF-beta(1) genotype and accelerated decline in lung function of patients with cystic fibrosis. Thorax 2000;55:459–62.

[29] Clancy RM, Backer CB, Yin X, et al. Cytokine polymorphisms and histologic expression in autopsy studies: Contribution of TNFα and TGFβ1 to the pathogenesis of autoimmune-associated congenital heart block. J Immunol 2003;171:3253–61.

[30] Werth VP, Zhang W, Dortzbach K, et al. Association of a promoter polymorphism of tumor necrosis factor-alpha with subacute cutaneous lupus erythematosus and distinct photoregulation of transcription. J Invest Dermatol 2000;115:726–30.

[31] Werth VP, Callen JP, Ang G, et al. Associations of tumor necrosis factor alpha and HLA polymorphisms with adult dermatomyositis: implications for a unique pathogenesis. J Invest Dermatol 2002;119:617–20.

[32] McGuire W, Hill AV, Allsopp CE, et al. Variation in the TNF-α promoter region associated with susceptibility to cerebral malaria. Nature 1994;371:508–10.

[33] Sullivan KE, Wooten C, Schmeckpeper BJ, et al. A promoter polymorphism of tumor necrosis factor alpha associated with systemic lupus erythematosus in African-Americans. Arthritis Rheum 1997;40:2207–11.

[34] Wilson AG, de Vries N, Pociot F, et al. An allelic polymorphism within the human tumor necrosis factor alpha promoter region is strongly associated with HLA A1, B8, and DR3 alleles. J Exp Med 1993;177:557–60.

[35] Clancy RM, Backer CB, Yin X, et al. Genetic association of cutaneous neonatal lupus with HLA class II and TNF-α: Implications for pathogenesis. Arthritis Rheum 2004;50:2598–603.

[36] Askanase AD, Friedman DM, Copel J, et al. Spectrum and progression of conduction abnormalities in infants born to mothers with anti-Ro/La antibodies. Lupus 2002;11:145–51.

[37] Jaeggi ET, Hamilton RM, Silverman ED, et al. Outcome of children with fetal, neonatal, or childhood diagnosis of isolated congenital atrioventricular block. J Am Coll Cardiol 2002;39: 130–7.

[38] Nield LE, Silverman ED, Taylor GP, et al. Maternal anti-Ro and anti-La antibody-associated endocardial fibroelastosis. Circulation 2002;105:843–8.

[39] Nield LE, Silverman ED, Smallhorn JF, et al. Endocardial fibroelastosis associated with maternal anti-Ro and anti-La antibodies in the absence of atrioventricular block. J Am Coll Cardiol 2002; 40:796–802.

[40] Glickstein JS, Buyon JP, Friedman D. The fetal PR interval: pulsed Doppler echocardiographic assessment. Am J Cardiol 2000;86:236–9.

[41] Glickstein J, Buyon J, Kim M, Friedman D, and the PRIDE investigators. The fetal Doppler mechanical PR interval: a validation study. Fetal Diagn Ther 2004;19:31–4.

[42] Waltuck J, Buyon JP. Autoantibody-associated congenital heart block: outcome in mothers and children. Ann Intern Med 1994;120:544–51.

[43] Blanford AT, Pearson Murphy BE. In vitro metabolism of prednisolone, dexamethasone, betamethasone, and cortisol by the human placenta. Am J Obstet Gynecol 1997;127:264–7.

[44] Kaaja R, Julkunen H. Prevention of recurrence of congenital heart block with intravenous immunoglobulin and corticosteroid therapy: comment on the editorial by Buyon et al. Arthritis Rheum 2003;48:280–1.

[45] Samuelsson A, Towers TL, Ravetch JV. Anti-inflammatory activity of IVIG mediated through the inhibitory Fc receptor. Science 2001;291:445–6.

[46] Saleeb S, Copel J, Friedman D, et al. Comparison of treatment with fluorinated glucocorticoids to the natural history of autoantibody-associated congenital heart block: Retrospective review of the Research Registry for Neonatal Lupus. Arthritis Rheum 1999;42:2335–45.

[47] Matsushita H, Higashino M, Sekizuka N, et al. Successful prenatal treatment of congenital heart block with ritodrine administered transplacentally. Arch Gynecol Obstet 2002;267:51–3.

[48] Neiman AR, Lee LA, Weston WL, et al. Cutaneous manifestations of neonatal lupus without heart block: characteristics of mothers and children enrolled in a national registry. J Pediatr 2002; 37:674–80.

[49] Askanase AD, Miranda-Carus ME, Tang X, et al. The presence of IgG antibodies reactive with components of the SSA/Ro-SSB/La complex in human breast milk: implications in neonatal lupus. Arthritis Rheum 2002;46:269–71.

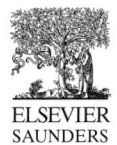

RHEUMATIC
DISEASE CLINICS
OF NORTH AMERICA

ELSEVIER
SAUNDERS

Rheum Dis Clin N Am 31 (2005) 315–328

# Newer Therapeutic Approaches for Systemic Lupus Erythematosus

## Ellen M. Ginzler, MD, MPH*, Olga Dvorkina, MD

*State University of New York–Downstate Medical Center, 450 Clarkson Avenue, Box 42, Brooklyn, NY 11203, USA*

Despite a 30-year drought in the approval of new agents for the treatment of systemic lupus erythematosus (SLE), a number of new clinical trials performed over the last decade provide promise that innovative therapies may soon be accepted for this complex disease. Some of these agents have multiple immuno-modulatory effects, whereas others have been designed to interfere with a specific immunologic process in the pathogenetic pathway of SLE activity. New modes of administering *standard of care* agents have also been studied in recent years. Particular attention has been paid not only to the efficacy of these new agents but also to their toxicity and patient tolerability.

## Immunomodulatory therapies

Renal disease continues to be the most common clinical manifestation of active SLE, and the one accounting for the most morbidity and mortality. In association with corticosteroids, immunosuppressive agents make up the primary regimens for both induction and maintenance therapy of lupus nephritis.

### Cyclophosphamide

For the past two decades, based on the randomized nonblinded trials performed at the National Institutes of Health (NIH), intravenous cyclophosphamide

---

* Corresponding author.
 *E-mail address:* ellen.ginzler@downstate.edu (E.M. Ginzler).

0889-857X/05/$ – see front matter © 2005 Elsevier Inc. All rights reserved.
doi:10.1016/j.rdc.2005.01.003　　　　　　　　　　　　　　　*rheumatic.theclinics.com*

(IVC) has been recognized as the standard of care for proliferative lupus nephritis (LN) in the United States [1]. Nevertheless, a significant improvement in progression to end-stage renal disease was observed only after 5 years from initiation of therapy, when IVC was compared with a regimen of prednisone alone or prednisone plus azathioprine. In addition, failure to achieve remission and relapses during maintenance therapy with IVC are well recognized [2,3]. A number of investigators have suggested that lack of efficacy may be related to racial, ethnic, and socioeconomic factors [4–7]. In a cohort by Dooley et al [4], IVC therapy for class IV LN in nonblack patients was associated with a subsequent 95% renal survival rate through 5 years of follow-up; however, renal survival in blacks declined progressively to 71% after 5 years. Among patients who have proliferative LN treated at Columbia Presbyterian, residence in a poor neighborhood was associated with doubling of serum creatinine, after adjustment for age, sex, creatinine, hypertension, cyclophosphamide (CYC) treatment, and race/ethnicity [5]. After further adjustment for poverty (residence by zip code) and insurance status, the risk of progression of renal insufficiency remained significant among Hispanics but not among African Americans. Response to treatment may also be less successful in children who have LN [8,9]. Based on these reports, consideration of a patient's sociodemographic status may be important in making a therapeutic decision.

Even in patients who respond well to CYC, both short and long-term toxicity is considerable, particularly with regard to infection, premature gonadal failure, and lymphoproliferative malignancies. The Euro-Lupus Nephritis Trial (ELNT) [10] was designed to minimize exposure to IVC with the goal of preserving efficacy. Ninety patients who have class IV LN were assigned by minimization technique to a regimen of either a high dose (6 monthly pulses followed by 2 quarterly pulses) or low dose (6 biweekly pulses of 500 mg) of IVC, followed in both treatment arms with oral azathioprine, 1 mg/kg/day [10]. Remissions of active nephritis occurred in 71% of the low-dose and 54% of the high-dose group; subsequent flares were noted in 27% and 29% during a median follow-up of 41 months. Severe infections were twice as frequent in the high-dose group. In extended follow-up to a median of 73 months, the cumulative probability of end-stage renal disease, doubling of serum creatinine, or death was not significantly different among patients in the low- and high-dose CYC groups [11]. A second renal biopsy was performed on 20 patients (11 low- and 9 high-dose) after a mean of 27 months. The activity index decreased significantly from baseline in both treatment groups, with no significant increase in chronicity index in either group. At long-term follow-up, 8 low-dose and 10 high-dose patients had progressed to permanent renal impairment and were classified in a poor long-term renal outcome group. In both treatment groups, an early reduction of 24-hour proteinuria was highly predictive of a good long-term renal outcome. Although the investigators concluded that data from the ELNT suggest a remission-inducing regimen of low-dose IVC to be equally effective as a high-dose regimen, they also point out that ELNT patients had clinically milder renal disease than did patients in the earlier NIH studies; the prevalence of renal impairment and nephrotic syndrome were 22% and 28%, respectively, in the ELNT, compared with 64% and 62% among NIH-treated patients [12].

Limited anecdotal data suggest that children refractory to IVC may tolerate and respond to a combined regimen of nine monthly infusions of IVC (750–1000 mg/m$^2$) and intravenous methotrexate (50–300 mg/m$^2$) given on the same day [13]. Clinical improvement persisted in five children despite discontinuation of immunosuppressive therapy, with mean prednisone dose reduced from 27.6 to 12.5 mg/day.

## Mycophenolate mofetil

In a search for an immunosuppressive agent with at least equivalent efficacy and improved toxicity and tolerability to CYC, investigators have turned to mycophenolate mofetil (MMF; CellCept). MMF is a reversible inhibitor of inosine monophosphate dehydrogenase, the rate-limiting step in purine synthesis, with a selective effect on lymphocytes and thereby less potential for hematologic toxicity. It is approved for prevention of allograft rejection and is therefore commercially available. Initially its use in patients who have SLE, usually with glomerulonephritis, was reserved for those who were unresponsive to steroids and CYC, or who had unacceptable toxicity to these agents (Table 1) [14–18]. Reported anecdotal series range in size from 10 to 21 patients, with follow-up extending up to 43 months. Some reports have noted differences in response to MMF based on the renal histologic type. Although most investigators report therapeutic efficacy in patients who have the proliferative forms of nephritis, conflicting results have been reported for membranous LN (MLN). Ferro et al [19] described 10 patients who had MLN treated for 1 year with MMF: proteinuria decreased significantly and 9 had a significant improvement in SLEDAI (Systemic Lupus Erythematosus Disease Activity Index) score. Among 13 patients who had MLN treated for 6 months with MMF by Spetie et al [20], complete or partial remission was achieved in 11. In a series of 11 patients, Diaz et al [21] reported efficacy of MMF in those who had proliferative nephritis, whereas patients who had MLN did not respond or relapsed. The pediatric experience of Buratti et al [22] was the reverse: 4 of 4 who had membranous histology had normalization of renal function, whereas all 3 children who had diffuse proliferative disease had deterioration in renal function during MMF therapy.

Four randomized nonblinded trials comparing MMF to CYC for LN have been reported. Two designed for the induction phase were performed at single centers. Chan et al [23] compared MMF to oral CYC in 42 patients who had class IV LN in Hong Kong. Treatment was continued for 1 year, with azathioprine substituted for CYC after 6 months. The efficacy of the two regimens was equivalent, with a high prevalence of complete response in both groups. Toxicity was not significantly different in the two groups. Hu et al [24] conducted a 6-month, open-label trial of 46 patients who had class IV LN, comparing MMF to IVC. They concluded that MMF was more effective than IVC, based

Table 1
Uncontrolled trials of mycophenolate mofetil for lupus glomerulonephritis

| Authors [Ref.] | No. of patients | MMF dose (g/d) | Renal features | Treatment duration | Response |
|---|---|---|---|---|---|
| Dooley et al [14] | 13 | 0.5–2.0 | All with nephritis | Mean 12.9 mo Range 3–24 mo | Significant improvement in proteinuria and serum creatinine |
| Gaubitz et al [15] | 10 | 1.5–2.0 | 4 with nephritis | Mean 11.2 mo Range 8–16 mo | Improvement in renal function, SLAM score, and steroid dose |
| Kingdon et al [16] | 13 | Median 1.0 | 2 membranous, 4 membranoproliferative, 7 proliferative | Median 25 mo up to 37 mo | Improvement in serum creatinine in 9/13, steroid-sparing in 8/10 |
| Karim et al [17] | 21 | 2.0 | 13 with worsening renal function | Median 14 mo Range 0.5–43 mo | Decreased proteinuria and SLEDAI, steroid-sparing |
| Kapitsinou et al [18] | 18 | 2.0 | 3 diffuse proliferative, 9 focal, 6 membranous | Mean 15.3 mo up to 31 mo | Complete remission in 10/18 and partial remission in 4, improved creatinine and proteinuria |

on significant differences in reduction in proteinuria, urinary red blood cells, anti-dsDNA titers, and improvement in renal histology on repeat biopsy.

Ginzler et al [25] recently reported the results of a multicenter nonblinded 6-month study of 140 patients who had LN (class III, IV, and V), randomized to either MMF or IVC for induction therapy of active nephritis. There was a highly significant difference in efficacy of the two regimens based on remission rate. Complete remission was achieved in 16 (23%) on MMF, compared with 4 (6%) on IVC; partial remission occurred in an additional 21 patients on MMF versus 17 on IVC.

Contreras et al [26] performed a study of sequential therapy in 59 patients who had proliferative LN in which induction with IVC was followed by maintenance therapy comparing three regimens (IVC, MMF, and azathioprine). Median follow-up was approximately 30 months, with primary end points of patient and renal survival. During maintenance therapy, there were 5 deaths (4 from CYC, 1 from MMF), and 5 patients progressed to chronic renal failure (3 from IVC, 1 from MMF, and 1 from azathioprine [AZA]). Event-free survival at 72 months was higher with MMF or AZA. Relapse-free survival was higher with MMF compared with IVC.

Subsequent anecdotal reports have described the efficacy of MMF for severe nonrenal lupus manifestations, including hemolytic anemia and pulmonary hemorrhage [27,28].

Considerable attention has been paid to the toxicity and tolerability of MMF, especially with regard to the issue of its potential as an alternative to IVC as a standard of care regimen for LN. The early anecdotal reports noted gastro-intestinal (GI) side effects, predominantly nausea and diarrhea [14,17,18], leuko-penia [14,17], and infection [14,17,18]. Riskalla et al [29] reported on 54 patients receiving MMF for a mean of 12.5 patient-months. Twenty-eight GI events were observed in 21 patients; 24 had a total of 37 infections, only 1 of which required hospitalization. Leukopenia occurred three times but did not require dose adjustment. In a prospective study of 42 patients receiving MMF for at least 9 months, Doria et al [30] observed adverse effects including infection in 5 patients, nausea in 4, abdominal pain in 3, diarrhea in 2, headache in 1, and leukopenia in 1. Therapy was discontinued due to side effects in 6 patients. In the multicenter comparison study of MMF to IVC, Ginzler et al [31] also noted that MMF was well tolerated and appeared to have better patient acceptance than IVC. Three deaths occurred, all in patients randomized to IVC and with severe manifestations of active lupus. Upper GI symptoms were common in both treatment groups, but nausea and diarrhea tended to be mild and self-limited on MMF, whereas 6 hospitalizations for dehydration after severe vomiting associated with IVC were noted. Infections were less frequent with MMF than IVC, particularly with regard to pyogenic infections, genital and skin herpes, and tinea. Hu et al [24] reported a lower rate of GI symptoms (26% versus 43%) and infections (17% versus 30%) with MMF versus IVC therapy. In the study by Contreras et al [26], adverse events including hospitalizations, amenorrhea, infections, and GI side effects were also significantly less frequent with

MMF compared with IVC. Most studies of MMF used doses of up to 2 g/day. In a multicenter study by Ginzler et al [31], the dose of MMF was increased progressively to a target of 3 g/day, or as tolerated by GI symptoms; 64% of the patients receiving MMF were able to tolerate this high dose.

*Leflunomide*

Leflunomide (Arava) is an inhibitor of de novo pyrimidine synthesis approved for treatment of rheumatoid arthritis (RA). Several small, uncontrolled open-label series have reported beneficial results in patients who have SLE, usually initiated because of steroid dependence. As with RA, most regimens began with a loading dose of 100 mg/day for 3 days, followed by 20 mg/day. In a pilot study including assessment of changes in European Consensus Lupus Study (ECLAM), anti-dsDNA C3, C4, and urinary protein excretion, Petera et al [32] treated 11 patients, 4 of whom completed a planned 24-week course. At last follow-up, mean ECLAM score decreased from $4.1 \pm 1.4$ to $3.3 \pm 2.1$. Changes in serologic parameters and proteinuria were not significant. Steroid doses were decreased in 4 patients and increased in 2. In a similar observational study of 18 patients treated for 2 to 3 months, Remer et al [33] reported subjective improvement in 10 of the 14 patients who did not discontinue the drug; 9 had a decrease in SLEDAI score. No serious adverse effects were noted. Petri [34] treated 20 patients who had SLE specifically for inflammatory arthritis, using a daily dose of 40 mg/day after the standard loading dose. Patients were seen monthly for 3 months, of which 6 had a complete response, which was sustained when the maintenance dose was subsequently decreased to 20 mg/day. Toxicity resulted in drug discontinuation in 4 patients (1 with rash, 2 with diarrhea, and 1 with liver function abnormalities). No controlled trials of leflunomide for SLE in general or for refractory arthritis have been reported.

**Biologic agents**

*T-cell activation, T-cell–B-cell interaction, and B-cell depletion*

In a comprehensive review of B cells as therapeutic targets for rheumatic disease, Looney et al [35] point out that B cells are critical to the development of SLE and ongoing disease activity even when they are unable to secrete autoantibodies. The development of new therapeutic agents has therefore focused on functions of B cells in taking up autoantigens and presenting them via specific cell surface immunoglobulins to T cells, subsequently affecting T-cell–dependent immune responses.

*Anti-CD20*

Among the newer biologic agents, anti-CD20 or rituximab (Rituxan) has received the most attention in recent years as a potential therapy for refractory

SLE. It is a chimeric monoclonal antibody directed against the CD20 receptor present on B lymphocytes. As an approved agent for the treatment of non-Hodgkin's B-cell lymphoma, it is commercially available. Several reports have been published since 2002, mostly of small case series noting therapeutic success for refractory lupus manifestations including central nervous system, and renal, vasculitic, and hematologic features [36–41]. Several open-label series have included larger numbers of patients with longer follow-up. Albert et al [42] used a regimen of four weekly infusions of rituximab in 9 patients who had active persistent SLE and visceral involvement refractory to at least one immuno-suppressive agent. Six of the patients improved clinically, with half remaining in remission at 6 to 9 months. Two patients developed human antichimeric antibodies. Anolik et al [43] reported a series of 19 patients, treated with either one infusion of 100 mg/m$^2$ rituximab, one infusion of 375 mg/m$^2$, or four weekly 375 mg/m$^2$ doses. Among the 16 patients who completed the protocol, 10 achieved full lymphocyte-B depletion with significant improvement in disease activity. In a single patient who had class IV nephritis, proteinuria resolved completely in 1 year and repeat renal biopsy showed complete resolution of previous proliferative pathology. Leandro et al [44] treated 6 patients who had lupus with a regimen including two weekly doses of 500 mg rituximab and 750 mg IVC plus high-dose oral prednisone. B-cell depletion was achieved in all patients persisting for 3 to 16 months. After 6 to 18 months, 5 patients remained in the study with clinical and laboratory improvement and no major side effects. Gunnarsson et al [45] also reported efficacy without serious adverse events of a combined regimen of rituximab and CYC in 11 female patients who had SLE who had failed therapy with conventional cytotoxic drugs including CYC.

*LJP 394*

LJP 394 or abetimus sodium (Riquent), was designed to prevent the recurrence of renal flares in patients with established nephritis by selectively reducing antibodies to dsDNA via antigen-specific tolerance. It is a synthetic composed of four deoxyribonucleotide sequences bound to a triethylene glycol backbone. In a large randomized blinded controlled study, 230 patients received either LJP 394 or placebo for 76 weeks [46]. The time to renal flare and the number of renal flares were not significantly different in the two treatment groups, and the trial was discontinued prematurely. Anti-dsDNA titers were found to decrease significantly more in the LJP 394 group, with concomitant increase in C3 levels. A subgroup analysis in patients who had high affinity antibodies against LJP 394 showed a longer time to renal flare, with fewer flares and a decreased requirement for subsequent treatment with IVC in the LJP 394 –treated compared with the placebo group. Side effects were similar in both groups. An additional randomized placebo-controlled phase 3 trial recruited 298 high-affinity antibody patients (145 LJP 394, 153 placebo). Changes in urine protein excretion were examined for those in the phase 2 and 3 studies who had 24-hour urine collections at baseline and at 1 year of follow-up. A statistically greater 50% reduction in proteinuria was observed in 23 of 52 (44.2%) patients in the LJP

394 group, compared with 11 of 61 (18.0%) in the placebo group [47]. Based on patient self-reports, health-related quality of life was significantly improved in the treated versus the placebo group [48].

*Anti–B-lymphocyte stimulator*

B-lymphocyte stimulator, or BlyS, is a member of the tumor necrosis factor (TNF) cytokine family, which is present on B cells. LymphoStat-B, a fully human monocolonal antibody to BlyS, was initially studied in murine lupus models, resulting in increased survival. A phase I single- and double-dose escalation trial in 57 stable patients who had SLE was recently completed [49]. Follow-up for 84 to 105 days posttreatment was performed. A significant reduction of peripheral B cells was observed, but no change in SLE activity was noted with this short drug exposure protocol. Enrollment in a phase II double-blind, placebo-controlled multicenter study has been completed. The treatment protocol will continue for 6 months.

*Costimulatory blockade*

Two distinct signals are necessary for T-cell–dependent B-cell responses, the first of which is binding of a T-cell receptor (TCR) to antigen, providing specificity to T-cell activation. Nonspecific signals occur with interactions between receptor-ligand pairs on T-cells and antigen-presenting cells. These functions provide a target for potential therapies that may inhibit T-cell–B-cell interactions. Efficacy of biologic agents with beneficial results in murine models of lupus has not yet been demonstrated in human lupus. Phase II clinical trials of two distinct preparations of anti-CD40 ligand, a humanized monoclonal antibody to the CD40 ligand that prevents interaction of CD40 on B cells with T-cell surface CD40 ligand, were unsuccessful. One trial was terminated prematurely because of an increased incidence of thromboembolic events [50], and the other failed to show efficacy compared with placebo [51]. The biologic agent CTLA4-Ig, a fusion protein derived from the extracellular domain of the cytotoxic T-lymphocyte antigen 4 and the Fc portion of IgG1, was designed to inhibit T-cell activation. Although it has been shown to improve proteinuria and prolong survival in murine lupus [52], controlled trials in human lupus are yet to be initiated.

*Cytokine inhibition*

The rationale for inhibition of proinflammatory cytokines in patients who have SLE was reviewed by Aringer and Smolen [53]. Studies of inhibition of interferon-γ, interleukin-6, and interleukin-18 have been reported in murine lupus, some with positive results, but experience in human SLE is lacking. Despite a study demonstrating decreased TNF-α secretion and successful amelioration of leukopenia, proteinuria, and immune complex deposition in an experimental mouse model treated with anti–TNF-α monoclonal antibody [54], no clinical trials of anti-TNF agents have been performed in patients who have SLE. Enthusiasm for this class of drugs may be diminished due to reports suggesting that they may be associated with the development of antinuclear antibodies or drug-induced lupuslike syndromes [55–58].

## Sex hormones

The importance of sex hormones in the pathogenesis of SLE, particularly with regard to the predominance of the disease in women of child-bearing age, has provided the rationale for studying these agents as potential therapies for SLE.

### Dehydroepiandrosterone

The rationale for treatment of SLE with male sex hormones is based on its marked female predominance and peak incidence in the child-bearing years. Although anecdotal uncontrolled studies suggested that the weak male androgen dehydroepoandrosterone (DHEA or prasterone) improved lupus symptoms and decreased steroid requirements, a significant difference in efficacy was not observed in a randomized controlled trial of prasterone, 100 mg or 200 mg/day, in 191 steroid-dependent (prednisone 10–30 mg/d for $\geq 12$ mo) female patients [59]. The protocol endpoint was sustained steroid tapering to $\leq 7.5$ mg pred-nisone/day over 7 to 9 months. The proportion of responders was highest in the 200-mg prasterone group (55%) and lowest in the placebo group (41%). In a subset analysis, prasterone was steroid-sparing in patients who had active lupus at study entry. In another randomized controlled trial comparing comparing prasterone 200 mg/day to placebo in 120 women treated for 24 weeks, a significant difference in the primary endpoint of change in SLAM (systemic lupus activity measure) score was not found, although significant differences were noted in the number of flares and patient visual analogue scores [60]. An increased incidence of acne was noted in both studies.

A potential added benefit of prasterone is its action in stabilizing or reversing osteoporosis. In a subset of patients in a controlled trial of 351 subjects, 55 underwent baseline bone mineral density assessments (31 placebo, 24 prasterone) [61]. At the lumbar spine there was a mean loss in bone density of $-1.1$ by T-score with a mean gain of 1.7 in the treatment group ($P = 0.003$). Bone density at the proximal femur ranged from a mean loss of 0.3 on placebo to a mean gain of 2.0 with prasterone treatment.

### Estrogen

In addition to finding new agents to treat active lupus or maintain remission, consideration must be given to determining whether drugs commonly used for other purposes in patients with SLE may have a deleterious effect on the course of their lupus. The SELENA (Safety of Estrogens in Lupus Erythematosus—

National Assessment trial investigated whether hormone replacement therapy (HRT), a component of preventive regimens for osteoporosis and cardiovascular disease, increases the flare rate in postmenopausal women who have inactive or stable-active lupus [62]. In a randomized, blinded protocol, 351 patients received conjugated estrogen and medroxyprogesterone HRT or placebo for 12 months. Severe flares were observed rarely, with no significant difference in rate between the HRT and placebo groups, although flares were more common in stable-active than inactive patients. On the other hand, mild–moderate flares were significantly more frequent in the HRT arm. Adverse events were seen almost exclusively in the HRT arm, including 1 death, 3 deep vein thromboses (1 on placebo), 1 stroke, and 1 thrombosis in an arteriovenous graft. Results of a parallel study of oral contraceptives versus placebo in premenopausal patients who have SLE have not yet been reported.

**Stem-cell transplantation and immunoablation**

Because it is believed that SLE exacerbations or chronic lupus activity are driven by continuous activation of autoreactive B and T lymphocytes, most general immunosuppressive drugs as well as the newer agents described here are designed to prevent pathogenetic autoantibody production. Nevertheless, total suppression of autoantibody production is rarely achieved. For this reason, immunoablation with high-dose immunosuppression followed by rescue with autologous hematopoietic stem-cell transplantation (HSCT) has been proposed as a mechanism to reverse the immune dysfunction in SLE. Various conditioning regimens before stem-cell reinfusion have been used, but most include high-dose CYC (200 mg/kg), along with antithymocyte globulin or rituximab. Traynor et al [63] described the clinical course following HSCT in 17 patients who had SLE and were refractory to conventional therapies, 15 of whom survived for a median of 36 months with a gradual but marked improvement in serologic and clinical manifestations with steroid requirements remaining in only 2. There were 2 deaths: 1 due to fungal sepsis before stem-cell replacement and 1 with central nervous system disease 4 months after HSCT. Relapses necessitating IVC therapy occurred in 2 patients at 30 and 40 months. The results of Lisukov et al [64] are less promising; 6 patients who had severe refractory lupus activity underwent HSCT, 3 of whom died within 2 months of transplant-related complications.

The need for stem-cell rescue after a conditioning regimen of high-dose immunosuppression has been questioned by some investigators. High-dose CYC is not myeloablative, and autoreactive lymphocytes may be reinfused at the time of stem-cell rescue, resulting in disease progression or early relapse [65]. Furthermore, pleuripotent stem cells contain a high concentration of aldehyde dehydrogenase, which protects them against the cytotoxic effects of CYC, which should allow marrow recovery without the need for stem-cell rescue. Bronson et al [66] compared very high-dose IVC (50 mg/kg × 4 d) to monthly IVC (750 mg/m2) in 51 patients and found a better patient-reported health status at

6 months in the high-dose group, as measured by short-form health survey SF-36. In an uncontrolled series of 14 patients treated with high-dose CYC, these investigators reported 5 long-term responses with significant improvement in steroid dose and SLEDAI score [67]. Gladstone et al [65] point out that the time to maximum response may take years and that posttreatment flares do not herald therapeutic failure.

## Summary

In recent years, advances in the treatment of SLE refractory to conventional therapy have been suggested in anecdotal series and some clinical trials. A number of promising agents have been studied only in murine models of SLE, and clinical trials are awaited. Rigorously conducted clinical trials must be completed to advance these studies to the point that new therapies for SLE will be approved.

## References

[1] Steinberg AD, Steinberg SC. Long-term preservation of renal function in patients with lupus nephritis receiving treatment that includes cyclophosphamide versus those treated with prednisone only. Arthritis Rheum 1991;34(8):945–50.

[2] Illei GG, Takada K, Parkin D. Renal flares are common in patients with severe proliferative lupus nephritis treated with immunosuppressive therapy: longterm followup of a cohort of 145 patients participating in randomized controlled studies. Arthritis Rheum 2002;46(4): 995–1002.

[3] Ioannidis JPA, Boki KA, Katsorida ME, et al. Remission, relapse, and re-remission of proliferative lupus nephritis treated with cyclophosphamide. Kidney Int 2000;57(1):258–64.

[4] Dooley MA, Hogan S, Jennette C, Falk R. Cyclophosphamide therapy for lupus nephritis: poor renal survival in black Americans. Kidney Int 1997;51(4):1188–95.

[5] Barr RG, Seliger S, Appel GB, et al. Prognosis in proliferative lupus nephritis: the role of socio-economic status and race/ethnicity. Nephrol Dial Transplant 2003;18(10):2039–46.

[6] Williams W, Bhagwandass A, Sargeant LA, Shah D. Severity of systemic lupus erythematosus with diffuse proliferative glomerulonephritis and the ineffectiveness of standard pulse intravenous cyclophosphamide therapy in Jamaican patient. Lupus 2003;12(8):640–5.

[7] Velasquez X, Verdejo U, Massardo L, et al. Outcome of Chilean patients with lupus nephritis and response to intravenous cyclophosphamide. J Clin Rheumatol 2003;9(1):7–14.

[8] Al Salloum AA. Cyclophosphamide therapy for lupus nephritis: poor survival in Arab children. Pediatr Nephrol 2003;18(4):357–61.

[9] Barbano G, Gusmano R, Damasio B, et al. Childhood-onset lupus nephritis: a single-center experience of pulse intravenous cyclophosphamide therapy. J Nephrol 2002;15(2):123–9.

[10] Houssiau FA, Vasconcelos C, D'Cruz D. Immunosuppressive therapy in lupus nephritis. The Euro-Lupus Nephritis Trial, a randomized trial of low-dose versus high-dose intravenous cyclophosphamide. Arthritis Rheum 2002;46(8):2121–31.

[11] Houssiau FA, Vasconcelos C, D'Cruz D, et al. Early response to immunosuppressive therapy predicts good renal outcome in lupus nephritis: lessons from the long-term follow-up of the Euro-Lupus Nephritis Trial. Arthritis Rheum, in press.

[12] Boumpas DT, Austin III HA, Vaughan EM, et al. Controlled trial of pulse methylprednisolone versus two regimens of pulse cyclophosphamide in severe lupus nephritis. Lancet 1992; 340(8822):741–5.

[13] Lehman TJ, Edelheit BS, Onel KB. Combined intravenous methotrexate and cyclophosphamide for refractory childhood lupus nephritis. Ann Rheum Dis 2004;63(3):321–3.

[14] Dooley MA, Cosio FG, Nachman PH, et al. Mycophenolate mofetil therapy in lupus nephritis: clinical observations. J Am Soc Nephrol 1999;10(4):833–9.

[15] Gaubitz M, Schorat A, Schotte H, et al. Mycophenolate mofetil for the treatment of systemic lupus erythematosus: an open pilot trial. Lupus 1999;8(9):731–6.

[16] Kingdon EJ, McLean AG, Psimenous E, et al. The safety and efficacy of MMF in lupus nephritis: a pilot study. Lupus 2001;10(9):606–11.

[17] Karim MY, Alba P, Cuadrado MJ, et al. Mycophenolate mofetil for systemic lupus erythematosus refractory to other immunosuppressive agents. Rheumatol 2002;41(8):876–82.

[18] Kapitsinou PP, Boletis JN, Skopouli FN, et al. Lupus nephritis: treatment with mycophenolate mofetil. Rheumatol 2004;43(3):377–80.

[19] Ferro ML, Karim MY, Abbs IC, et al. Mycophenolate mofetil: a potential treatment for reducing proteinuria associated with membranous lupus nephritis. Arthritis Rheum 2003;48(9):S588.

[20] Spetie DN, Tang Y, Rovin BH, et al. Mycophenolate (MMF) therapy of SLE membranous nephropathy (MN). Presented at the 7th International Lupus Congress, New York, May 2004.

[21] Diaz C, Baron MA, Camps MT, et al. Lupus nephritis treatment with mycophenolate mofetil. Clinical study of eleven patients. Presented at the 7th International Lupus Congress, New York, May 2004.

[22] Buratti S, Szer IS, Spencer CH, et al. Mycophenolate mofetil treatment of severe renal disease in pediatric onset systemic lupus erythematosus. J Rheumatol 2001;28(9):2103–8.

[23] Chan TM, Li FK, Tang CSO, et al. Efficacy of mycophenolate mofetil in patients with diffuse proliferative lupus nephritis. N Engl J Med 2002;343(16):1156–62.

[24] Hu W, Liu Z, Chen H, et al. Mycophenolate mofetil vs cyclophosphamide therapy for patients with diffuse proliferative lupus nephritis. Chin Med J 2002;115(5):705–9.

[25] Ginzler EM, Aranow C, Buyon J, et al. A multicenter study of mycophenolate mofetil (MMF) vs. intravenous cyclophosphamide (IVC) as induction therapy for severe lupus nephritis (LN): preliminary results. Arthritis Rheum 2003;48(9):S647.

[26] Contreras G, Pardo C, Leclercq B, et al. Sequential therapies for proliferative lupus nephritis. N Engl J Med 2004;350(10):971–80.

[27] Alba P, Karim MY, Hunt BJ. Mycophenolate mofetil as a treatment for autoimmune hemolytic anemia in patients with systemic lupus erythematosus and antiphospholipid syndrome. Lupus 2003;12(8):633–5.

[28] Samad AS, Lindsley CB. Treatment of pulmonary hemorrhage in childhood systemic lupus erythematosus with mycophenolate mofetil. South Med J 2003;96:705–7.

[29] Riskalla MM, Somers EC, Fatica RA, McCune WJ. Tolerability of mycophenolate mofetil in patients with systemic lupus erythematosus. J Rheumatol 2003;30(7):1508–12.

[30] Doria A, Frassi M, Della Libera S, et al. Prospective study on tolerability and efficacy of mycophenolate mofetil (MMF) in SLE. Arthritis Rheum 2003;48(9):S587.

[31] Ginzler EM, Aranow C, Merrill JT, et al. Toxicity and tolerability of mycophenolate mofetil (MMF) versus intravenous cyclophosphamide (IVC) in a multicenter trial as induction therapy for lupus nephritis (LN). Arthritis Rheum 2003;48(9):S586.

[32] Petera P, Mander B, Manger K, et al. A pilot study of leflunomide in systemic lupus erythematosus (SLE). Arthritis Rheum 2000;43(9):S241.

[33] Remer CF, Weisman MH, Wallace DJ. Benefits of leflunomide in systemic lupus erythematosus: a pilot observational study. Lupus 2001;10(7):480–3.

[34] Petri M. High dose Arava in lupus. Arthritis Rheum 2001;44(9):S280.

[35] Looney JR, Anolik J, Sanz I. B cells as therapeutic targets for rheumatic diseases. Curr Opin Rheumatol 2004;16(3):180–5.

[36] Saito K, Nawata M, Nakayamada S, et al. Successful treatment with anti-CD20 monoclonal

antibody (rituximab) of life-threatening refractory systemic lupus erythematosus with renal and central nervous system involvement. Lupus 2003;12(10):798–800.

[37] Saigal K, Valencia IC, Cohen J, Kerdel FA. Hypocomplementemic urticarial vasculitis with angioedema, a rare presentation of systemic lupus erythematosus: rapid response to rituximab. J Am Acad Dermatol 2003;49(5 Suppl):S283–5.

[38] Perrotta S, Locatelli F, La Manna A, et al. Anti-CD20 monoclonal antibody (rituximab) for life-threatening autoimmune hemolytic anemia in a patient with systemic lupus erythematosus. Brit J Hematol 2002;116(2):465–7.

[39] Weide R, Heymans J, Pandorf A, Koppler H. Successful long-term treatment of systemic lupus erythematosus with rituximab maintenance therapy. Lupus 2003;12(10):779–82.

[40] Yamazaki M, Takami A, Asakura H, Nakao S. Rituximab reduces antiphosphlipid antibody (APA) titers and improves hypercoagulability in patients with antiphospholipid syndrome. Presented at the America Society of Hematology. Philadelphia, Pennsylvania, 2002. Abstract #1027.

[41] Fra GP, Avanzi GC, Bartoli E. Remission of refractory lupus nephritis with a protocol including rituximab. Lupus 2003;12(10):783–7.

[42] Albert DA, Khan SR, Stansberry J, et al. A phase I trial of rituximab (anti-CD20) for treatment of systemic lupus erythematosus. Presented at the American College of Rheumatology Annual Meeting. Orlando, Florida, October 2003. Presentation #LB9.

[43] Anolik JH, Campbell D, Felgar R, et al. B lymphocyte depletion in the treatment of systemic lupus (SLE): phase i/ii trial of rituximab (Rituxan) in SLE. Arthritis Rheum 2002; 46(9):S717.

[44] Leandro MJ, Ehrenstein MR, Edwards JCW, et al. Treatment of refractory lupus nephritis with B lymphocyte depletion. Arthritis Rheum 2003;48(9):S378.

[45] Gunnarsson I, Henriksson EW, Sundelin B, et al. Rituximab plus cyclophosphmaide in severe SLE: promising results in 11 patients who failed conventional immunosuppressive therapy. Presented at the 7th International Lupus Congress, New York, May 2004.

[46] Alarcon-Segovia D, Tumlin AJ, Furie R, et al. LJP 394 for the prevention of renal flare in patients with systemic lupus erythematosus. Arthritis Rheum 2003;48(2):442–54.

[47] Tumlin JA, Cardiel MH, Furie RA, et al. Reductions in 24 hour urine protein levels associated with treatment of lupus patients with LJP 394 in two randomized placebo controlled double-blind clinical trials. Presented at the 7th International Lupus Congress, New York, May 2004.

[48] Strand V, Aranow C, Cardiel MH, et al. Improvement in health-related quality of life in systemic erythematosus patients enrolled in a randomized clinical trial comparing LJP 394 treatment with placebo. Lupus 2003;12(9):677–86.

[49] Furie R, Stohl W, Ginzler E, et al. Safety, pharmacokinetic and pharmacodynamic results of a phase I single and double dose-escalation study of LymphoStat-B (human monoclonal antibody to BlyS) in SLE patients. Arthritis Rheum 2003;48(9):S377.

[50] Boumpas DT, Furie R, Manzi S, et al. A short course of BG9588 (anti-CD40 ligand antibody) improves serologic activity and decreases hematuria in patients with proliferative lupus glomerulonephritis. Arthritis Rheum 2003;48(3):719–27.

[51] Kalunian KC, Davis Jr JC, Merrill JT, et al. Treatment of systemic lupus erythematosus by inhibition of T cell costimulation with anti-CD154: a randomized, double-blind, placebo-controlled trial. Arthritis Rheum 2002;46(12):3251–8.

[52] Daikh D, Wofsy D. Cutting edge: reversal of murine lupus nephritis with CTLA4-Ig and cyclophosphamide. J Immunol 2001;166:2913–6.

[53] Aringer M, Smolen JS. Tumour necrosis factor and other proinflammatory cytokines in systemic lupus erythematosus: a rationale for therapeutic intervention. Lupus 2004;13(5):344–7.

[54] Segal R, Dayan M, Zinger H, Mozes E. Suppression of experimental systemic lupus erythematosus (SLE) in mice via TNF inhibition by an anti-TNFalpha monoclonal antibody and by pentoxiphylline. Lupus 2001;10(1):23–31.

[55] Shakoor N, Michalska M, Harris CA, Block JA. Drug-induced systemic lupus erythematosus associated with etanercept therapy. Lancet 2000;359(9306):579–80.

[56] Debandt M, Vittecoq O, Descamps V, et al. Anti-TNF-α-induced systemic lupus erythematosus. Clin Rheumatol 2003;22(1):56–61.

[57] Ali Y, Shah S. Infliximab-induced systemic lupus erythematosus. Ann Intern Med 2002;137(7): 625–6.

[58] Charles PJ, Smeenk RJ, De Jong J, et al. Assessment of antibodies to double-stranded DNA induced in rheumatoid arthritis patients following treatment with infliximab, a monoclonal antibody to tumor necrosis factor α: findings in open-label and randomized placebo-controlled trials. Arthritis Rheum 2000;43(11):2383–90.

[59] Petri M, Lahita RG, van Vollenhoven RF, et al. Effects of prasterone on corticosteroid requirements of women with systemic lupus erythematosus. Arthritis Rheum 2002;46(7):1820–9.

[60] Chang D-M, Lan J-L, Lin H-Y, Luo S-F. Dehydroepiandrosterone treatment of women with mild-to-moderate systemic lupus erythematosus. Arthritis Rheum 2002;46(11):2924–7.

[61] Petri MA, Mease PJ, Merrill JT, et al. Lupus disease activity and bone mineral density in women with active lupus: results of a double-blind, multicenter trial comparing prasterone with placebo. Presented at the 7th International Congress on SLE. New York, New York, May 2004.

[62] Buyon JP, Petri M, Kim M, et al. Estrogen/cyclic progesterone replacement is associated with an increased rate of mild/moderate but not severe flares in SLE patients in the SELENA trial. Presented at the American College of Rheumatology Annual Meeting. Orlando, Florida, October 2003. Presentation #LB10.

[63] Traynor AE, Barr WG, Rosa RM, et al. Hematopoietic stem cell transplantation for severe and refractory lupus. Analysis after five years and fifteen patients. Arthritis Rheum 2002; 46(11):2917–23.

[64] Lisukov IA, Sizkova SA, Kulagin AD, et al. High-dose immunosuppression with autologous stem cell transplantation in severe refractory systemic lupus erythematosus. Lupus 2004;13: 89–94.

[65] Gladstone DE, Prestrud AA, Pradhan A, et al. High-dose cyclophosphamide for severe systemic lupus erythematosus. Lupus 2003;11(7):405–10.

[66] Bronson K, Petri M, Brodsky R, Jones R. High-dose cyclophosphamide is preferable to monthly IV cyclophosphamide at six months. Arthritis Rheum 2003;48(9):S588.

[67] Petri M, Jones RJ, Brodsky RA. High-dose cyclophosphamide without stem cell transplant in systemic lupus erythematosus. Arthritis Rheum 2003;48(9):166–73.

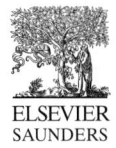
ELSEVIER
SAUNDERS

RHEUMATIC
DISEASE CLINICS
OF NORTH AMERICA

Rheum Dis Clin N Am 31 (2005) 329–354

# Premature Atherosclerosis in Systemic Lupus Erythematosus

Mandana Nikpour, MBBS, FRACP[a],
Murray B. Urowitz, MD, FRCP(C)[b,c,*],
Dafna D. Gladman, MD, FRCP(C)[a,b]

[a]University of Toronto Lupus Clinic, Toronto Western Hospital, ON, Canada
[b]University of Toronto, Toronto, ON, Canada
[c]Centre of Prognosis Studies in the Rheumatic Diseases, Toronto Western Hospital,
Toronto, ON, Canada

Systemic lupus erythematosus (SLE), a chronic multisystem autoimmune disease, was first described in medical literature in the 1800s. Centuries on, although the pathogenesis and etiologic associations of SLE are yet to be elucidated fully, significant advances have been made in defining the spectrum of clinical manifestations and the prognosis of this disease. The advent of corticosteroids in the 1950s dramatically altered the short-term prognosis of patients who have SLE from frequently fatal, with less than 50% survival at 5 years, to 93% 5-year and 85% 10-year survival [1]. Early diagnosis and the use of other immunosuppressive and immunomodulatory agents such as the antimalarials, as well as better management of complications such as infection, have also contributed to the reduction in early mortality.

With improved long-term survival, longitudinal cohort studies have served to determine prognostic factors and disease outcome in the corticosteroid era. The *bimodal* pattern of mortality in SLE was first suggested by case series and later confirmed in prospective cohort studies. It was shown that many patients who survive early complications of organ failure and sepsis later develop premature coronary artery disease (CAD). In this evidence-based review, the objec-

This work was supported by the Geoff Carr Lupus Fellowship from the Ontario Lupus Association.
* Corresponding author. Centre of Prognosis in the Rheumatic Diseases, Toronto Western Hospital, 399 Bathurst Street, 1E 409 East Wing, Toronto, ON, M5T 2S8, Canada.
*E-mail address:* m.urowitz@utoronto.ca (M.B. Urowitz).

tives are to define the magnitude of the problem of premature atherosclerosis (AS) in SLE and to evaluate the strength of association of risk factors determined to date. The authors focus on the emerging role of new modalities for noninvasive assessment of vascular health in patients who have SLE and offer a strategy for screening and management of those at risk of CAD. The article concludes by discussing important questions that remain to be answered and future directions for research.

## Systemic lupus erythematosus and coronary artery disease: epidemiologic evidence of association

The first cases suggesting an association between SLE and atherosclerotic CAD were reported in the 1960s [2]. In 1976, Urowitz et al [3] described the bimodal pattern of mortality in SLE based on a case series of 11 deaths among 81 patients followed for 5 years at the University of Toronto Rheumatic Disease Unit. Six of the 11 deaths occurred within the first year after diagnosis in patients who had active disease. In four of the six *early* deaths, a major septic episode contributed to the death. In the five patients who died late in the course of the disease, all had a myocardial infarct (MI) close to the time of death and in four patients MI was the primary cause of death. Subsequently, a case series described premature CAD with onset of symptoms before the age of 35 years in six women with SLE [4]. A larger case series published in 1985 and a case-control autopsy study in 1987 further supported these observations [5,6]. The first large prospective SLE cohort was established in Toronto, Canada in 1970, and the mortality data for 665 patients followed to 1993 in this clinic were reported in 1995 [1]. In the duration of follow-up, 124 (18.6%) patients died. In 31 (25%) the cause of death was an acute vascular event, congestive heart failure or sudden death. These causes accounted for 17% of early deaths within 5 years compared with 30% of *late* deaths beyond 5 years of diagnosis. In addition, in the 40 autopsies performed in this cohort, moderate to severe AS of the major vessels was found in 21 (54%) regardless of the cause of death. The prevalence of symptomatic CAD in more recently established lupus cohorts in Baltimore (8.3%) and Pittsburgh (6.6%) is similar to the Toronto lupus cohort (8.9%) [1,7–9]. Although there are some differences in the demographic composition of these large cohorts, the mean age at the first CAD event is similar at 48 to 49 years.

In addition to data from cohorts followed in a tertiary setting, a community based study by Ward using the California Discharge Database found that women with SLE between 18 and 44 years were more likely than age-matched controls to have been admitted to hospital with MI (odds ratio [OR], 2.27; 95% CI, 1.08 to 3.46), congestive heart failure (OR, 3.8; 95% CI, 2.41 to 5.19) and stroke (OR, 2.05; 95% CI, 1.17 to 2.93) [10]. In this study it was estimated that MI, heart failure, and stroke were overall 8.5, 13.2, and 10.1 times, respectively, more likely in women with SLE than in the general population.

Studies of incidence rates of coronary events in women with SLE have shown a significantly raised rate ratio of MI and angina in women with SLE compared with age matched controls. Manzi et al [8] compared the age-specific incidence rates of MI and angina in women with SLE (3522 person years) seen at the university of Pittsburgh Medical Center from 1980 to 1993 with women in the Framingham Offspring Study (17,519 person years). Women with lupus in the 35- to 44-year age group were over 50 times more likely to have an MI than women of similar age in the Framingham Offspring Study (rate ratio 52.43, 95% CI 21.6 to 98.5). Overall two thirds of all *first* cardiac events after the diagnosis of lupus were in women under the age of 55 years. When the annual incidence of MI among lupus patients attending the Toronto lupus clinic was compared with background population rates for the province of Ontario, the rate of MI in the lupus cohort was 5 per 1000 patients compared with 1 per 1000 patients in the general population for 1993 to 1994. Furthermore the mean age of MI in the lupus clinic was 49 years compared with the peak incidence in the general population of 65 to 74 years (unpublished observations). Based on these studies the annual incidence of MI in SLE is estimated to be 0.5% to 1.5%.

Collectively studies to date confirm that women with SLE have a significantly increased relative risk of MI compared with women in the general population and that the onset of CAD in SLE is premature with loss of premenopausal protection.

**Atherosclerosis in noncoronary vessels: a link with coronary artery disease**

AS often affects multiple vessel territories in the same patient. Studies have shown that in patients who have diabetes, a classic risk factor for cardiovascular disease, AS in one vessel territory is a risk factor for presence of AS in other vascular territories [11]. Similarly in patients who do not have diabetes, coronary and cerebral arterial disease often coexist with small studies showing up to 20% to 40% prevalence of silent cardiac ischemia in patients who have a history of stroke, whereas larger studies have shown that 2% to 5% of patients who have acute stroke have fatal cardiac-related events in the short term after stroke [12]. In the Toronto cohort, 25 new strokes unrelated to cerebral lupus occurred among 1087 patients over a mean follow-up of 8.9 years, giving a prevalence of stroke of 2.3% [13]. Only a small number of patients who had had stroke had antiphospholipid antibodies (aPL), indicating that atherosclerotic cerebrovascular disease was the likely culprit in the majority of cases. In a case (n = 66) control (n = 33) study, premenopausal women with SLE (aPL positive and aPL negative) had an increased prevalence of carotid or femoral plaque compared with healthy controls (5.3% versus 1% of vessels affected, $P < 0.05$) [14]. Conventional predictors of AS including lipid variables did not account for this difference. In this study neither anticardiolipin (aCL) nor anti-B$_2$GPI antibodies were associated with AS. Manzi et al [15] determined the prevalence of carotid plaque in 175 women with SLE, mean age 44.9 ± 11.5 years. Twenty-six women (15%) had a previous arterial event (10 coronary, 11 cerebrovascular, and five both); 70 (40%) had carotid plaque. In logistic regression models, independent determinants of plaque were older age, higher systolic blood pressure, higher levels of low-density lipoprotein (LDL) cholesterol, prolonged treatment with prednisone, and a previous coronary event. Moreover, older age, elevated systolic blood pressure, and a previous coronary event were independently associated with increased severity of plaque ($P < 0.01$). Roman et al [16,17] determined the prevalence and correlates of carotid plaque in 197 patients who had lupus compared with 197 age- and sex-matched controls. Eight patients had pre-existing clinical CAD and 17 patients had clinical cerebrovascular disease. Carotid plaque was more prevalent in SLE patients than controls (37.1% versus 15.2%, $P < 0.001$, relative risk 2.4, 95% CI 1.7 to 3.6). When data were analyzed according to decade of life, the relative risk of carotid plaque was 5.6 times as high among patients less than 40 years of age as among controls in this age group, but small numbers in each age group precluded the difference from being statistically significant. Patients who had plaque were more likely to have pre-existing CAD (angina or MI), but not clinical cerebrovascular disease, than patients who did not have plaque.

In the Toronto lupus cohort of 563 patients followed prospectively from 1970 to 1987, 10 patients had symptomatic peripheral vascular disease (PVD) [18]. When these patients were matched for age, sex, and baseline demographics with lupus patients who did not have a history of symptomatic PVD, the only risk factors for developing PVD were longer duration of SLE and longer duration of use of steroids. Anticardiolipin antibodies, smoking, hyperlipidemia, and hypertension were not significantly different in patients who had PVD compared with those who did not have PVD. Eight of the 10 patients who had PVD had coexistent CAD or a history of transient ischemic attacks (TIA). The overall prevalence of clinical AS (coronary, cerebral, and peripheral) in the Toronto lupus cohort is 13% [13].

Perfusion reserve was compared in the lower limbs of 25 female patients who had SLE and were asymptomatic for PVD, with 25 healthy age-matched patients, using thallium-201 ($^{201}$Tl) lower limb muscle perfusion scanning [19,20]. Patients who had SLE had significantly lower limb perfusion reserves than matched controls (75.3 ± 8.9% versus 99.6 ± 9.0%; $P < 0.05$). Using a similar technique of radionuclide scanning (xenon-133 muscle washout), Lin et al [21] showed significantly reduced muscle perfusion in patients who had SLE and were asymptomatic for PVD compared with controls. When the 34 patients were divided into two groups based on normal versus abnormal myocardial perfusion scanning, there was significantly reduced muscle perfusion in the 18 SLE patients who had abnormal myocardial perfusion compared with 16 patients who had normal myocardial perfusion. The investigators concluded that muscle perfusion in the lower extremities of SLE patients who do not have symptoms or signs of PVD is significantly decreased and related to abnormal myocardial perfusion.

Collectively these studies indicate that women with SLE have two to six times the relative risk of cerebral vascular disease and an increased relative risk of peripheral vascular disease. In addition, some patients who have carotid or femoral plaque or reduced limb perfusion reserve are asymptomatic with no history of stroke or limb ischemia. Importantly, in patients who have SLE, AS in carotid and peripheral arteries is frequently associated with coexistent CAD.

## Subclinical atherosclerosis in systemic lupus erythematosus: prevalence and methods of detection

Many patients who have SLE have subclinical AS with no history of MI or stroke. Detection of subclinical AS is not only important in determining the true prevalence of AS in SLE but also provides a window of opportunity for prevention of subsequent ischemic events. In addition, studying the natural history of subclinical disease may provide valuable insight in to means of attenuating risk and enhancing protective factors for adverse future outcomes.

### Autopsy studies

Bulkley and Roberts [22] described the cardiac findings in a case series of 36 autopsies performed in corticosteroid-treated patients who had SLE. Eight patients were found to have atherosclerotic narrowing of one or more coronary arteries, with only four of these (50%) having a history of MI. Similar observations were made in 40 autopsies performed among 124 deaths, which occurred over 23 years of follow-up in the Toronto lupus cohort [1]. Moderate to severe AS of the major coronary vessels was found in 21 (54%) regardless of the cause of death.

### Noninvasive imaging techniques

With recent technological advances a number of noninvasive imaging techniques have been used to detect subclinical disease of the coronary arteries. Whereas conventional coronary angiography allows direct examination of coronary vessel anatomy for the presence of occlusive plaque, noninvasive imaging techniques detect the hemodynamic defects caused by vascular disease or measure surrogate markers of coronary AS such as calcification of coronary vessel wall or presence of carotid plaque.

### Carotid ultrasound

Carotid arterial plaque, defined as a focal protrusion of more than 50% of surrounding vessel wall, is not only indicative of cerebrovascular disease but is also a surrogate marker of prevalent cardiovascular disease [23]. In a cross-sectional study of 214 women without clinical cardiovascular disease enrolled in the Pittsburgh Lupus Registry, B-mode ultrasound was used to detect carotid plaque [24]. Sixty-eight (32%) of the women had at least one focal plaque defined as maximum intima–media thickness (M-IMT) > 1.3 mm. In another study of 78 women with SLE without clinical atherosclerotic disease the prevalence of plaque was 17%, whereas a thickened intima (IMT > 0.9 mm) was seen in 28% [25].

Ultrasonic biopsy (U-B) is a refinement of B-mode ultrasound, allowing noninvasive assessment of alterations in the morphology of the posterior wall and atherosclerotic plaques in the common carotid (CCA) and common femoral (CFA) arteries. This technique allows detection of early changes that occur in the vessel wall before the development of plaque, such as lumen–intimal interface disruption. High-grade changes (class D; plaque without hemodynamic disturbance and class E; stenotic plaque) have been shown to correlate with ischemic changes on cardiac stress testing in asymptomatic individuals [26]. Wolak et al [27] used this technique to identify AS in the CCA and CFA of patients who had SLE (n = 51) and matched controls (n = 51). Twenty-eight percent of SLE patients had at least a single class D-F lesion in one of the four vessels tested, compared with 10% in the control group ($P$ = 0.02). Only six of 14 patients who had SLE and high-grade lesions had a history of stroke.

*Myocardial perfusion scintigraphy*

Hosenpud et al [28] first suggested in 1984 that myocardial perfusion defects might be common in patients who have SLE. They selected 26 patients who had SLE irrespective of cardiac history to undergo exercise $^{201}$Th–myocardial scintigraphy. Ten (38.5%) patients had reversible or fixed defects. Later Bruce et al [29] determined the prevalence of myocardial perfusion abnormalities among 133 women who had SLE. A dual-isotope (DIMPI) single photon emission CT (SPECT) technique with $^{201}$Th as well as technetium-99m ($^{99m}$Tc)–sestamibi was used to minimize breast artifact and enhance specificity [30]. After dipyridamole-induced stress, a perfusion defect was detected in 41 (35%) patients who had no history of CAD. Eleven of 13 (85%) patients who had a history of angina or MI had perfusion defects. Overall 52 (40%) patients had an abnormality of myocardial perfusion. Sella et al [31] performed SPECT $^{99m}$Tc-sestamibi myocardial scanning at rest and after dipyridamole-induced stress in 82 patients who had SLE who had no history of CAD. Twenty-three (28%) patients had perfusion defects. Based on these studies the prevalence of perfusion defects in patients who had SLE without clinical CAD is 28% to 35%.

*Electron-beam computed tomography*

Electron-beam computed tomography (EBCT) used to measure coronary artery calcification is a sensitive and specific marker for the presence of obstructive CAD [32]. In asymptomatic adults, EBCT of the coronary arteries has been shown to predict CAD–related death and nonfatal MI and the need for revascularization procedures at 3 to 4 years [33]. In addition, in patients undergoing angiography the extent of coronary artery calcification (CAC) on EBCT measured by the CAC score has been shown to be highly predictive of future cardiac events, adding prognostic information [34].

Asanuma et al [35] used EBCT to screen for the presence of coronary artery calcification in 65 patients who had SLE and 69 control subjects with similar baseline demographics. Patients and controls with a history of cardiovascular disease were excluded. CAC was more frequent in patients who had lupus (20 [30.8%]) than in controls (6 [8.7%]), $P = 0.002$. The mean CAC score was also significantly higher in patients compared with controls.

In summary, despite differences in the technique used, recent cross-sectional and case-control studies have consistently demonstrated the prevalence of subclinical CAD in SLE to be 30% to 40%. In a therapeutic context, diagnostic modalities used to detect asymptomatic CAD may have a place in the algorithm used to screen patients for risk of future ischemic events.

## Factors associated with coronary artery disease in systemic lupus erythematosus: interplay between disease, therapy, and conventional cardiovascular risk factors

Defining risk factors associated with premature AS in SLE is fundamental to understanding the pathogenesis of this complication and prevention of ischemic events and cardiovascular mortality in this disease. The large population-based Framingham Study has identified major risk factors for the development of CAD in the general population [36,37]. These risk factors include hypertension, hypercholesterolemia (> 5.2 mmol/L), low HDL cholesterol (< 0.9 mmol/L), current smoking, diabetes mellitus, and family history of premature CAD. The classic Framingham risk formula based on these risk factors may be used to predict an individual's absolute risk of cardiovascular events at 10 years. To date several studies have confirmed that traditional Framingham risk factors do not fully account for accelerated AS in SLE. In a retrospective cohort analysis, Rahman et al [38] compared the prevalence of traditional cardiovascular risk factors (hypertension, hypercholesterolemia, diabetes, smoking, family history) in 35 patients who had SLE (27 women, eight men) that developed CAD during the course of their illness, with 397 age- and sex-matched non-SLE controls (83 women, 314 men) who had premature CAD (< 60 years of age at time of first event and angiographically documented CAD). The sexes were analyzed separately. Women who had SLE had significantly fewer CAD risk factors per cardiac event than female controls (2.0 ± 0.77 versus 2.9 ± 1.19, $P = 0.0008$). Similarly men who had SLE had significantly fewer CAD risk factors than the comparison group (1.87 ± 0.83 versus 2.73 ± 0.99, $P = 0.016$). Esdaile and colleagues [39] sought to determine to what extent the increase in risk of cardiovascular disease in SLE could not be explained by common risk factors.

The participants at two SLE registries were assessed retrospectively for the presence of cerebral and cardiac vascular outcomes. For each patient the probability of the given outcome was estimated based on the individual's risk profile and the Framingham multiple logistic regression model. After controlling for traditional risk factors at baseline, the increase in relative risk for all CAD events was 7.5 (95% CI 5.1 to 10.4) and the relative risk for stroke was 7.9 (95% CI 4.0 to 13.6). The investigators concluded that there is a substantial statistically significant increase in CAD and stroke in patients who had SLE that cannot be fully explained by traditional Framingham risk factors alone.

*What are the risk factors associated with coronary artery disease in systemic lupus erythematosus?*

Due to the low prevalence of SLE (1:2,000), most AS risk factor studies in this disease are limited by small numbers of affected patients [40]. Differences in the racial and ethnic composition of large SLE cohorts may confound the findings of risk factor studies (57% blacks in the Baltimore cohort versus 7% blacks in the Toronto cohort) [1,9]. Despite these limitations, it has been shown that conventional risk factors, in particular hyperlipidemia, are in fact independently associated with accelerated AS in SLE.

Three large studies of cohorts in Baltimore, Pittsburgh, and Toronto have examined the risk factors for CAD in patients who had SLE [7–9,13]. In the prospective study of 229 patients from the Baltimore cohort, one or more CAD event(s) occurred in 19 (8.3%) patients over 4 years of follow-up [9]. In multivariate analysis, compared with subjects who did not have CAD, patients who did were more likely to be older at diagnosis of SLE (37.1 versus 28.9 years, $P = 0.004$), have a longer mean duration of SLE (12.3 versus 7.2 years, $P < 0.0001$), have a longer mean duration of prednisone use (14.3 versus 7.2 years, $P < 0.0001$), have a higher mean cholesterol (271.2 versus 214.9 mg/dL, $P < 0.0001$), and have a history of hypertension (OR 3.5, 95% CI 1.3 to 9.6) or antihypertensive use (OR 5.5, 95% CI 1.8 to 17.2). In this study there were no significant associations with other known CAD risk factors such as smoking, diabetes, family history of CAD, race, or sex.

In the Pittsburgh cohort of 498 women, 33 cardiovascular events were identified that followed the diagnosis of SLE [8]. In multivariate analysis older age at lupus diagnosis (39.0 versus 34.0 years, $P = 0.02$), longer duration of lupus (13.0 versus 10.0 years, $P = 0.01$), longer duration of corticosteroid use (11.0 versus 7.0 years, $P = 0.002$), hypercholesterolemia (18.0% versus 4.0%, $P = 0.003$), and postmenopausal status (48.0% versus 29.0%, $P = 0.03$) were more common in women who had SLE with a cardiovascular event than in those who did not. In a Cox proportional hazards model controlling for age, lupus disease duration (rate ratio [RR] = 0.83, 95% CI 0.74 to 0.94), hyper-cholesterolemia (RR = 3.35, 95% CI 1.34 to 8.36), and older age at lupus diagnosis (RR = 1.21, 95% CI 1.09 to 1.35) were the three variables significantly associated with cardiovascular events.

When the Toronto cohort was reviewed in 2004, among 1087 patients, 144 atherosclerotic vascular events (AVE)—cardiac, cerebral, or peripheral—were identified that occurred after the first clinic visit [13]. When the patients who had AVE were matched for sex, date of first clinic visit, age at first clinic visit, and duration of follow-up, with 144 patients who had SLE and no AVE, hypertension (66.6% versus 46.5%, $P = 0.001$), smoking (53.5% versus 38.9%, $P = 0.01$), and elevated cholesterol (85.4% versus 76.3%, $P = 0.01$) were significant risk factors for AVE. In multivariate analysis vasculitis (RR = 2.28, 95% CI: 1.2 to 3.94, $P = 0.003$), neuropsychiatric disease (RR = 2.16, 95% CI: 1.29 to 3.64, $P = 0.004$) and presence of more than one traditional cardiovascular risk factor (RR = 1.75, 95% CI: 1.32 to 2.32, $P = 0.0001$) were significantly associated with AVE.

Other studies examining risk factors for CAD in SLE have defined the prevalence of AS in the study population on the basis of carotid ultrasound and myocardial perfusion scintigraphy in absence of or in addition to documented ischemic events. Studies by Bruce et al [29], Manzi et al [15], and Sella et al [31] have been referred to earlier. In the study by Bruce et al [41], factors associated with an abnormal myocardial perfusion scan (DIMPI) included current hypertension (BP > 140/90 mmHg), elevated cholesterol ever, and elevated total cholesterol:high-density lipoprotein (HDL) cholesterol ratio. In the study by Sella et al [31], 30 of the 90 female SLE patients who had no history of CAD had myocardial perfusion defects on scanning. Of these, 21 agreed to undergo coronary angiography, where atherosclerotic lesions were identified in 8 of the 21 patients. Hypertension and postmenopausal status were significantly associated with abnormal angiographic findings. In the study by Manzi et al [15], carotid plaque and IMT, surrogate measures of coronary AS, were determined by B-mode ultrasound in 179 women who had SLE of whom 26 had previous arterial events. Independent determinants of plaque were older age, higher systolic blood pressure, higher LDL cholesterol at the time of study, prolonged treatment with prednisone, and a previous coronary event. Older age, elevated pulse pressure, a previous coronary event, and higher SLICC (Systemic Lupus International Collaborative Clinics) damage score were independently related to increased IMT. In a similar study of 78 patients who had SLE without clinical AS disease, Doria et al [25] found a thickened carotid artery intima in 22 (28%) patients and plaque in 13 (17%) on duplex sonography. In multivariate analysis, age and cumulative prednisone dose were associated with carotid abnormalities, whereas age and hypertension during the study period (as defined by systolic BP > 140 or diastolic BP > 90 mmHg or use of antihypertensive drugs) correlated with higher mean and maximum IMT. Selzer et al [24] undertook a cross-sectional study of 214 women who did not have clinical cardiovascular disease enrolled in the Pittsburgh Lupus Registry. B-mode ultrasound was used to measure carotid plaque and IMT and Doppler probes were used to collect pulse-wave velocity waveforms from the carotid and femoral arteries as a measure of aortic stiffness. Independent determinants of plaque included older age, higher systolic blood pressure, lower HDL, and antidepressant use. Independent determinants of the highest quartile of IMT were older age, higher pulse pressure, lower albumin, elevated C-reactive protein (CRP), high cholesterol, and high glucose. Aortic stiffness was associated with older age, higher systolic BP, higher C3 level, lower white blood cell count, higher insulin levels, and renal disease.

Overall it is worth noting that large cohort studies that have defined AS based on clinical criteria (such as previous MI) have consistently found that older age at diagnosis of SLE and high cholesterol are risk factors for ischemic events, whereas smaller studies looking at subclinical disease have found currently elevated blood pressure to be a risk factor for AS in SLE. This may reflect the possibility that modalities used to detect subclinical disease may be demonstrating earlier lesions associated with altered vessel physiology. These early lesions may be dynamic and acutely influenced by increased shear forces seen with elevated arterial blood pressure at the time of study. However, if early lesions such as increased carotid IMT are indeed precursors to occlusive plaques, sustained hypertension is potentially a modifiable risk factor for the development of atherosclerotic lesions in SLE.

Hypercholesterolemia has been shown in three large cohort studies to be a significant risk factor for CAD in SLE [8,9,13]. However, the definition of hypercholesterolemia has not been consistent across all studies. Bruce et al [42] examined the natural history of hypercholesterolemia, defined as cholesterol $> 5.2$ mmol/L, in the first 3 years of disease in an inception cohort of patients who had SLE and determined the influence of hypercholesterolemia on the subsequent development of CAD-related events. A total of 133 patients was identified as having been seen in the clinic within 1 year of diagnosis and reviewed at least once a year after diagnosis. Patients were divided in to three groups: normal cholesterol (fasting serum cholesterol $< 5.2$ mmol/L throughout the period of study), sustained hypercholesterolemia (at least one elevated reading in each of the first 3 years of follow-up), and variable hypercholesterolemia (total cholesterol $> 5.2$ mmol/L in no more than 2 of the first 3 years of follow-up). There was a significantly higher proportion of CAD-related events in the group with sustained hypercholesterolemia than in the normal or variable groups (27.8% versus 3% versus 6.4%, $P = 0.003$). In multiple logistic regression analysis the best predictors of sustained hypercholesterolemia were cumulative dose of steroid (OR 1.11/g, 95% CI 1.05–1.2, $P < 0.001$), lack of antimalarial therapy (antimalarial OR 0.08, 95% CI 0.02–0.25, $P < 0.001$), and age of onset of SLE $> 35$ years (OR 6.46, 95% CI 1.70–28.73, $P = 0.006$).

In addition to hypercholesterolemia, other lipid abnormalities have also been described in SLE, including elevated very-low-density lipoprotein (VLDL) and triglycerides and low HDL (the *lupus pattern*) [43]. Although more pronounced in patients who have active disease, these abnormalities have been observed even among patients who had quiescent disease [43]. Female SLE patients also have raised levels of small, dense LDL subfractions compared with healthy controls. In population-based studies these lipid abnormalities have been shown to be associated with increased risk of CAD [44].

*Disease-related factors and their association with coronary artery disease in systemic lupus erythematosus*

The study by Roman et al [17] demonstrated a role for disease-related factors in atherogenesis in SLE. In this study, independent predictors of carotid plaque in patients who had SLE were a longer duration of disease, a higher SLICC/AC damage index score, a lower incidence of cyclophosphamide use, and the absence of anti-Smith antibodies. Although the disease-activity-index score was not significantly different in those with and without plaque, the results suggested that less exposure to therapy might itself be a risk factor, indicating that uncontrolled disease activity may be the hidden culprit. Furthermore, the damage index is a marker of the cumulative severity of disease. The study by Manzi et al [15] also showed an independent association between higher SLICC damage scores and increased carotid IMT.

Most lupus cardiovascular risk factor studies to date have not examined the role of disease activity measured using validated indices such as the SLEDAI (Systemic Lupus Erythematosus Disease Activity Index). Two prospective cohort studies have shown that longer mean duration of prednisone use, a possible surrogate marker for disease activity over time, is a risk factor for CAD events in SLE [8,9]. Furthermore, hypercholesterolemia, a known risk factor for CAD in SLE is seen more commonly, along with a more atherogenic lipid profile in patients who have active untreated disease [43]. However, disease activity in SLE varies over time and is influenced by a number of factors including therapy. In addition, validated indices of disease activity may not reflect persistent active disease in some descriptors. To summarize disease activity over the course of illness, the adjusted mean SLEDAI (AMS) has been derived [45]. The AMS is a measure of the area under the curve of SLEDAI-2K (a modification of SLEDAI reflecting persistent active disease in all descriptors) over time [46]. The AMS has been shown to be strongly associated with mortality and CAD in SLE. For each unit increase in AMS the hazard ratio (HR) for CAD has been shown to increase by 10% (HR 1.10, 95% CI: 1.02–1.18, $P = 0.012$) [47].

## Novel risk factors for coronary artery disease in systemic lupus erythematosus

There has been much interest in identification of novel risk factors for CAD. Although many such risk factors have been proposed, most have yet to be linked conclusively to CAD in patients who have SLE, or indeed, in the general population.

*Homocysteine*

The association between homocysteine and premature AS was first noted in familial hyperhomocysteinemia. Homocysteine has been shown to have toxic effects on the endothelium and to promote vascular smooth muscle cell growth [48]. The Physicians' Health Study and the Framingham Heart Study have shown that high homocysteine levels are associated with increased relative risk of CAD and stroke [49,50].

Petri et al [51] examined the association between plasma homocysteine concentration and atherothrombotic events in 337 patients (311 women of whom 54% were African American) with SLE in the Hopkins lupus cohort comprising 1619 person-years of follow-up. The end-points of stroke and arterial or venous thrombotic events were prospectively defined. In this study homocysteine levels were significantly higher in men than women and in patients with serum creatinine greater than 88.4 mmol/L, those taking prednisone, and in those with evidence of lupus anticoagulant activity. After adjustment for these and established cardiovascular risk factors such as hypercholesterolemia and hypertension, total plasma homocysteine concentration greater than 14.1 mmol/L was an independent risk factor for thromboembolic stroke (OR 2.44 [1.04–5.75], $P = 0.04$) and arterial thromboses overall, including MI and limb ischemia (OR 3.49 [0.97–12.54], $P = 0.05$), but not venous thromboses.

In the Toronto Risk Factor Study, elevated homocysteine level (> 15 μmol/L) was seen more commonly in patients who had SLE than in matched controls (11.6% versus 0.8%, $P<0.01$) [44]. Although supplementation with folic acid has been shown to reduce elevated levels of homocysteine, to date there is insufficient evidence on the efficacy of this intervention in reducing the incidence of CAD or cerebrovascular events among patients who had SLE or in the general population [52]. Furthermore, although it is generally agreed that the upper limit of normal serum homocysteine is 15 μmol/L, there are no consensus guidelines as to the level of homocysteine that requires treatment in patients who have SLE. Nevertheless, homocysteine is a potentially modifiable risk factor for stroke and arterial thrombosis in SLE.

*C-reactive protein*

CRP level, measured using an assay with high sensitivity in the lower range, has been shown to predict the risk of MI and stroke among healthy young men. In the Physicians' Health Study of 543 healthy men followed for an average of 8 years, baseline plasma concentration of CRP was higher among men who went on to have MI (1.51 versus 1.13 mg/L; $P<0.001$) or ischemic stroke (1.38 versus 1.13 mg/L; $P = 0.02$) [53]. Men in the quartile with the highest CRP values had three times the risk of MI and two times the risk of ischemic stroke of men in the lowest quartile. Similarly in the Women's Health Study, baseline CRP concentration was shown to be an independent risk factor for cardiovascular disease, even among low-risk subgroups of women with no other conventional cardiovascular risk factors [54].

In contrast, most studies to date have not shown CRP to be an independent risk factor for prevalent vascular disease in SLE as determined by carotid, aortic, or femoral ultrasound [15,55]. Similarly in a prospective cohort of 78 patients who had SLE followed for 5 years, CRP was not found to be an independent predictor for development of subclinical AS detected by ultrasound measurement of carotid IMT [25]. However, in a recent cross-sectional study of 214 women enrolled in the Pittsburgh lupus registry who did not have clinical cardiovascular disease, women with carotid plaque had significantly higher median CRP levels than women without plaque [24]. In contrast in the same study there was no significant association between high CRP level and aortic vascular stiffness measured using pulse-wave velocity. Overall these partially conflicting results may reflect the fact that CRP may be elevated in patients who have SLE due to disease itself or infective complications. Single random measurements of CRP may therefore be less useful in predicting cardiovascular risk in patients who have SLE. Prospective studies are needed to determine the role of CRP measurement in predicting the risk of new coronary events.

*Other novel risk factors*

Numerous other possible risk factors for CAD are currently under investigation. These include intercellular adhesion molecule-1 (ICAM-1), vascular adhesion molecule-1 (VCAM-1), and E- and P-selectin. These molecules mediate adhesion and transmigration of leukocytes across the vascular endothelium, a step critical to the initiation and progression of the inflammatory process in atherogenesis [56]. Elevated plasma concentration of soluble ICAM-1 has been shown to be significantly associated with increased risk of future MI in apparently healthy men and a predictor of future cardiovascular events in healthy postmenopausal women [57,58]. Soluble VCAM-1 has also been shown to be associated with the presence and extent of atherosclerotic peripheral arterial vascular disease (pAVD) determined angiographically in patients who have symptoms of pAVD [59]. However, no studies to date have examined the association between soluble adhesion molecules and cardiovascular disease in SLE. Soluble CD40L has also been identified as a possible atherogenic mediator. In a prospective, nested case-control study of healthy middle-aged women participating in the Women's Health Study, after adjustment for usual cardiovascular risk factors, women with CD40L concentrations above the 95th percentile of the control distribution (> 3.71 ng/mL) had a significantly increased relative risk of developing future cardiovascular events (RR 2.8; 95% CI 0.9 to 8.0, $P = 0.05$) [60]. Although to date no studies have examined the link between elevated soluble CD40L and premature AS in SLE, it is possible that soluble CD40L implicated in the pathogenesis of SLE also plays a role in the pathogenesis of the atherosclerotic complications frequently seen in this disease.

A pathogenic role for antiendothelial cell antibodies (AECAs) has been proposed by studies showing that monoclonal or purified antiendothelial cell IgG antibodies, derived from patients who have SLE and vasculitis bind and activate human endothelium in vitro, inducing the expression of adhesion molecules and release of endothelium-derived mediators [61–63]. Whereas AECA may play a pathogenic role in SLE, more likely they are an epiphenomenona reflecting widespread unrecognized vessel injury despite the absence of clinically apparent vasculitis in patients with active disease. Whether plasma levels of AECA measured in the active phase of disease are predictive of future cardiovascular risk is yet to be determined.

Atherogenic and atheroprotective lipoproteins have also been a focal point of interest in AS complicating SLE. Small studies comparing SLE patients with normal controls have shown elevated levels of apolipoprotein-B (apoB) in corticosteroid-treated patients [64]. Recent prospective epidemiologic studies have demonstrated apoB to be superior to other lipid indices in estimating the risk of vascular disease in the general population [65]. The magnitude of risk conferred by atherogenic lipoproteins in SLE is unknown and at present not routinely measured in risk stratification.

## Role of antiphospholipid antibodies in atherogenesis in systemic lupus erythematosus

Antiphospholipid antibodies (aPLs) are the hallmark of the antiphospholipid syndrome, which is characterized by arterial and venous thrombosis. Up to 47% of patients who have SLE have elevated levels of aPL [66]. High levels of aPLs have been linked to MI in young patients in several prospective studies [67–69] and shown to be an independent risk factor for MI and cardiac death in middle-aged men [70,71]. Studies have also shown a link between anti-B2GPI antibodies and ischemic heart disease and stroke [72–74]. Many of the ischemic events observed in patients who have SLE and aPLs are presumably mediated by the associated coagulopathy, and there is evidence that such patients may present with MI despite angiographically normal coronary arteries [75–77]. However, in addition to their prothrombotic properties, aPLs may also be proatherogenic by promoting the uptake of oxidized LDL into macrophages [78]. This is discussed in depth elsewhere in this issue. At present further epidemiologic data are required to determine whether the proatherogenic properties of aPLs render them independent risk factors for AS in patients who have SLE.

## New tools for cardiovascular risk profiling and their use in systemic lupus erythematosus

With advances in the understanding of vessel physiology and applications of ultrasound technology, there has been a trend away from invasive angiographic assessment of flow-limiting coronary lesions toward measuring earlier changes in structural and functional aspects of vessels potentially amenable to reversal with intervention.

*External vascular ultrasound*

The endothelium is thought to play a central role in the pathogenesis of AS [79]. Several techniques of assessing endothelial function, all measuring endothelial cell response to pharmacologic or physiologic stimulation, have been validated in the nonlupus population. Intracoronary Doppler ultrasound, measuring coronary blood flow in response to stimuli such as acetylcholine, is considered to be the best assessment of endothelial function [80]. However, this technique is limited by its invasiveness and seldom used. Brachial artery high-resolution external ultrasound is a widely used, noninvasive measure of endothelial function [81,82]. This technique measures endothelium-dependent nitric oxide (NO)–mediated vasodilation in response to ischemia induced by inflating a blood pressure cuff in the upper arm or the forearm. The dilation seen in response to postischemic hyperemia is presented as percentage vessel dilation compared with baseline diameter. Endothelium-dependent brachial artery flow-mediated vasodilation (FMD) is blunted in patients who had endothelial dysfunction of the coronary arteries and in patients who have documented CAD [83]. Although this technique is noninvasive and quick, its drawbacks include poor reproducibility and the need for ultrasonographic expertise [84].

Lima et al [85] compared endothelial function in 69 premenopausal women who had SLE with 35 age- and sex-matched controls using external vascular ultrasound and a forearm cuff. FMD was significantly impaired in patients who had SLE compared with controls (5.0 ± 5.0% versus 12.0 ± 6.0%, $P < 0.001$), even in patients who did not have cardiovascular risk factors. The FMD in patients who had SLE was not related to disease duration, cumulative prednisone dose, antimalarial use, aPLs, hypertension, Raynaud's phenomenon, SLE disease activity, or vasculitis. In another study, El-Magadmi et al [86] examined endothelial function in 62 women who had SLE versus 38 healthy women. FMD was significantly impaired in patients who had lupus versus controls (median 3.6% versus 6.9%, $P < 0.01$). In multiple regression analysis, where all classic cardiovascular risk factors were retained and all subjects included, systolic blood pressure ($P = 0.019$) and SLE itself ($P = 0.017$) were significantly associated with impaired FMD.

The authors have examined endothelial function in 92 women who had SLE but not clinical CAD [87]. In this study, impaired FMD was defined based on mean minus one standard deviation FMD measured in 15 healthy premenopausal women studied under identical experimental conditions using an upper arm cuff. A total of 21 (22.8%) women who had SLE had impaired FMD. Older age (50.7 ± 10.9 versus 43.2 ± 12.1 years, $P = 0.02$) and menopausal status (71.4% versus 35.2%, $P = 0.003$) at the time of study as well as hypertension (BP > 140/90 mmHg on three or more occasions or use of antihypertensives) in the 3 years before the study (57.1% versus 31.0%, $P = 0.04$) were significantly associated with impaired FMD. Factors at the time of study, such as statin or hormone replacement therapy, did not significantly influence FMD. Overall, despite some differences in technique (upper arm versus forearm cuff) and study design, most studies to date have shown a high prevalence of endothelial dys-function in patients who have SLE.

If endothelial dysfunction is indeed a precursor to atheromatous CAD in SLE, how does its presence correlate with myocardial perfusion? In the Toronto endothelial dysfunction study [88], myocardial perfusion scanning as well as FMD was performed in 92 women with SLE, without clinical CAD. Overall there was poor agreement between the two tests (kappa 0.21, 95% CI: 0.1–0.41). There are several possible explanations for this discordance. An abnormal FMD with normal MPS is in keeping with the hypothesis that endothelial dysfunction is a precursor to myocardial ischemia, whereas normal FMD with abnormal MPS may reflect external influences such as disease factors or therapy at the time of study, which may lead to pseudonormalization of FMD. Furthermore these two modalities may be assessing different aspects of vascular function, for example macro- versus microvascular function that may not be governed by the same regulatory mechanisms. The preliminary findings of this study indicate that brachial FMD and myocardial perfusion scintigraphy may be independent investigations in assessing the cardiovascular health of patients who have SLE and that they should not be used interchangeably.

Increased carotid IMT, also assessed by external vascular ultrasound is associated with an increased risk of MI and stroke in men and women without a history of cardiovascular disease [89,90]. In the study by El-Magadmi et al [86], IMT showed a negative correlation with percent FMD ($r = -0.37$, $P < 0.01$). However, only the patients who had SLE and not the controls had IMT measurement performed. In the case-control study by Roman et al [17], IMT in women with lupus was less than the control group ($0.61 \pm 1.16$ mm versus $0.67 \pm 0.14$ mm, $P < 0.001$), even though these patients had more plaque than controls (37.1% versus 15.2%, $P < 0.001$). This result suggests that in patients who have SLE, carotid IMT may not be as reliable a marker of AS as in the general population.

Brachial FMD, carotid IMT, and other noninvasive techniques for mea-suring endothelial function or early vascular changes, although shown to correlate with subclinical AS and future AS events in the general population, have not yet been shown to predict future events in patients who have SLE.

## Continuum of vascular disease in systemic lupus erythematosus and the concept of nonocclusive coronary artery disease

In the study by Sella et al [31], only 8 of 21 patients with myocardial per-fusion defects and no history of CAD had coronary plaques identified on angiography. The investigators have also noted similar findings where of 21 patients with perfusion defects on MPS (10 of whom were symptomatic for CAD), 14 (67.0%) had no occlusive lesions on angiography [91]. In a descriptive study of 35 patients who had SLE and underwent coronary angiography in the course of routine clinical care in a 25-year interval at the Toronto lupus clinic,

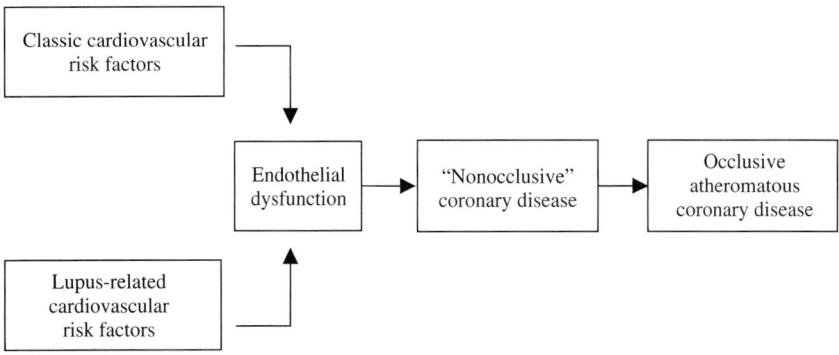

Fig. 1. The continuum of vascular disease in SLE.

30 patients were symptomatic for angina, MI, or congestive heart failure. A total of 13 (43%) of the 30 symptomatic patients had no significant lesions of proximal or distal coronary arteries on conventional angiography (ongoing study: Coronary Angiographic Findings in SLE, M. Nikpour, MBBS, FRACP, D.D. Gladman, MD, D. Ibanez, MSc, MB, et al, 2005). These results suggest mechanisms of ischemia other than occlusive plaques. Endothelial dysfunction and coronary vasospasm have been proposed as possible alternate mechanisms. Conventional angiography, however, does not allow imaging of the coronary microvasculature where the pathophysiology may lie. The prognosis in these cases of nonocclusive CAD is unknown. It is possible, however, that the natural history of such cases may not be benign as exemplified by the 13 patients in our study who had documented coronary syndromes. It may also be postulated that if endothelial dysfunction is a precursor to atherosclerotic CAD, then nonocclusive CAD forms an intermediary step in the evolution to full-blown occlusive CAD (Fig. 1).

## An approach to screening patients who had systemic lupus erythematosus for risk of future ischemic events

As discussed, several conventional cardiovascular risk factors have been shown to be associated with the development of clinical CAD in prospective cohort studies. All patients who have SLE should, therefore, be regularly screened for the presence of cardiovascular risk factors. The first tier of screening must include obtaining history in relation to smoking and measurement of body weight, blood pressure, serum cholesterol (including HDL and LDL), triglycerides, and blood glucose, as well as CRP and homocysteine.

Endothelial dysfunction, a postulated precursor to AS in SLE, is thought to be the result of the interplay between disease-specific and nonspecific risk factors. Although the risk factors for CAD in SLE have not been fully defined, assessment of endothelial function, an integrated index of all putative and protective factors, is a potentially useful screening tool, even in patients where no classical cardiovascular risk factors have been identified. We therefore propose that in a second tier of screening, one or more validated noninvasive methods of assessing endothelial function be used to evaluate the vascular health of patients who have SLE. This information has potential therapeutic implications in light of emerging evidence for reversibility of endothelial dysfunction with certain therapeutic agents such as angiotensin-converting enzyme inhibitors (ACEIs) [92,93]. At this stage it is not known whether one technique for evaluating endothelial function should be favored over others in patients who have SLE. Furthermore, the frequency of testing has not been defined. The need for technicians, specifically trained in the performance of these tests, however, may prohibit the use of these modalities in many centers.

The third tier of screening includes modalities such as myocardial perfusion scanning used to detect subclinical CAD. Detection of subclinical CAD would identify candidates for more aggressive secondary prevention of cardiovascular risk factors.

## Modifying risk factors for coronary artery disease in systemic lupus erythematosus

In the Toronto Risk Factor Study, a prospective cohort-control study of 250 women who had SLE without clinical CAD, compared with 250 age-matched controls, hypertension (RR 2.59, 95% CI 1.79–3.75, $P = 0.001$), and diabetes (RR 6.00, 95% CI 1.36–26.53, $P = 0.0066$) were significantly more common among patients who had SLE [44]. SLE patients also had higher levels of VLDL cholesterol and total triglycerides, and higher levels of homocysteine. Premature menopause, sedentary lifestyle, and an at-risk body habitus (BMI $> 27.0$ kg/m$^2$ or waist:hip ratio $> 0.85$) were also more prevalent in patient who had SLE. After 4 to 6 years of follow-up, 26 new atherosclerotic vascular events (AVEs) were noted in the cohort group. When the risk factor profile of patients who had SLE with vascular events was compared with patients who had SLE without vascular events, individual risk factors were not predictive of new AVEs, indicating that all modifiable risk factors should be addressed in all patients who have SLE [94]. In a quality improvement study undertaken through the Toronto Lupus Clinic, 24 patients were identified with MI or angina who had 2 years of follow-up before their event. Risk factors and interventions undertaken were identified by review of case notes. Whereas treating physicians performed well in optimizing the control of SLE, minimizing steroid dose, and managing hypertension, other risk factors such as hypercholesterolemia, hyperglycemia, smoking, and obesity were less favorably managed [95]. In addition, it has been shown that poor patient awareness of the problem of CAD in SLE may contribute to the low use of cardiovascular preventive practices [96].

Intervention studies have shown benefit in cholesterol reduction in high-risk nonlupus populations. The recommended target level of cholesterol in adults is based on the number of cardiovascular risk factors present [97]. As patients who have SLE are at increased risk of CAD due to the disease itself, they should probably be viewed as starting with one risk factor. Other potentially modifiable risk factors should also be addressed including treatment of hypertension with antihypertensives and lowering of elevated homocysteine levels with folic acid. Physicians must also address risk factors that may be modifiable using nonpharmacologic or behavioral strategies such as smoking cessation, weight reduction, and physical exercise. It must be noted however, that more studies are needed to assess the role of specific interventions in reducing the incidence of CAD-related events in patients who have SLE. Also, the interaction between risk factors in patients who have lupus is unknown and it is possible that risk factors may behave synergistically. In the Toronto lupus cohort of 1087 patients, those with AVE occurring after entry to clinic had significantly more hypertension, smoking, and hypercholesterolemia than those with no history of AVE [13]. In multivariate logistic regression analysis, in those where one Framingham risk factor was present, the presence of any additional risk factor increased the relative risk of AVE by 75% (RR 1.75, CI 1.32–2.32, $P$ = 0.0001). This highlights the importance of a detailed and comprehensive cardiovascular risk evaluation in SLE and suggests that the ideal targets for blood pressure and lipids may in fact need to be lower in patients who have SLE than the general population, especially where multiple traditional cardiovascular risk factors coexist.

*Antimalarials and effects on lipid metabolism*

There is evidence that antimalarial drugs reduce serum cholesterol and LDL levels, elevate HDL cholesterol, and when taken concomitantly with steroids can reduce serum cholesterol by up to 10% over 3 to 6 months [98–102]. In the study of an inception cohort of patients who had SLE, only 20% of patients who had sustained hypercholesterolemia over the first 3 years of follow-up were taking antimalarials, suggesting that in clinical practice, antimalarials should be more widely considered in management of SLE [42].

*Reversal of endothelial dysfunction*

Modena et al [93] studied 400 postmenopausal women with hypertension and impaired brachial FMD. After 6 months of optimal therapy for blood pressure control, FMD improved (FMD increased to > 10%) in 250 patients but remained abnormal in 150 patients. After an average of 67 months of therapy, patients in whom FMD remained impaired had significantly more cardiovascular events than patients whose endothelial function improved with treatment. Overall this landmark study suggested that endothelial dysfunction may be reversible, that endothelial function testing may identify individuals that may benefit from intervention, and that serial testing may be useful in determining long-term response to treatment [103]. The validity of this hypothesis warrants further investigation in controlled trials. Although amelioration of endothelial dysfunction in patients who have SLE has yet to be shown to correlate with improved cardiovascular outcome, the use of agents that improve endothelial function is a strategy that is potentially complementary to the treatment of individual risk factors.

Statins have been shown to improve endothelial dysfunction independently of their lipid-lowering effects, even in patients who have normal cholesterol levels [104]. This effect is thought to be due to the increase in NO production induced by these agents. The ACE inhibitor enalapril and the calcium channel blocker amlodipine have both been shown to slow progressive carotid IMT in patients who have type 2 diabetes [105,106]. However, the endothelial effects of antihypertensives may not be equivalent [107,108]. The use of statins, calcium channel blockers, and agents that block the angiotensin pathway in patients who have SLE with endothelial dysfunction merits investigation.

**Summary**

The association between SLE and premature CAD has been well established. Longitudinal cohort studies have estimated the prevalence of CAD in SLE to be at least 10%. However, despite variations in the technique used, the prevalence of subclinical CAD is close to 35%, indicating that the burden of this complication is in fact greater than may at first appear. Clinicians must therefore have a low threshold for cardiac evaluation in patients who have SLE, including premenopausal women who present with cardiac symptoms.

Although the risk factors for the development of CAD in SLE have yet to be fully defined, some classical cardiovascular risk factors, namely hypercholesterolemia and hypertension, have been shown to be significantly associated with CAD events and subclinical CAD. Evidence points to SLE itself as an independent risk factor for premature CAD, possibly through immune-mediated mechanisms that are common to the pathogenesis of both SLE and AS. The development of new measurement tools to summarize disease activity and other possible risk factors over the course of illness may prove useful in deciphering the exact nature of and the interaction between risk factors. Noninvasive ultrasound-based techniques used to detect endothelial dysfunction, a proposed precursor to CAD, are new modalities that may be used to stratify patients who have SLE for risk of CAD. The identification of novel risk factors may also aid risk stratification.

Clearly, many questions remain to be answered. The mechanism and prognosis of subclinical myocardial perfusion defects in absence of occlusive atheromatous coronary artery lesions are yet to be determined. The place of ultrasound-based assessment of endothelial function in screening is yet to be defined. And the threshold for treatment of known cardiovascular risk factors in patients who have SLE is still to be delineated. Although many agree that there is sufficient justification for aggressive treatment of classic CAD risk factors with statins, ACE inhibitors, and other pharmacologic agents, there is currently no available evidence to relate the use of these agents to a reduction in the incidence of CAD events in patients who have SLE. Furthermore, there are currently no evidence-based guidelines for the use of lipid-lowering agents, antiplatelets, and ACEIs in patients without classic cardiovascular risk factors but with evidence of endothelial dysfunction or subclinical CAD. The concept of substituting bio-markers such as FMD or IMT as surrogates for clinical end-points in therapeutic trials also merits further exploration.

Premature AS may be a price we pay for improved short-term survival in SLE. Defining pathogenic mechanisms, risk factors, and screening strategies offers hope of therapeutic intervention aimed at reducing the incidence, morbidity, and mortality associated with this complication.

# References

[1] Abu-Shakra M, Urowitz MB, Gladman DD, Gough J. Mortality studies in systemic lupus erythematosus. Results from a single center. I. Causes of death. J Rheumatol 1995;22(7): 1259–64.

[2] Aravanis C, Toutouzas P, Yatzidis I. Fatal myocardial infarction in lupus erythematosus. Report of a case of a young female patient. Vasc Dis 1964;1(5):258–60.

[3] Urowitz MB, Bookman AA, Koehler BE, et al. The bimodal mortality pattern of systemic lupus erythematosus. Am J Med 1976;60(2):221–5.

[4] Homcy CJ, Liberthson RR, Fallon JT, et al. Ischemic heart disease in systemic lupus erythematosus in the young patient: report of six cases. Am J Cardiol 1982;49(2):478–84.

[5] Fukumoto S, Tsumagari T, Kinjo M, Tanaka K. Coronary atherosclerosis in patients with systemic lupus erythematosus at autopsy. Acta Pathol Jpn 1987;37(1):1–9.

[6] Rubin LA, Urowitz MB, Gladman DD. Mortality in systemic lupus erythematosus: the bimodal pattern revisited. Q J Med 1985;55(216):87–98.

[7] Gladman DD, Urowitz MB. Morbidity in systemic lupus erythematosus. J Rheumatol 1987;14(13 Suppl):223–6.

[8] Manzi S, Meilahn EN, Rairie JE, et al. Age-specific incidence rates of myocardial infarction and angina in women with systemic lupus erythematosus: comparison with the Framingham Study. Am J Epidemiol 1997;145(5):408–15.

[9] Petri M, Perez-Gutthann S, Spence D, Hochberg MC. Risk factors for coronary artery disease in patients with systemic lupus erythematosus. Am J Med 1992;93(5):513–9.

[10] Ward MM. Premature morbidity from cardiovascular and cerebrovascular diseases in women with systemic lupus erythematosus. Arthritis Rheum 1999;42(2):338–46.

[11] Kaarisalo MM, Immonen-Raiha P, Marttila RJ, et al. The risk of stroke following coronary revascularization—a population-based long-term follow-up study. Scand Cardiovasc J 2002; 36(4):231–6.

[12] Adams RJ, Chimowitz MI, Alpert JS, et al. Coronary risk evaluation in patients with transient ischemic attack and ischemic stroke: a scientific statement for healthcare professionals from the Stroke Council and the Council on Clinical Cardiology of the American Heart Association/American Stroke Association. Stroke 2003;34(9):2310–22.

[13] Urowitz MB, Gladman DD, Ibanez D. Atherosclerotic vascular events in a single large lupus cohort: prevalence and risk factors [abstract 1570]. Arthritis Rheum 2004;50(9 Suppl):S594.

[14] Vlachoyiannopoulos PG, Kanellopoulos PG, Ioannidis JP, et al. Atherosclerosis in premenopausal women with antiphospholipid syndrome and systemic lupus erythematosus: a controlled study. Rheumatology (Oxford) 2003;42(5):645–51.

[15] Manzi S, Selzer F, Sutton-Tyrrell K, et al. Prevalence and risk factors of carotid plaque in women with systemic lupus erythematosus. Arthritis Rheum 1999;42(1):51–60.

[16] Roman MJ, Salmon JE, Sobel R, et al. Prevalence and relation to risk factors of carotid atherosclerosis and left ventricular hypertrophy in systemic lupus erythematosus and antiphospholipid antibody syndrome. Am J Cardiol 2001;87(5):663–6.

[17] Roman MJ, Shanker BA, Davis A, et al. Prevalence and correlates of accelerated atherosclerosis in systemic lupus erythematosus. N Engl J Med 2003;349(25):2399–406.

[18] McDonald J, Stewart J, Urowitz MB, Gladman DD. Peripheral vascular disease in patients with systemic lupus erythematosus. Ann Rheum Dis 1992;51(1):56–60.

[19] Cosson E, Paycha F, Tellier P, et al. Lower-limb vascularization in diabetic patients. Assessment by thallium-201 scanning coupled with exercise myocardial scintigraphy. Diabetes Care 2001; 24(5):870–4.

[20] Hsu HB, Sun SS, Chen JJ, et al. Usefulness of thallium-201 muscle scan to investigate perfusion reserve in the lower limbs of patients with systemic lupus erythematosus. Rheumatol Int 2004;24(5):291–3.

[21] Lin CC, Ding HJ, Chen YW, et al. High prevalence of asymptomatically poor muscle perfusion of lower extremities measured in systemic lupus erythematosus patients with abnormal myocardial perfusion. Rheumatol Int 2004;24(4):227–9.

[22] Bulkley BH, Roberts WC. The heart in systemic lupus erythematosus and the changes induced in it by corticosteroid therapy. A study of 36 necropsy patients. Am J Med 1975;58(2):243–64.

[23] Burke GL, Evans GW, Riley WA, et al. Arterial wall thickness is associated with prevalent cardiovascular disease in middle-aged adults. The Atherosclerosis Risk in Communities (ARIC) Study. Stroke 1995;26(3):386–91.

[24] Selzer F, Sutton-Tyrrell K, Fitzgerald SG, et al. Comparison of risk factors for vascular disease in the carotid artery and aorta in women with systemic lupus erythematosus. Arthritis Rheum 2004;50(1):151–9.

[25] Doria A, Shoenfeld Y, Wu R, et al. Risk factors for subclinical atherosclerosis in a prospective cohort of patients with systemic lupus erythematosus. Ann Rheum Dis 2003;62(11):1071–7.

[26] Belcaro G, Barsotti A, Nicolaides AN. Ultrasonic biopsy—a non-invasive screening technique to evaluate the cardiovascular risk and to follow up the progression and the regression of arteriosclerosis. Vasa 1991;20(1):40–50.

[27] Wolak T, Todosoui E, Szendro G, et al. Duplex study of the carotid and femoral arteries of patients with systemic lupus erythematosus: a controlled study. J Rheumatol 2004;31(5): 909–14.

[28] Hosenpud JD, Montanaro A, Hart MV, et al. Myocardial perfusion abnormalities in asymptomatic patients with systemic lupus erythematosus. Am J Med 1984;77(2):286–92.

[29] Bruce IN, Burns RJ, Gladman DD, Urowitz MB. Single photon emission computed tomography dual isotope myocardial perfusion imaging in women with systemic lupus erythematosus. I. Prevalence and distribution of abnormalities. J Rheumatol 2000;27(10):2372–7.

[30] Berman DS, Kiat H, Friedman JD, et al. Separate acquisition rest thallium-201/stress technetium-99m sestamibi dual-isotope myocardial perfusion single-photon emission computed tomography: a clinical validation study. J Am Coll Cardiol 1993;22(5):1455–64.

[31] Sella EM, Sato EI, Barbieri A. Coronary artery angiography in systemic lupus erythematosus patients with abnormal myocardial perfusion scintigraphy. Arthritis Rheum 2003;48(11): 3168–75.

[32] Nallamothu BK, Saint S, Bielak LF, et al. Electron-beam computed tomography in the diagnosis of coronary artery disease: a meta-analysis. Arch Intern Med 2001;161(6):833–8.

[33] Arad Y, Spadaro LA, Goodman K, et al. Prediction of coronary events with electron beam computed tomography. J Am Coll Cardiol 2000;36(4):1253–60.

[34] Keelan PC, Bielak LF, Ashai K, et al. Long-term prognostic value of coronary calcification detected by electron-beam computed tomography in patients undergoing coronary angiography. Circulation 2001;104(4):412–7.

[35] Asanuma Y, Oeser A, Shintani AK, et al. Premature coronary-artery atherosclerosis in systemic lupus erythematosus. N Engl J Med 2003;349(25):2407–15.

[36] Wilson PW, Castelli WP, Kannel WB. Coronary risk prediction in adults (the Framingham Heart Study). Am J Cardiol 1987;59(14):91G–4G.

[37] Wilson PW, D'Agostino RB, Levy D, et al. Prediction of coronary heart disease using risk factor categories. Circulation 1998;97(18):1837–47.

[38] Rahman P, Urowitz MB, Gladman DD, et al. Contribution of traditional risk factors to coronary artery disease in patients with systemic lupus erythematosus. J Rheumatol 1999;26(11): 2363–8.

[39] Esdaile JM, Abrahamowicz M, Grodzicky T, et al. Traditional Framingham risk factors fail to fully account for accelerated atherosclerosis in systemic lupus erythematosus. Arthritis Rheum 2001;44(10):2331–7.

[40] Gladman DD. Epidemiology of systemic lupus erythematosus. In: Lahita RG, editor. Systemic lupus erythematosus. 4th edition. San Diego (CA): Elsevier Academic Press; 2004. p. 697–709.

[41] Bruce IN, Gladman DD, Ibanez D, Urowitz MB. Single photon emission computed tomography dual isotope myocardial perfusion imaging in women with systemic lupus erythematosus. II. Predictive factors for perfusion abnormalities. J Rheumatol 2003;30(2):288–91.

[42] Bruce IN, Urowitz MB, Gladman DD, Hallett DC. Natural history of hypercholesterolemia in systemic lupus erythematosus. J Rheumatol 1999;26(10):2137–43.

[43] Borba EF, Bonfa E. Dyslipoproteinemias in systemic lupus erythematosus: influence of disease, activity, and anticardiolipin antibodies. Lupus 1997;6(6):533–9.

[44] Bruce IN, Urowitz MB, Gladman DD, et al. Risk factors for coronary heart disease in women with systemic lupus erythematosus: the Toronto Risk Factor Study. Arthritis Rheum 2003; 48(11):3159–67.

[45] Ibanez D, Urowitz MB, Gladman DD. Summarizing disease features over time: I. Adjusted mean SLEDAI derivation and application to an index of disease activity in lupus. J Rheumatol 2003;30(9):1977–82.

[46] Gladman DD, Ibanez D, Urowitz MB. Systemic lupus erythematosus disease activity index 2000. J Rheumatol 2002;29(2):288–91.

[47] Ibanez D, Gladman DD, Urowitz MB. Adjusted Mean SLEDAI-2K (AMS) in Outcome Prediction in SLE [Abstract 400]. Arthritis Rheum 2004;50(9 Suppl):S199.

[48] Tsai JC, Perrella MA, Yoshizumi M, et al. Promotion of vascular smooth muscle cell growth by homocysteine: a link to atherosclerosis. Proc Natl Acad Sci USA 1994;91(14):6369–73.

[49] Bostom AG, Rosenberg IH, Silbershatz H, et al. Nonfasting plasma total homocysteine levels and stroke incidence in elderly persons: the Framingham Study. Ann Intern Med 1999; 131(5):352–5.

[50] Stampfer MJ, Malinow MR, Willett WC, et al. A prospective study of plasma homocyst(e)ine and risk of myocardial infarction in US physicians. JAMA 1992;268(7):877–81.

[51] Petri M, Roubenoff R, Dallal GE, et al. Plasma homocysteine as a risk factor for atherothrombotic events in systemic lupus erythematosus. Lancet 1996;348(9035):1120–4.

[52] Booth GL, Wang EE. Preventive health care, 2000 update: screening and management of hyperhomocysteinemia for the prevention of coronary artery disease events. The Canadian Task Force on Preventive Health Care. CMAJ 2000;163(1):21–9.

[53] Ridker PM, Cushman M, Stampfer MJ, et al. Inflammation, aspirin, and the risk of cardiovascular disease in apparently healthy men. N Engl J Med 1997;336(14):973–9.

[54] Ridker PM, Buring JE, Shih J, et al. Prospective study of C-reactive protein and the risk of future cardiovascular events among apparently healthy women. Circulation 1998;98(8): 731–3.

[55] Selzer F, Sutton-Tyrrell K, Fitzgerald S, et al. Vascular stiffness in women with systemic lupus erythematosus. Hypertension 2001;37(4):1075–82.

[56] Hope SA, Meredith IT. Cellular adhesion molecules and cardiovascular disease. Part I. Their expression and role in atherogenesis. Intern Med J 2003;33(8):380–6.

[57] Ridker PM, Hennekens CH, Roitman-Johnson B, et al. Plasma concentration of soluble intercellular adhesion molecule 1 and risks of future myocardial infarction in apparently healthy men. Lancet 1998;351(9096):88–92.

[58] Ridker PM, Hennekens CH, Buring JE, Rifai N. C-reactive protein and other markers of

inflammation in the prediction of cardiovascular disease in women. N Engl J Med 2000; 342(12):836–43.

[59] Peter K, Nawroth P, Conradt C, et al. Circulating vascular cell adhesion molecule-1 correlates with the extent of human atherosclerosis in contrast to circulating intercellular adhesion molecule-1, E-selectin, P-selectin, and thrombomodulin. Arterioscler Thromb Vasc Biol 1997; 17(3):505–12.

[60] Schonbeck U, Varo N, Libby P, et al. Soluble CD40L and cardiovascular risk in women. Circulation 2001;104(19):2266–8.

[61] Carvalho D, Savage CO, Isenberg D, Pearson JD. IgG anti-endothelial cell autoantibodies from patients with systemic lupus erythematosus or systemic vasculitis stimulate the release of two endothelial cell-derived mediators, which enhance adhesion molecule expression and leukocyte adhesion in an autocrine manner. Arthritis Rheum 1999;42(4):631–40.

[62] Del Papa N, Conforti G, Gambini D, et al. Characterization of the endothelial surface proteins recognized by anti-endothelial antibodies in primary and secondary autoimmune vasculitis. Clin Immunol Immunopathol 1994;70(3):211–6.

[63] Yazici ZA, Raschi E, Patel A, et al. Human monoclonal anti-endothelial cell IgG-derived from a systemic lupus erythematosus patient binds and activates human endothelium in vitro. Int Immunol 2001;13(3):349–57.

[64] Ettinger Jr WH, Hazzard WR. Elevated apolipoprotein-B levels in corticosteroid-treated patients with systemic lupus erythematosus. J Clin Endocrinol Metab 1988;67(3):425–8.

[65] Walldius G, Jungner I. Apolipoprotein B and apolipoprotein A-I: risk indicators of coronary heart disease and targets for lipid-modifying therapy. J Intern Med 2004;255(2):188–205.

[66] Abu-Shakra M, Gladman DD, Urowitz MB, Farewell V. Anticardiolipin antibodies in systemic lupus erythematosus: clinical and laboratory correlations. Am J Med 1995;99(6):624–8.

[67] Levine SR, Salowich-Palm L, Sawaya KL, et al. IgG anticardiolipin antibody titer >40 GPL and the risk of subsequent thrombo-occlusive events and death. A prospective cohort study. Stroke 1997;28(9):1660–5.

[68] Maaravi Y, Raz E, Gilon D, Rubinow A. Cerebrovascular accident and myocardial infarction associated with anticardiolipin antibodies in a young woman with systemic lupus erythematosus. Ann Rheum Dis 1989;48(10):853–5.

[69] Zuckerman E, Toubi E, Shiran A, et al. Anticardiolipin antibodies and acute myocardial infarction in non-systemic lupus erythmatosus patients: a controlled prospective study. Am J Med 1996;101(4):381–6.

[70] Vaarala O. Antiphospholipid antibodies and myocardial infarction. Lupus 1998;7(Suppl 2): S132–4.

[71] Wu R, Nityanand S, Berglund L, et al. Antibodies against cardiolipin and oxidatively modified LDL in 50-year-old men predict myocardial infarction. Arterioscler Thromb Vasc Biol 1997;17(11):3159–63.

[72] Farsi A, Domeneghetti MP, Fedi S, et al. High prevalence of anti-beta2 glycoprotein I antibodies in patients with ischemic heart disease. Autoimmunity 1999;30(2):93–8.

[73] Fiallo P, Tomasina C, Clapasson A, Cardo PP. Antibodies to beta(2)-glycoprotein I in ischemic stroke. Cerebrovasc Dis 2000;10(4):293–7.

[74] Tanne D, Triplett DA, Levine SR. Antiphospholipid-protein antibodies and ischemic stroke: not just cardiolipin any more. Stroke 1998;29(9):1755–8.

[75] Kattwinkel N, Villanueva AG, Labib SB, et al. Myocardial infarction caused by cardiac microvasculopathy in a patient with the primary antiphospholipid syndrome. Ann Intern Med 1992;116(12 Pt 1):974–6.

[76] Murphy JJ, Leach IH. Findings at necropsy in the heart of a patient with anticardiolipin syndrome. Br Heart J 1989;62(1):61–4.

[77] Rangel A, Lavalle C, Chavez E, et al. Myocardial infarction in patients with systemic lupus erythematosus with normal findings from coronary arteriography and without coronary vasculitis—case reports. Angiology 1999;50(3):245–53.

[78] Sherer Y, Shoenfeld Y. Antiphospholipid antibodies: are they pro-atherogenic or an epiphenomenon of atherosclerosis? Immunobiology 2003;207(1):13–6.

[79] Ross R. Atherosclerosis—an inflammatory disease. N Engl J Med 1999;340(2):115–26.

[80] Zeiher AM, Drexler H, Wollschlager H, Just H. Endothelial dysfunction of the coronary microvasculature is associated with coronary blood flow regulation in patients with early atherosclerosis. Circulation 1991;84(5):1984–92.

[81] Corretti MC, Plotnick GD, Vogel RA. Technical aspects of evaluating brachial artery vasodilatation using high-frequency ultrasound. Am J Physiol 1995;268(4 Pt 2):H1397–404.

[82] Corretti MC, Anderson TJ, Benjamin EJ, et al. Guidelines for the ultrasound assessment of endothelial-dependent flow-mediated vasodilation of the brachial artery: a report of the International Brachial Artery Reactivity Task Force. J Am Coll Cardiol 2002;39(2):257–65.

[83] Anderson TJ, Uehata A, Gerhard MD, et al. Close relation of endothelial function in the human coronary and peripheral circulations. J Am Coll Cardiol 1995;26(5):1235–41.

[84] Hardie KL, Kinlay S, Hardy DB, et al. Reproducibility of brachial ultrasonography and flow-mediated dilatation (FMD) for assessing endothelial function. Aust N Z J Med 1997; 27(6):649–52.

[85] Lima DS, Sato EI, Lima VC, et al. Brachial endothelial function is impaired in patients with systemic lupus erythematosus. J Rheumatol 2002;29(2):292–7.

[86] El-Magadmi M, Bodill H, Ahmad Y, et al. Systemic lupus erythematosus: an independent risk factor for endothelial dysfunction in women. Circulation 2004;110(4):399–404.

[87] Nikpour M, Urowitz MB, Gladman DD, et al. Prevalence and risk factors for endothelial dysfunction in systemic lupus erythematosus [Abstract F39]. Arthritis Rheum 2004;50(12): 4093–4.

[88] Nikpour M, Urowitz MB, Gladman DD, et al. Relationship between myocardial perfusion scintigraphy and brachial artery endothelial function in systemic lupus erythematosus [Abstract F27]. Arthritis Rheum 2004;50(12):4089–90.

[89] O'Leary DH, Polak JF, Kronmal RA, et al. Carotid-artery intima and media thickness as a risk factor for myocardial infarction and stroke in older adults. Cardiovascular Health Study Collaborative Research Group. N Engl J Med 1999;340(1):14–22.

[90] van der Meer IM, Bots ML, Hofman A, et al. Predictive value of noninvasive measures of atherosclerosis for incident myocardial infarction: the Rotterdam Study. Circulation 2004; 109(9):1089–94.

[91] Nikpour M, Urowitz MB, Gladman DD, et al. Relationship Between scintigraphic myocardial perfusion defects and coronary angiographic findings in patients with SLE [Abstract F28]. Arthritis Rheum 2004;50(12):4090.

[92] Mancini GB. Role of angiotensin-converting enzyme inhibition in reversal of endothelial dysfunction in coronary artery disease. Am J Med 1998;105(1A):40S–7S.

[93] Modena MG, Bonetti L, Coppi F, et al. Prognostic role of reversible endothelial dysfunction in hypertensive postmenopausal women. J Am Coll Cardiol 2002;40(3):505–10.

[94] Urowitz MB, Gladman DD, Ibanez D. Atherosclerotic vascular events in a risk factor study from a single center: prevalence and risk factors [Abstract 1569]. Arthritis Rheum 2004; 50(9 Suppl):S594.

[95] Bruce IN, Gladman DD, Urowitz MB. Detection and modification of risk factors for coronary artery disease in patients with systemic lupus erythematosus: a quality improvement study. Clin Exp Rheumatol 1998;16(4):435–40.

[96] Petri M, Spence D, Bone LR, Hochberg MC. Coronary artery disease risk factors in the Johns Hopkins Lupus Cohort: prevalence, recognition by patients, and preventive practices. Medicine (Baltimore) 1992;71(5):291–302.

[97] Third Report of the National Cholesterol Education Program (NCEP) Expert Panel on detection, evaluation, and treatment of high blood cholesterol in adults (adult treatment panel iii) final report. Circulation 2002;106(25):3143–421.

[98] Borba EF, Bonfa E. Longterm beneficial effect of chloroquine diphosphate on lipoprotein profile in lupus patients with and without steroid therapy. J Rheumatol 2001;28(4):780–5.

[99] Hodis HN, Quismorio Jr FP, Wickham E, Blankenhorn DH. The lipid, lipoprotein, and apolipoprotein effects of hydroxychloroquine in patients with systemic lupus erythematosus. J Rheumatol 1993;20(4):661–5.

[100] Rahman P, Gladman DD, Urowitz MB, et al. The cholesterol lowering effect of antimalarial drugs is enhanced in patients with lupus taking corticosteroid drugs. J Rheumatol 1999; 26(2):325–30.

[101] Tam LS, Gladman DD, Hallett DC, et al. Effect of antimalarial agents on the fasting lipid profile in systemic lupus erythematosus. J Rheumatol 2000;27(9):2142–5.

[102] Wallace DJ, Linker-Israeli M, Metzger AL, Stecher VJ. The relevance of antimalarial therapy with regard to thrombosis, hypercholesterolemia and cytokines in SLE. Lupus 1993; 2(1 Suppl):S13–5.

[103] Kuvin JT, Karas RH. Clinical utility of endothelial function testing: ready for prime time? Circulation 2003;107(25):3243–7.

[104] Tsiara S, Elisaf M, Mikhailidis DP. Early vascular benefits of statin therapy. Curr Med Res Opin 2003;19(6):540–56.

[105] Hosomi N, Mizushige K, Ohyama H, et al. Angiotensin-converting enzyme inhibition with enalapril slows progressive intima-media thickening of the common carotid artery in patients with non-insulin-dependent diabetes mellitus. Stroke 2001;32(7):1539–45.

[106] Koshiyama H, Tanaka S, Minamikawa J. Effect of calcium channel blocker amlodipine on the intimal-medial thickness of carotid arterial wall in type 2 diabetes. J Cardiovasc Pharmacol 1999;33(6):894–6.

[107] Rajzer M, Klocek M, Kawecka-Jaszcz K. Effect of amlodipine, quinapril, and losartan on pulse wave velocity and plasma collagen markers in patients with mild-to-moderate arterial hypertension. Am J Hypertens 2003;16(6):439–44.

[108] Stanton AV, Chapman JN, Mayet J, et al. Effects of blood pressure lowering with amlodipine or lisinopril on vascular structure of the common carotid artery. Clin Sci (Lond) 2001;101(5): 455–64.

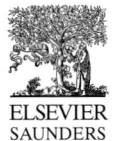

ELSEVIER
SAUNDERS

Rheum Dis Clin N Am 31 (2005) 355–362

RHEUMATIC
DISEASE CLINICS
OF NORTH AMERICA

# Inflammation and Accelerated Atherosclerosis: Basic Mechanisms

Andrea Doria, MD[a], Yaniv Sherer, MD[b], Pier L. Meroni, MD[c], Yehuda Shoenfeld, MD[b],*

[a]*Division of Rheumatology, Department of Medical and Surgical Science, University of Padua, Via Giustiniani 2, 35128 Padua, Italy*
[b]*Department of Medicine B, Sackler Faculty of Medicine, Center for Autoimmune Diseases, Chaim Sheba Medical Center, Tel-Aviv University, Tel-Hashomer 52621, Israel*
[c]*Allergy and Clinical Immunology Unit, Department of Internal Medicine, IRCCS Istituto Auxologico Italiano, University of Milan, Via G. Spagoletto 32, 10249 Milan, Italy*

The last decade was characterized by a revolution achieved in the therapy of many of the autoimmune rheumatic diseases (AIRDs), leading to decreased morbidity and mortality. The dramatic change was caused by the more efficient use of existing therapies or the use of novel biological agents including anti-cytokine monoclonal antibodies, fusion molecules, and peptides having neutralizing and immunomodulatory effects. These approaches enabled reduction in the doses of corticosteroids and immunosuppressants used, drugs associated with major and severe adverse effects. With these changes, novel factors have emerged determining the prognosis of AIRD. One of those factors is the accelerated atherosclerosis (AS) recorded in almost all AIRDs (ie, systemic lupus erythematosus [SLE], rheumatoid arthritis, Sjogren's syndrome, systemic sclerosis, and vasculitis). Another aspect unraveled during the previous decade is the autoimmune nature of AS [1–4].

Atherosclerosis is a multifactorial process that commences as early as childhood but usually clinically manifests itself later in life. Atherosclerosis increasingly is considered to be an immune-mediated process of the vascular

* Corresponding author.
*E-mail address:* shoenfel@post.tau.ac.il (Y. Shoenfeld).

0889-857X/05/$ – see front matter © 2005 Elsevier Inc. All rights reserved.
doi:10.1016/j.rdc.2005.01.006
*rheumatic.theclinics.com*

system. The presence of macrophages and activated lymphocytes within athero-sclerotic plaques supports the concept of AS as an immuno-mediated inflam-matory disorder [5]. Inflammation can be implicated in AS by means of different mechanisms, such as secondary to autoimmunity, infectious diseases and general inflammatory state. This article summarizes knowledge of the pathogenic mecha-nisms in AIRD as risk factors for accelerated AS.

## Immune cellular components in atherosclerosis

Cells of the immune system can be found within AS plaques, suggesting that they have a role in the atherogenic process. Their migration and activation within the plaques can be secondary to various stimuli such as infectious agents. These cells probably aggravate AS, as $CD4^+$ and $CD8^+$ T-cell depletion reduced fatty streak formation in C57BL/6 mice [6]. In addition, following crossing of ApoE knockout mice with immunodeficient scid/scid mice, the offspring had a 73% reduction in aortic fatty streak lesions compared with the immunocompetent apoE mice. Moreover, when $CD4^+$ T cells were transferred from the immuno-competent to the immunodeficient mice, they increased lesion area in the latter by 164% [7]. Associated findings were infiltration of the transferred T cells into the atherosclerotic lesions.

It is not surprising therefore that similar to autoimmune diseases, the cellu-lar components within atherosclerotic plaques secrete various cytokines includ-ing interleukin (IL)-1, IL-2, IL-6, IL-8, IL-12, IL-10, tumor necrosis factor alpha (TNF-$\alpha$), interferon gamma (INF-$\gamma$), and platelet-derived growth factor (PDGF) [4].

A cellular immune response specifically directed against heat shock pro-teins (HSPs), oxidized low-density lipoproteins (ox-LDL) and β2-glycoprotein-I (β2GPI) has been reported, suggesting a direct involvement of these molecules in the atherosclerotic process [1–3].

β2GPI is the main target antigen recognized by antiphospholipid antibodies (aPLs) frequently present in AIRD patients. It can be found in human athero-sclerotic lesions obtained from carotid endarterectomies and expressed abun-dantly within the subendothelial regions and the intimal–medial border of human atherosclerotic plaques and colocalizing with $CD4^+$ lymphocytes [8]. Upon transfer of lymphocytes obtained from β2GPI-immunized LDL receptor-deficient mice into syngeneic mice, the recipients exhibited larger fatty streaks compared with mice that received lymphocytes from control mice. T-cell depletion, how-ever, failed to induce this effect [9]. Therefore, T cells specific for β2GPI are capable of increasing AS, suggesting that β2GPI is a target autoantigen in AS. This study demonstrates that T cells reacting with a specific autoantigen can aggravate AS. There are probably many more such cell lines reacting with specific antigens that can modulate AS, either by aggravating or decreasing its extent (pro- or antiatherogenic) [10].

## Immune humoral components in atherosclerosis

Several autoantibodies are associated with AS and its manifestations in people. Animals provide good models for studying the effect of these autoantibodies on AS. Active immunization of LDL receptor-deficient mice with anticardiolipin antibodies (aCLs: the hallmark of antiphospholipid syndrome [APS], an autoimmune procoagulant syndrome that affects many SLE patients) resulted in development of high titers of mouse aCL and increased AS compared with controls [11]. Immunization of mice with β2GPI resulted in pronounced cellular and humoral response to β2GPI, with high titers of anti-β2GPI antibodies concomitant with larger atherosclerotic lesions that contained abundant CD4$^+$ cells [12,13].

ox-LDL is the type of LDL that is more likely to undergo uptake by macrophages, which turn into the foam cells characterizing the atherosclerotic lesions. Anti-ox-LDL antibodies are present in patients with AS and AIRD and in healthy individuals [14].

In multivariate analyses, anti–ox-LDL autoantibodies discriminated better between patients with peripheral vascular disease and control subjects than did any of the different lipoprotein analyses. There was also a tendency for higher autoantibody levels in patients with more extensive atherosclerotic lesions [15].

The autoantibodies to ox-LDL were investigated in several AIRD groups, including patients with systemic sclerosis [16,17] systemic vasculitides [14,18], and SLE [17,18]. The antibody levels were higher in each of those patient groups than in normals. There was a correlation between the total level of immunoglobulins and the level of antibodies against ox-LDL, while no correlation was demonstrated between the levels of the total immunoglobulin and the levels of antibodies to unrelated antigens (Epstein Barr virus and purified protein derivative). This finding suggests that the increasing total immunoglobulin levels in SLE patients are selective for some specific antibodies including autoantibodies against ox-LDL [17,18].

Although in people these autoantibodies are associated with manifestations and extent of AS in most studies, immunization with ox-LDL in animal models was followed by induction of anti-ox-LDL antibodies but surprisingly with suppression rather than aggravation of early atherogenesis [19]. These results support the presence of different types of anti–ox-LDL antibodies, some of which might be protective against AS [20]. This also may be true regarding aCL, as in a recent study, those antibodies that cross-react with native and ox-LDL succeeded in decreasing rather than aggravating the extent of AS [21].

These discrepancies may be explained by the presence of several types of autoantibodies that are measured together, namely protective and pathogenic autoantibodies [20]. It is possible that upon immunization with ox-LDL, the immune system acts by producing anti–ox-LDL antibodies, which help to clear the high levels of ox-LDL, thus being protective. On the other hand, upon oxidation of LDL, other autoantibodies directed toward other parts of the ox-LDL particle are produced, and these aid in uptake of ox-LDL by macrophages, turning them into foam cells within the atherosclerotic plaque (ie, pathogenic).

## Endothelium as an additional key player in atherosclerosis

Two main pathogenic hypotheses have been suggested to explain the athero-sclerotic plaque formation: the injury hypothesis and the lipid hypothesis [22]. In both cases, endothelium has been suggested to play a pivotal role in all the phases of the atherosclerotic process, given its ability to regulate vessel tone and interfere with inflammatory processes and coagulation [23].

In the early and intermediate stages, endothelial cells (ECs) activated by ox-LDL or other triggers up-regulate adhesion molecules, thereby favoring monocyte adhesion and transmigration. At the same time, EC perturbation leads to proinflammatory cytokine (chemokine) secretion, which activates monocytes and ultimately facilitates the foam cell formation [22]. When activated, ECs express class II major histocompatibility complex (MHC) molecules and might serve as nonprofessional antigen presenting cells (APCd) [24]. In this way, they might cooperate with the professional APC of the vascular-associated lymphoid tissue in mounting the adaptive immune responses to endogenous (eg, ox-LDL, HSP, or β2GPI) or exogenous (infectious antigens) molecules that have been proposed as playing a role in the early phases of the atherosclerotic process [1–3].

Endothelium activation appears also to be important in favoring fibroblast and smooth muscle cell proliferation and migration through the secretion of growth factors in the intermediate steps of plaque formation [22]. The same growth factors and the pro-inflammatory cytokines (and chemokines) themselves cooperate in macrophage activation with the consequent secretion of metal-loproteases able to increase the matrix turnover and eventually lead to plaque instability [22].

The final event that produces the clinical cardiovascular manifestations is the plaque rupture and subsequent thrombus formation (atherothrombosis). Interest-ingly, EC are involved largely in hemostasis and, once perturbed, they display a procoagulant phenotype [23]. The up-regulation of tissue factor (TF) expression and the impairment of the fibrinolytic system in perturbed ECs have been suggested to play major roles in favoring the thrombus formation on the ruptured plaques [22].

On the other hand, in AIRD, endothelium itself is also a target for several circulating immune mediators that might induce a cell perturbation potentially able to facilitate the atherosclerotic process.

Complement (C) activation by circulating immune complexes or by other mechanisms might induce endothelial damage by activated products of the C cascade or even the cell membrane insertion of the membrane attack complex (MAC). The latter phenomenon was reported to result in the release of an array of growth factors and cytokines that induces proliferation, inflammation, and thrombus formation in the vascular walls [25]. These events might cooperate in all the different steps of the atherosclerotic process. C deposition has been reported in the atherosclerotic lesions recently, raising its potential role in the plaque formation [26].

Antiendothelial cell antibodies (AECAs) reacting with yet unknown EC membrane constituents have been described in sera from different AIRD [27]. In most cases, AECAs were shown to induce a proinflammatory and a procoagulant phenotype in EC monolayers in vitro [27]. It is useful to speculate on the potential role of these autoantibodies in perturbing the endothelium, thus favoring the occurrence of the accelerated AS reported in AIRD. In accordance with such a hypothesis is the demonstration of AECA in primary AS or in patients displaying conditions at risk for AS [28–30].

Besides the pure antiendothelial antibodies, other autoantibodies have been reported to react with ECd because of their ability to recognize their own antigens planted on the EC membranes. This is the case for the anti-dsDNA antibodies that can react with DNA-histone complexes adhering on EC membranes through electric charge interactions [27,31]. The binding of anti-dsDNA antibodies to their own antigens adhered on the cell membranes has been shown to induce EC activation in vitro [27,31]. A similar effect has been described when aPL is incubated with human EC monolayers in vitro. Antiphospholipid antibodies react with plasma PL-binding proteins; among them the most important one is represented by $\beta$2GPI. $\beta$2GPI was found to be expressed on ECs obtained from different anatomical localizations in in vitro and in vivo studies. The binding of the autoantibodies to adhered $\beta$2GPI has been suggested to induce a cell signaling that ends with the expression of an endothelial proinflammatory and procoagulant phenotype. Interestingly, such an effect was reported in in vivo experimental models also, suggesting that it might be one of the actual pathogenic mechanisms for the thrombophilic state associated with the persistent presence of aPL [32]. Antiphospholipid antibodies frequently are detected in AIRD and might contribute to the plaque formation through their endothelial proinflammatory effect and to the athero-thrombosis, owing to their procoagulant ability.

Moreover, most AIRDs are characterized by a chronic systemic inflammatory state with elevated plasma levels of proinflammatory cytokines and chemokines. As reported in patients with primary AS, a chronic inflammatory state is suggested to represent a risk factor for plaque formation and a condition that favors its instability and rupture [33]. Being in close contact with the blood and expressing specific cell membrane receptors, the endothelium represents one of the most available cell targets for the circulating cytokines. The final result is a further EC perturbation.

In line with the endothelium perturbation mediated by several circulating immune mediators is the demonstration of an impaired endothelium-dependent vasodilation in AIRD patients [34]. Such impairment is related to the reduction in vasodilator bioavailability (mainly nitric oxide), and it has been associated with the propensity of an individual to develop atherosclerotic disease [34].

## Immunomodulation of atherosclerosis

Several experimental studies emphasize that immunomodulation can affect AS and thus provide hope for the development of similar therapies for people. These options recently have been summarized [35]. Among them, several approaches have been shown to be effective: treatment with antibodies against CD40 ligand [36], induction of oral tolerance to autoantigens associated with AS [37], manipulation of the cytokine network in AS (upregulating the antiatherogenic cytokines and blockade of proatherogenic cytokines), and gene therapy [35]. There is also evidence for the use of statins and intravenous immunoglobulin (IVIg) as therapeutic tools to immunomodulate the atherosclerotic process [38,39].

Statins, beyond their ability to reduce serum cholesterol levels, display clear anti-inflammatory and immunomodulatory effects by reducing monocyte adhesion to EC and endothelial secretion of cytokines and MHC class II expression [38,40].

Intravenous immunoglobulins have many immunoregulatory and anti-inflammatory properties and have shown the ability to reduce plaque development in a model of murine AS [41]. Looking at mechanisms specifically relevant in AS, it has been reported that IVIgs contain anti-idiotypic activity against anti–ox-LDL antibodies [42], and they are able to reduce metaloproteinase-9 (MMP-9) activity [39]; moreover IVIgs include a subset of natural antiendothelial antibodies that, opposite to pathologic AECA, directly modulate endothelial function, reducing proinflammatory and prothrombotic properties of resting EC and inhibiting cytokine and metalloprotease secretion by EC activated with proinflammatory stimuli [43]. Finally IVIgs reduce cytokine secretion and the membrane expression of adhesion molecules on EC stimulated with TNF-$\alpha$ and ox-LDL, and inhibit one of the pathways of internalization of ox-LDL in EC [44].

## Summary

The studies described in this article support a role for immunologic–inflammatory mechanisms in the pathogenesis of atherosclerosis. This immunologic–inflammatory state is evident in many autoimmune diseases, but also in the general population lacking an overt autoimmune disease. The ability to immunomodulate atherosclerosis (currently only experimental) should lead to future research into the mechanisms and treatment of atherosclerosis, the leading cause of death in the Western world.

## References

[1] Shoenfeld Y. Atherosclerosis and the immune system: is atherosclerosis an autoimmune disease? Seminars in Clinical Immunology 2000;1:5–6.

[2] Shoenfeld Y, Sherer Y, Haratz D. Atherosclerosis as an infectious, inflammatory and auto-immune disease. Trends Immunol 2001;22:293−5.

[3] Sherer Y, Shoenfeld Y. Atherosclerosis: is atherosclerosis a cellular or humoral mediated auto-immune disease? Ann Rheum Dis 2002;61:97−9.

[4] George J, Harats D, Shoenfeld Y. Inflammatory and immune aspects of atherosclerosis. Isr Med Assoc J 1999;1:112−6.

[5] Ross R. Atherosclerosis — an inflammatory condition. N Engl J Med 1999;340:115−26.

[6] Emeson EE, Shen ML, Bell CG, et al. Inhibition of atherosclerosis in CD4 T-cell-depleted and nude (nu/nu) C57BL/6 hyperlipidemic mice. Am J Pathol 1996;149:675−85.

[7] Zhou X, Nicoletti A, Elhage R, et al. Transfer of CD4 + T cells aggravates atherosclerosis in immunodeficient apolipoprotein E knockout mice. Circulation 2000;102:2919−22.

[8] George J, Harats D, Gilburd B, et al. Immunolocalization of β2-glycoprotein I (apolipoprotein H) to human atherosclerotic plaques: potential implications for lesion progression. Circulation 1999; 99:2227−30.

[9] George J, Harats D, Gilburd B, et al. Adoptive transfer of beta-2-glycoprotein-I-reactive lym-phocytes enhances early atherosclerosis in LDL receptor-deficient mice. Circulation 2000;102: 1822−7.

[10] George J, Afek A, Gilburd B, et al. Cellular and humoral immune responses to heat shock pro-tein both involved in promoting fatty-streak formation in LDL-deficient mice. J Am Coll Cardiol 2001;38:900−5.

[11] George J, Afek A, Gilburd B, et al. Atherosclerosis in LDL-receptor knockout mice is ac-celerated by immunization with anticardiolipin antibodies. Lupus 1997;6:723−9.

[12] Afek A, George J, Shoenfeld Y, et al. Enhancement of atherosclerosis in beta-2-glycoprotein I-immunized apolipoprotein E-deficient mice. Pathobiology 1999;67:19−25.

[13] George J, Afek A, Gilburd B, et al. Induction of early atherosclerosis in LDL-receptor-deficient mice immunized with beta2-glycoprotein I. Circulation 1998;98:1108−15.

[14] Wu R, Lefvert AK. Autoantibodies against oxidized low density lipoproteins (oxLDL): charac-terization of antibody isotope, subclass, affinity and effect on the macrophage uptake of oxLDL. Clin Exp Immunol 1995;102:174−80.

[15] Bergmark C, Wu R, de Faire U, et al. Patients with early onset of peripheral vascular disease have high levels of autoantibodies against oxidized low-density lipoproteins. Arterioscler Thromb Vasc Biol 1995;15:441−5.

[16] Wu R, Shoenfeld Y, Matucci M, et al. Nontraditional factors vary in patients with autoimmune diseases. Clin Invest Med, in press.

[17] Wu R, Svenungsson E, Gunnarsson I, et al. Antibodies against lysophosphatidylcholine and oxidized LDL in-patients with SLE. Lupus 1999;8:142−50.

[18] Wu R, Svenungsson E, Gunnarsson I, et al. Antibodies to adult human endothelial cells cross-react with oxidized LDL and β2-glycoprotein I in SLE. Clin Exp Immunol 1999;115:561−6.

[19] George J, Afek A, Gilburd B, et al. Hyperimmunization of apo-E mice with homologous malondialdehyde low-density lipoprotein suppresses early atherogenesis. Atherosclerosis 1998; 138:147−52.

[20] Wu R, Dearing L, Matsuura E, et al. Are anti-oxLDL antibodies pathogenic or protective? Circulation 2004;110:2252−8.

[21] Nicolo D, Goldman BI, Monestier M. Reduction of atherosclerosis in low-density lipoprotein receptor-deficient mice by passive administration of antiphospholipid antibody. Arthritis Rheum 2003;48:2974−8.

[22] Lusis AJ. Atherosclerosis. Nature 2000;407:233−41.

[23] Cines DB, Pollak ES, Buck CA, et al. Endothelial cells in physiology and in the pathophysiology of vascular disorders. Blood 1998;91:3527−61.

[24] Rothermel AL, Wang Y, Schechner J, et al. Endothelial cells present antigens in vivo. BMC Immunol 2005;16:5−24.

[25] Acosta J, Qin X, Halperin J. Complement and complement regulatory proteins as potential molecular targets for vascular diseases. Curr Pharm Des 2004;10:203−11.

[26] Niculescu F, Rus H. The complement activation in atherosclerosis. Immunol Res 2004;30: 73–80.

[27] Meroni PL, Raschi E, Testoni C, et al. Functional heterogeneity of pathogenic anti-endothelial antibodies. In: Shoenfeld Y, Harats D, Wick G, editors. Atherosclerosis and autoimmunity. Amsterdam: Elsevier; 2001. p. 211–20.

[28] George J, Meroni PL, Gilburd B, et al. Antiendothelial cell antibodies in patients with coronary atherosclerosis. Immunol Lett 2000;73:23–7.

[29] Farsi A, Domeneghetti MP, Brunelli T, et al. Activation of the immune system and coronary artery disease: the role of antiendothelial cell antibodies. Atherosclerosis 2001;154:429–36.

[30] Faulk WP, Rose M, Meroni PL, et al. Antibodies to human endothelial cells identify myocardial damage and predicts development of coronary artery disease in patients with transplanted hearts. Hum Immunol 1999;60:826–32.

[31] Lai KN, Leung JC, Lai KB, et al. Upregulation of adhesion molecules on endothelial cells by anti-DNA autoantibodies in systemic lupus erythematosus. Clin Immunol Immunopathol 1996;81:229–38.

[32] Meroni PL, Raschi E, Testoni C, et al. Endothelial cell activation by antiphospholipid antibodies. Clin Immunol 2004;112:169–74.

[33] Libby P, Ridker P, Maseri A. Inflammation and atherosclerosis. Circulation 2002;105:1135–43.

[34] Bonetti PO, Lilach OL, Lerman A. Endothelial dysfunction. A marker of atherosclerotic risk. Arterioscler Thromb Vasc Biol 2003;23:168–75.

[35] Sherer Y, Shoenfeld Y. Immunomodulation for treatment and prevention of atherosclerosis. Autoimmun Rev 2002;1:21–7.

[36] Toubi E, Shoenfeld Y. The role of DC40–CD154 interactions in autoimmunity and the benefit of disrupting this pathway. Autoimmunity 2004;37:457–64.

[37] Harats D, Yacov N, Gilburd B, et al. Oral tolerance with heat shock protein 65 attenuates *Mycobacterium tuberculosis*-induced and high-fat-diet-driven atherosclerotic lesions. J Am Coll Cardiol 2002;7:1333–8.

[38] Shovman O, Levy Y, Gilburd B, et al. Anti-inflammatory and immunomodulatory properties of statins. Immunol Res 2002;25:271–85.

[39] Shapiro S, Shoenfeld Y, Gilburd B, et al. Intravenous gamma globulin inhibits the production of matrix metalloproteinase-9 in macrophages. Cancer 2002;95:2032–7.

[40] Meroni PL, Luzzana C, Ventura D. Anti-inflammatory and immunomodulating properties of statins. An additional tool for the therapeutic approach of systemic autoimmune diseases? Clin Rev Allergy Immunol 2002;23:263–77.

[41] Nicoletti A, Kaveri S, Caligiuri G, et al. Immunoglobulin treatment reduces atherosclerosis in apo E knockout mice. J Clin Invest 1998;102:910–8.

[42] Wu R, Shoenfeld Y, Sherer Y, et al. Anti-idiotypes to oxidized LDL antibodies in intravenous immunoglobulin preparations—possible immunomodulation of atherosclerosis. Autoimmunity 2003;36:91–7.

[43] Ronda N, Leonardi S, Orlandini G, et al. Natural antiendothelial cell antibodies (AECA). J Autoimmun 1999;13:121–7.

[44] Ronda N, Bernini F, Giacosa R, et al. Normal human IgG prevents endothelial cell activation induced by TNFα and oxidized low-density lipoprotein atherogenic stimuli. Clin Exp Immunol 2003;133:219–26.

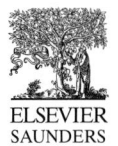

RHEUMATIC
DISEASE CLINICS
OF NORTH AMERICA

ELSEVIER
SAUNDERS

Rheum Dis Clin N Am 31 (2005) 363–385

# Osteoporosis in Systemic Lupus Erythematosus Mechanisms

Chin Lee, MD*, Rosalind Ramsey-Goldman, MD, DrPH

*Division of Rheumatology, Feinberg School of Medicine, Northwestern University,
240 East Huron Street, McGaw Pavilion 2300, Chicago, IL 60611, USA*

Osteoporosis is an important and preventable condition associated with systemic lupus erythematosus (SLE) [1]. The incidence of SLE has increased, but disease survival has improved over the last several decades in some patient groups [2–4], although not all [5]. Accordingly, clinicians have placed a growing emphasis on prevention and treatment of SLE-related comorbidities, such as osteoporosis [6]. Previous cross-sectional and longitudinal studies offer epidemiologic evidence for reduced bone mineral density (BMD) and increased fracture risk in patients who have SLE. Bone loss in lupus is likely a multifactorial process, and both traditional and SLE-related risk factors for osteoporosis have been implicated. In this article, the current epidemiologic information on reduced BMD, fracture data, associated risk factors, and clinically relevant strategies to minimize bone loss and reduce fracture risk in the SLE population are discussed.

## Epidemiology

*Bone mineral density in systemic lupus erythematosus*

According to the suggested World Health Organization (WHO) classification criteria for osteoporosis, SLE patients have lower BMD than do aged-matched

This work was supported by Grants from the National Institutes of Health (K24-AR 02138, P60-AR48098, P60-AR 30692, T32-AR 07611, K12-RR017707), the Arthritis Foundation Clinical Science Grant, Lupus Foundation of Illinois, Arthritis Foundation Greater Chicago Chapter, and unrestricted educational grants from Proctor & Gamble Pharmaceuticals and Merck & Co., Inc.

* Corresponding author.
*E-mail address:* c-lee17@northwestern.edu (C. Lee).

controls [7–11]. The estimated prevalence of osteoporosis among those who have SLE ranges from 4% to 23%, whereas osteopenia ranges from 25% to 46% [8,11–21]. However, most prior studies examining bone loss in SLE primarily include white women [7–9,11,12,16,21–23], and data on bone health in men and nonwhite women who have SLE are comparatively sparse.

Premenopausal women who have longstanding SLE and corticosteroid exposure have significantly lower BMD at the spine and hip as compared with normal controls in cross-sectional studies [7–9,11,24]. Similar findings of lower BMD at both the spine and hip have been observed in investigations including both pre- and postmenopausal women who have SLE. However, women in such studies generally have longstanding disease (>5 years) and history of corticosteroid use [14,15]. In a study consisting of 20 premenopausal women who have early disease (mean disease duration of less than 6.5 months) and no corticosteroid use, Teichmann and coworkers [24] reported significantly lower BMD at the spine, but not at the hip. Additionally, in 15 premenopausal women who have new onset SLE without prior corticosteroid use, Pons and colleagues [12] found no significant difference for the hip or spine in BMD when compared with controls.

Only a handful of studies have assessed BMD in a modest number of men [8,15,25–28]. Formiga and colleagues [26] reported no significant reduction in BMD at either the hip or lumbar spine in 20 men who have SLE as compared with normal healthy controls, even though the patients had or were currently using corticosteroids. In a subsequent study assessing BMD exclusively in men who have SLE, Bhattoa and colleagues [28] noted no differences in BMD at the lumbar spine, femoral neck, or distal forearm (radius) as compared with age- and sex-matched controls. Based on the WHO criteria for osteoporosis, 17.4% of the men had osteoporosis at the lumbar spine, whereas 4.3% and 13.0% had osteoporosis at the femoral neck and distal forearm (radius), respectively, and the frequencies of osteopenia at all three anatomic sites were even higher. But there were only two fractures reported by men in the study. Unlike many cross-sectional studies evaluating BMD in SLE that include mostly women, the men in the Bhattoa study were relatively older with a mean age of 45.6 years. Furthermore, although all but two men had received or were currently using corticosteroids, no correlation was seen between BMD at any anatomic site with either daily or cumulative corticosteroid dosage [28].

The prevalence of osteoporosis in SLE varies across different racial groups. Among white women who have SLE, the prevalence ranges from 12% to 16%. In contrast, prevalence is estimated to be 4% to 6% in Chinese women who have SLE [29]. Similarly, the frequency of osteoporosis at the lumbar spine in a group of premenopausal Thai women who have SLE was 1.4%, which was also comparatively lower than the published prevalence of osteoporosis in white women who have SLE [23]. Although the prevalence of osteoporosis in African American women who have SLE is higher than in women who do not have SLE, and comparable to that in white women who have SLE [30], African American women having lupus appear to be at greater risk for osteopenia and osteoporosis at the lumbar spine than white women [31]. An analysis of 75 African American women from the Chicago Lupus Database found 44% of the women to have osteoporosis at the spine, which was significantly higher than in white women [31]. Additionally, 32.9% and 6.4% of African Americans also had osteoporosis at the hip and distal forearm, respectively [31]. Variation in the prevalence of osteoporosis among different racial groups may be partially attributable to dissimilarities in inherent calcium metabolism, severity of SLE, as well as the cumulative exposure to specific disease therapies, such as corticosteroids [29].

The nature of bone loss in SLE is likely heterogeneous [32], involving both trabecular and cortical bone at the hip, spine, and forearm [7,9,13]. Although most studies agree that SLE subjects have reduced BMD, discrepancies exist with respect to the type of bone (cortical or trabecular) and anatomic site (hip, spine, or forearm) affected. Overall, findings from most cross-sectional studies point to lower BMD at both the spine and hip among those who have SLE as compared with control groups. Subjects who have early and less severe SLE appear to have minimal change in BMD at the spine and hip [19]. Moreover, subjects who have established disease tend to have lower BMD at the lumbar spine, whereas BMD at the hip appears to be somewhat less affected (Table 1) [7–9]. In contrast, there is minimal information with regard to BMD at the distal forearm in SLE subjects, and presently no reports have found reduced BMD at this anatomic site [27,28]. Prior studies have also evaluated BMD at other anatomic sites, including the hand [13,27]. Kalla and colleagues [13] observed significant thinning of the metacarpal cortices in SLE subjects as compared with controls, but this finding was not related to either disease duration or corticosteroid use, and the metacarpal bone mass was normal.

In currently available longitudinal studies, the findings of reduced BMD in SLE have been inconsistent and vary according to anatomic site (Table 2). The first longitudinal study of premenopausal women who have SLE found significantly lower BMD at the lumbar spine and femur as compared with age-matched controls at baseline, but failed to find any notable changes in BMD at either site among 21 women followed over a 3-year period [12]. In a subsequent study, Hansen and collaborators [27] reported BMD Z-scores, which represent the difference between the subject's BMD and the normal BMD for those of the same age, sex, and race, divided by the standard deviation of healthy controls, for 31 women and 5 men. At 2 years follow-up, there were significant reductions in BMD Z-scores at the femoral neck and third metacarpal bone, but not at the lumbar spine or distal forearm, for females only. Likewise, Kipen and colleagues [22] found no significant changes in BMD at the lumbar spine and femoral neck in 32 premenopausal women who had SLE over 3 years. Although the investigators observed no differences for yearly change in BMD between corticosteroid and noncorticosteroid-exposed women, subjects receiving more than 7.5 mg of corticosteroid per day experienced a reduction in spine BMD, whereas individuals receiving less than 7.5 mg of corticosteroids per day experienced an increase in their spine BMD [22]. In the most recent longitu-

Table 1
Cross-sectional data available on bone mineral density in systemic lupus erythematosus

| First author, year [Ref.] | Non-SLE control group | SLE patients (n) | Sex | Menop. status | Mean age for SLE group (±SD y) | Mean SLE duration (±SD mo or y) | Corticost. exposure | Expression of BMD | Spine | Hip[a] | Distal forearm |
|---|---|---|---|---|---|---|---|---|---|---|---|
| Dhillon, 1990 [33] | + | 12 | F | NA | 35.0 ± 8.5 | NA | (+) | g/cm² | ↔[b] | NA | NA |
| Dhillon, 1990 [33] | + | 10 | F | NA | 34.0 ± 10.8 | NA | (+) | g/cm² | ↔[b] | NA | NA |
| Kalla, 1993 [7] | + | 46 | F | Pre- | 31.0 ± 7.0 | 76.0 ± 66.0 mo | (+) | g/cm² | ↓[b] | ↓[b] | NA |
| Formiga, 1995 [8] | + | 74 | F | Pre- | 30.8 ± 6.5 | 86.4 ± 60.7 mo | (+) | g/cm² | ↓[b] | ↓[b] | NA |
| Pons, 1995 [12] | + | 15 | F | Pre- | 29.9 ± 9.1 | 0.0 ± 0.0 mo | (−) | g/cm² | ↔[b] | ↔[b] | NA |
| Pons, 1995 [12] | + | 43 | F | Pre- | 30.6 | 67.5 ± 45.2 mo | (+) | g/cm² | ↔[b] | ↔[b] | NA |
| Houssiau, 1996 [9] | + | 47 | F | Pre- | 33.0 ± 8.0 | ≥ 6.0 mo | (+) | g/cm² | ↓[b] | ↓[b] | NA |
| Formiga, 1996 [26] | + | 20 | M | NA | 37.0 ± 12.9 | 63.7 ± 70.4 mo | (+) | g/cm² | ↔[b] | ↔[b] | NA |
| Kipen, 1997 [14] | − | 97 | F | Pre-/post- | 44.2 ± 14.9 | 8.4 ± 7.0 y | (+) | g/cm² | ↔ | ↓ | NA |
| Trapani, 1998 [10] | + | 20 | M/F | Juvenile | 13.7 ± 5.3 | NA | (±) | Z & T-scores | ↔ | NA | ↔ |
| Hansen, 1998 [27] | − | 36 | M/F | Pre-/post- | 39.0 | 11.0 y | (±) | Z-score | ↔ | ↓[b] | NA |
| Sinigaglia, 1999 [11] | + | 84 | F | Pre- | 30.5 ± 7.5 | 7.0 ± 5.8 y | (+) | Z-score | ↓[b] | ↓[b] | NA |
| Jardinet, 2000 [16] | − | 35 | F | Pre- | 30.0 ± 9.0 | 11.0 ± 7.0 y | (±) | Z-score | ↓[b] | ↓[b] | NA |
| Gilboe, 2000 [15] | + | 75 | M/F | Pre-/post- | 45.0 | 8.1 y | (±) | g/cm² | ↓[b] | ↓[b] | NA |
| Teichmann, 1999 [24] | + | 20 | F | Pre- | 38.7 ± 4.9 | < 6.5 ± 4.5 mo | (−) | g/cm² | ↓[b] | ↔ | NA |
| Teichmann, 1999 [24] | + | 35 | F | Pre- | 59.7 ± 6.2 | NA | (+) | g/cm² | ↓[b] | ↓[b] | NA |
| Bhattoa, 2001 [28] | + | 23 | M | NA | 45.6 | 11.9 ± 6.9 y | (±) | g/cm² | ↔[b] | ↔[b] | ↔[b] |
| Redlich, 2000 [21] | + | 30 | F | Pre- | 33.0 | 79.0 mo | (+) | g/cm², Z- & T-scores | NA | NA | NA |
| Uaratanawong, 2003 [23] | − | 44 | F | Pre- | 34.0 ± 7.9 | 17.1 ± 25.8 mo | (−) | g/cm² | NA | NA | NA |
| Uaratanawong, 2003 [23] | − | 74 | F | Pre- | 31.8 ± 8.1 | 30.3 ± 31.6 mo | (+) | g/cm² | ↓ | ↓ | NA |

*Abbreviations:* Corticost., corticosteroid; F, female; M, male; Menop., menopausal; NA, data not available or not assessed in this study; +, corticosteroid-exposed patients; −, corticosteroid-naïve patients; (±), corticosteroid-exposed and -naïve patients.

[a] Hip represents changes in total hip, total femur, femoral neck, trochanter or Ward's triangle.

[b] Compared to normal control group.

Table 2
Longitudinal data available on bone mineral density in SLE

| First author, year [Ref.] | Mean duration of follow-up mo (±SD) | Non-SLE control group | SLE patients (n) | Sex | Menop. status | Mean age for SLE group (±SD y) | SLE mean duration (±SD mo or y) | Corticost. exposure | Expression of BMD | Lumbar spine | Hips[a] | Distal forearm |
|---|---|---|---|---|---|---|---|---|---|---|---|---|
| Pons, 1995 [12] | 36.6 ± 12.7 | + | 21 | F | Pre- | NA | NA | (+) | g/cm² | ↔[b] | ↔[b] | NA |
| Formiga, 1996 [26] | 18.0 | – | 25 | F | Pre- | 31.7 | 91.0 ± 64.0 mo | (+) | g/cm² | ↔[b] | ↔[b] | NA |
| Hansen, 1998 [27] | 24.0 | – | 36 | M/F | Pre-/post- | 39.0 | 11.0 y | (±) | Z-score | ↔[c] | ↓[c] | ↔[c] |
| Trapani, 1998 [10] | 12.0 | + | 20 | M/F | Juvenile | 13.7 ± 5.3 | NA | (±) | g/cm² | ↔[b] | NA | NA |
| Kipen, 1999 [22] | 36.0 | – | 32 | F | Pre- | 35.2 ± 1.5[d] | 7.0 ± 0.8 y[d] | (±) | Z-score | ↔ | ↔ | NA |
| Jardinet, 2000 [16] | 21.0 ± 11.0 | – | 35 | F | Pre- | 30.0 ± 9.0 | 11.0 ± 7.0 y | (±) | g/cm² | ↓[e] | ↔[e] | NA |

*Abbreviations*: Corticost., corticosteroid; F, female; M, male; Menop., menopausal; NA, data not available or not assessed in this study; +, corticosteroid-exposed patients; –, corticosteroid-naïve patients; (±), corticosteroid-exposed and -naïve patients.

[a] Hip represents changes in total hip, total femur, femoral neck, trochanter, or Ward's triangle.

[b] Compared to baseline.

[c] Compared to normal control group.

[d] Mean age ± standard error of the mean (SEM).

[e] Represents percent change in BMD per year as compared with no change.

dinal investigation, Jardinet and coworkers [16] observed significantly lower BMD Z-scores at the lumbar spine and total hip in 35 premenopausal women who have SLE as compared with age-matched controls at baseline, but repeated BMD measurements at a mean period of 21 months showed significant bone loss only at the spine. In a subset analysis of women who have diminished spine BMD in this study, only those taking more than 7.5 mg of daily glucocorticoids experienced a reduction in bone mass.

*Fractures in systemic lupus erythematosus*

In comparison to available BMD data, information on factures in SLE patients is more limited. Most early cross-sectional studies did not observe or report fractures in SLE [7,33]. However, a higher occurrence of fractures in women who have SLE has been found in more recent investigations. In a study examining a cohort of SLE subjects from two centers, Petri [25] reported fractures occurring in 22 of 364 individuals in adulthood. The most common sites of fracture included the hip, femur, vertebra, and rib.

A large population-based cohort of SLE women providing data on self-reported fractures, 12.3% of 702 women who have SLE reported at least one fracture after being diagnosed with disease. When compared with a historic population-based group of women of similar age, women who have SLE experienced fractures five times more frequently than expected. Moreover, nearly half of all fractures occurred in SLE women younger than 50 years old or before menopause [34]. This finding is notable given that fractures are the leading cause of morbidity in postmenopausal women over age 55 in the general population [35]. Duration of glucocorticoid use was an independent factor related to the time from lupus diagnosis to fracture occurrence in this study [34].

A more recent study found that 9% of 242 subjects who have SLE experienced nontraumatic fractures from the time of disease onset. Of these individuals, 1 in 5 was osteoporotic, 1 in 7 was osteopenic, whereas 1 in 22 had normal BMD at the spine and femoral neck [1]. Both older age at SLE diagnosis and longer duration of glucocorticoid use appear to be associated with fractures in SLE patients [1,34].

**Risk factors of systemic lupus erythematosus–related osteoporosis**

The original WHO classification was developed for assessing postmenopausal white women [36]. Thus, in premenopausal women, nonwhites, and men who have SLE, BMD assessment alone may not be adequate for establishing a diagnosis of osteoporosis and identifying patients at higher risk for fractures. However, recognizing risk factors for osteoporosis (eg, corticosteroid use) in the setting of low BMD matched for age, sex, and ethnicity may more appropriately stratify individuals at risks for future fractures [37].

*Traditional risk factors*

The traditional risk factors associated with osteoporosis in SLE are typically associated with osteoporosis in the general population: female sex, older age ($\geq 65$ years of age), white or Asian race, low body weight (below 127 pounds), a personal or maternal history of fracture, early menopause, and lifestyle factors, including smoking, a diet low in calcium and vitamin D, and excessive alcohol consumption. Other traditional risk factors include specific medications, such as long-term use of thyroid hormone, and factors increasing likelihood for falls (Box 1) [38–41]. Although older age is related to fractures in SLE and non-SLE women, the mean age at the time of first symptomatic fracture is 48.2 years for those who have SLE, which is somewhat younger than those who do not have disease [34]. Additionally, although African American

---

**Box 1. Traditional and systemic lupus erythematosus–related risk factors for low bone mineral density and osteoporosis**

*Traditional risk factors*

- Female sex
- Women age >65 years
- White or Asian
- Low body weight (<127 lbs)
- Personal or maternal history of fragility fracture
- Early menopause (<40 years of age)
- Recurrent falls
- Low physical activity
- Current smoking
- Low dietary calcium or vitamin D
- Excessive alcohol use (>2 drinks/day)

*Systemic lupus erythematosus–related risk factors*

- Active disease or frequent SLE flares
  Early SLE onset may prevent reaching optimal peak bone mass
  Symptoms related to SLE may prevent physical activity
  Hypogonadism due to active SLE
- Sun exposure and nonuse of sunscreens
- Chronic glucocorticoid use (>3 months)
- Therapy-related premature menopause (eg, cyclophosphamide)
- Therapy associated with low bone mineral density (eg, anticonvulsant, low molecular weight heparin, suppressive levels of thyroid hormone)

women are traditionally viewed as being at lower risk for osteoporosis, the African American race does not appear to be protective for fracture in the setting of SLE [31].

*System lupus erythematosus–related risk factors*

In addition to the traditional risk factors, specific SLE-related risk factors have been identified or suspected to be associated with lower BMD and increased risk for osteoporosis and fractures among those with SLE. These risk factors may be intrinsic to SLE or be related to disease treatment (see Box 1). The epidemiologic information, biochemical bone markers, and histomorphometric bone data from murine models point to a relationship between SLE activity and lower BMD; however, the specific pathogenesis of osteoporosis due to SLE per se has yet to be elucidated [11,42]. In SLE, increased inflammatory mediators and cytokines, such as interleukin (IL)-6, IL-1, tumor necrosis factor (TNF)-$\alpha$, and receptor activator of nuclear factors $\kappa\beta$ ligand (RANKL) may create a milieu suitable for promoting accelerated bone remodeling and reducing BMD [43–46]. Currently, there is greater interest over the osteoprotegerin (OPG) and RANKL and RANK system as it appears to be an important regulator of bone metabolism. RANKL–RANK interaction is necessary for osteoclast differentiation and activation, whereas OPG can prevent RANKL binding to RANK and in turn inhibit osteoclast formation. In addition to the role of OPG–RANKL–RANK system in bone metabolism, this system also appears to be important in regulating immunity, but details linking bone loss in the setting of SLE, a prototypical condition of dysregulated immunity, presently remain unclear [47].

Data supporting SLE as a potential risk factor for bone loss come from studies demonstrating lower BMD in SLE women without prior glucocorticoid exposure than in healthy controls [7,9]. For instance, an association between cumulative disease damage, but not disease activity, and lower BMD not attributable to glucocorticoid use alone has been reported [11]. But this finding is inconsistent across published studies [14,22,27]. Other investigations have shown a relationship between longer disease duration and reduced BMD [12]. SLE patients with longer disease, however, may have higher cumulative corticosteroid exposure, which may account for lower levels of BMD seen in SLE [14]. Cumulative disease damage, disease activity, and duration of SLE were not found to be associated with lower BMD at the lumbar spine and femoral neck by Kipen and colleagues [14]; subjects in this particular study, however, had relatively mild disease as the overall disease damage due to SLE was low.

Active SLE has been associated with ovarian dysfunction, including transient and premature menopause, which may account for low BMD observed in some young SLE women of reproductive age that appears to be independent of glucocorticoid exposure [9,48,49]. It is important to recognize such patients since these women are at increased risk for developing osteoporosis later in life [8].

Although a less direct cause of bone loss, reduced physical activity due to fatigue and musculoskeletal symptoms, such as arthritis not uncommonly experienced by SLE patients, may also contribute to the development of osteoporosis. The benefits of exercise on maintaining BMD in women with low BMD are known [50]. Prospective data suggest regular exercise defined as a minimum of 40 minutes of aerobic exercise three times per week may be a protective factor for bone loss at the femoral neck in SLE patients receiving glucocorticoids [22].

Avoiding sunlight and using a topical sunscreen are commonly recommended to minimize the occurrence of SLE flares or exacerbation of disease symptoms. But this practice can potentially result in vitamin D deficiency, another risk factor for bone loss. Exposure to ultraviolet light allows dermal conversion of 7-dehydrocholesterol to an inert form of vitamin D, an important regulator of serum calcium levels. Subsequent hydroxylation in the liver and kidney leads to the production of the biologically active 1,25-dihydroxy-vitamin D, which in turn aids in both the intestinal absorption of dietary calcium and the maturation of osteoclasts that mobilize calcium from bone. Additionally, renal disease in SLE may disrupt production of active vitamin D and consequently lead to bone loss [51].

Specific therapies to manage SLE can affect bone mass via different mechanisms. The deleterious effects of glucocorticoids on bone and the increased risk for osteoporosis and fractures are well recognized in SLE and other rheumatic conditions [52,53] and seem to be independent of BMD status and prior fragility fractures [54]. The ability of glucocorticoids to induce bone loss and increase fracture risk occurs through both direct and indirect mechanisms. Glucocorticoids can inhibit osteoblastogenesis and promote apoptosis of osteoblasts and osteocytes, key cells in bone formation [55].

Glucocorticoid use in SLE patients is associated with lower BMD in cross-sectional studies, and both higher cumulative and daily dosages of glucocorticoids appear to be predictive of reduced BMD in longitudinal investigations [25]. Previous studies have documented reduced BMD either at the spine or hip among subjects who have SLE previously treated with glucocorticoids compared with healthy controls [12,14,29] in trabecular [32] and cortical bone [11]. Cumulative glucocorticoid dose has been associated with lower spine BMD in individuals who have SLE when compared with those who did not use glucocorticoid [9]. Furthermore, the duration of corticosteroid use, peak dose, and current use of corticosteroids have all been linked to diminished BMD at the spine and hip in SLE patients. Kipen and coworkers [14] found that corticosteroid use remained significantly associated with lower BMD even after accounting for age, body mass index, cumulative disease damage, disease activity, and duration of disease. However, not all studies have shown a similar relationship between glucocorticoid use in SLE, including dose or duration of use, and lower BMD at the lumbar spine or femoral neck [8,13]. Absence of a relationship in some reports may be partially attributable to a relatively small number of SLE subjects studied [37]. Other possible explanations may be that most longitudinal studies also include premenopausal women, thus minimizing the potential effect of bone loss due to menopause, bone loss may have occurred earlier in SLE, or bone loss in early disease may have been a result of initial exposure to corticosteroids, such that there are limited changes in BMD noted over time in some longitudinal studies [22].

Immunosuppressive therapies can also lead to ovarian dysfunction and indirectly reduce BMD. Cyclophosphamide, an important immunosuppressive agent used to treat organ or life-threatening SLE, is capable of inducing premature menopause [56,57] and is a disease-related risk factor for bone loss. Cyclosporine has been associated with osteoclast activation, osteoblast suppression, and retardation of bone formation. Low BMD seen with cyclosporine use has been reported primarily in posttransplant patients [58]. Nevertheless, cyclosporine remains a therapeutic option in SLE, and its use should be viewed as a potential risk factor for bone loss. High-dose methotrexate administration in the treatment of oncology patients has been associated with bone loss and fractures, but long-term administration and doses used to treat SLE have no reported adverse effects on BMD [59].

Bone loss can also be promoted by prolonged use of the anticoagulant therapy heparin. In some SLE patients, anticoagulants are required to manage hypercoagulable states, such as antiphospholipid antibody syndrome. Although oral anticoagulants such as warfarin or coumadin are usually the treatment of choice, they are contraindicated in pregnancy because of their associated risk for teratogenicity. Pregnant women who have SLE and secondary antiphospholipid syndrome are often treated with heparin to minimize their risk for miscarriage. Unfractionated heparin can reduce cancellous bone by promoting osteoclastic bone destruction and reducing osteoblastic activity. Patients on long-term unfractionated heparin may have up to a 30% reduction in BMD, and 2% to 3% of individuals may experience symptomatic vertebral fractures [60]. On the other hand, low molecular weight heparin seems to have less deleterious effect on bone than unfractionated heparin when used in SLE women during pregnancy [61].

Anticonvulsant therapy may be required for symptomatic treatment of seizures in patients who have neuropsychiatric SLE [62]. Chronic administration of anticonvulsants is an independent risk factor for lower BMD and has been associated with increased fractures. Although the mechanism by which anticonvulsants lead to these abnormalities is unclear, they may accelerate vitamin D metabolism, resulting in decreased calcium absorption, and cause secondary hyperparathyroidism and decreased BMD. Although no study has specifically assessed the potential bone loss with anticonvulsant use in SLE, chronic use of such drugs in SLE patients remains another factor that may contribute to bone loss [45].

## Evaluation of osteoporosis in systemic lupus erythematosus

Many of the current strategies for monitoring and diagnosing osteoporosis in the general population also apply to those who have SLE (Fig. 1). Loss of

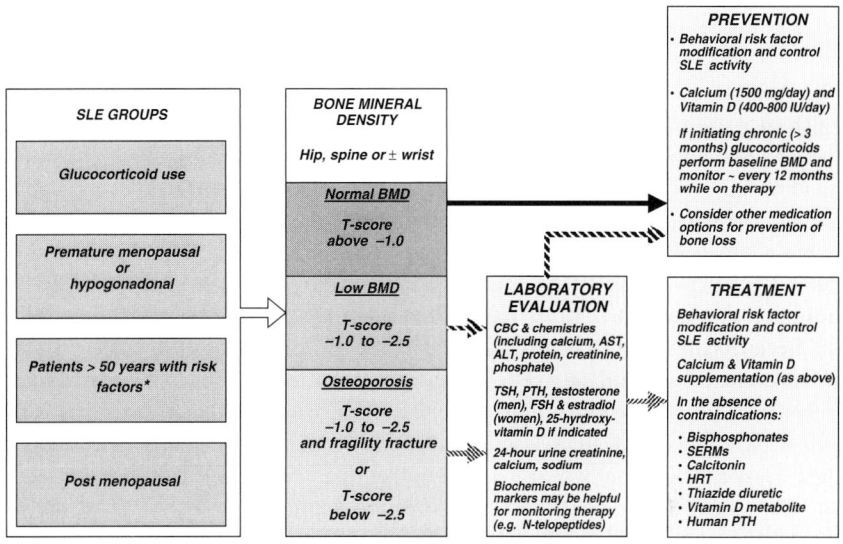

Fig. 1. Evaluation and management of bone health in systemic lupus erythematosus patients.

height and spinal kyphosis are late physical findings consistent with underlying osteoporosis, and the former has been a predictor of future fractures. Despite the potential for technical limitations, osteopenia identified on thoracic lumbar spine films can occur when there is loss of approximately 20% to 40% of bone mass [63]. SLE patients presenting with either physical or radiographic findings suggestive of underlying bone loss should prompt further investigation. In a study assessing factors associated with referral for BMD measurement in SLE, Pineau and coworkers [64] reported that patients receiving dual energy radiographic absorptiometry tended to have more traditional risks factors for osteoporosis, including older age and a higher proportion of patients were postmenopausal. Additionally, patients who had SLE undergoing BMD measurement had greater disease activity and damage, higher mean dose of corticosteroids, and a larger proportion had renal disease and ever used immunosuppressants.

Early detection of bone loss or low bone mass can be achieved by performing a BMD measurement. Because of the heterogeneity of bone loss in SLE, BMD measurement at both the spine and hip should be performed, and assessment of the distal forearm can provide further information. BMD measurements should be obtained at approximately 2-year intervals as this should allow for determination of a significant change. Differences of 2% to 3% at the lumbar spine and 4% to 6% at the hip are viewed as significant [63]. However, those at higher risk for new or recurrent fractures, such as individuals on glucocorticoid therapy or those with prior fragility fractures, can have a significant change in BMD over a shorter time interval, and obtaining BMD measurements as frequently as every 6 to 12 months may be warranted.

Despite the utility of BMD measurement as a means for assessing fracture risk, approximately 60% to 80% of bone strength is accounted by BMD, whereas the remaining 20% to 40% of bone strength is related to a number of factors, such as bone microarchitecture, underlying microfactures, bone turnover, all of which are components of bone quality. Suboptimal bone quality may not be evident based on BMD alone, and factures may occur even at BMD levels higher than expected. In a recent large longitudinal study, 82% of postmenopausal, white women who do not have SLE having BMD T-scores of −2.5 or less sustained fractures at 1 year [65]. Such data support the practice of interpreting BMD results in the context of other risk factors that may predispose to fractures [66].

Because the WHO classification using BMD for diagnosis of osteoporosis was originally developed for postmenopausal white women, this classification scheme may not be entirely applicable to premenopausal women, men, and non-whites who have SLE [67]. In premenopausal women, the diagnosis of osteoporosis in premenopausal women should not be made on the basis of densitometric criteria alone. When BMD measurements are applied in the clinical setting of lupus, the corresponding Z-scores, rather than T-scores, may need to be considered when interpreting the results, and osteoporosis may be diagnosed if there is reduced BMD with secondary causes or with risk factors for fracture. Additionally, the Z-scores should be adjusted for ethnicity. In men aged 65 years and older, the T-scores should be applied and osteoporosis diagnosed if the T-score is at or below −2.5, using a male reference database. For men between the ages of 50 and 65 years, the T-scores may be applied and a diagnosis of osteoporosis made if both the T-score is at or below −2.5 in the presence of other risk factors for fractures. On the other hand, osteoporosis may be diagnosed in men of any age with low BMD and secondary causes of low BMD (eg, glucocorticoid therapy, hypogonadism, hyperparathyroidism). For nonwhites, the previous guidelines may be followed, but the Z-scores, rather than T-scores, should be used to determine *low bone density*, defined as two standard deviations below the mean [37].

Women who have SLE and low bone density should be assessed for underlying secondary causes of osteoporosis, other than bone loss due to medications, which may be correctable (Box 2). The initial laboratory evaluation should include a complete blood count with differential, serum chemistries, including calcium, alkaline phosphatase, creatinine, as well as a thyroid stimulating hormone and parathyroid hormone levels. Additional tests, such as bone-specific alkaline phosphatase, serum hormone levels (eg, testosterone, follicular stimulating hormone), and urinary electrolytes can be assessed if clinically appropriate [68]. With respect to bone biochemical markers, lower levels of osteocalcin, a marker associated with bone formation, and elevated serum carboxyterminal cross-linked telopeptide of type I collagen, indicative of bone resorption, have been observed in SLE patients, suggesting bone loss due to disease [21,27]. Yet, other studies have found no appreciable correlation between bone biochemical markers with bone loss in SLE [14,28]. Inconsistency in the predictive value of bone biochemical markers for lowering of BMD in SLE patients may be

---

**Box 2. Secondary causes of bone loss not related to medications**

- Hypogonadism
- Hypercortisolism
- Renal disease
- Malabsorptive states
- Primary hyperparathyroidism
- Thyrotoxicosis
- Growth hormone deficiency
- Osteomalacia
- Connective tissue disorders (other than systemic lupus erythematosus)
- Hypophosphatasia
- Mastocytosis
- Myeloproliferative disorders
- Hepatic disorders
- Inflammatory bowel disease
- Hypercalcemia
- Osteogenesis imperfecta

---

due to the relatively small numbers of subjects evaluated in published studies. Since bone biochemical markers reflect the dynamic nature of bone turnover, multiple measurements over time may better predict future changes in BMD and may indeed be useful in monitoring SLE patients. Further study will help define the clinical utility of bone biochemical markers in management of bone health in SLE. Similarly, active investigation of the potential role of cytokines and inflammatory mediators likely involved in the pathogenesis of osteoporosis in SLE is ongoing, and at present, their clinical applicability is yet undefined.

**Prevention and treatment of osteoporosis in systemic lupus erythematosus**

Initial preventive measures consist of behavioral modification of both traditional and SLE-related risk factors when possible (see Fig. 1). Minimizing frequency and severity of SLE disease activity is in itself a treatment goal, but it may also have long-term benefit on bone health. Beyond modification of risk factors, specific therapeutic agents available for prevention and treatment of bone loss in SLE patients are discussed later.

*Calcium and vitamin D*

Calcium supplementation alone has been shown to have a modest but statistically significant positive effect on BMD at one or more skeletal sites in both perimenopausal and postmenopausal women [69]. In a double-blinded randomized, placebo-controlled study investigating the prevention of glucocorticoid-induced osteoporosis in a group of subjects who had a variety of inflammatory diseases, including SLE, there was no significant difference in percent change in BMD at 36 months between vitamin D plus 1000 mg per day of calcium versus placebo [70]. However, recent meta-analyses have found a benefit of calcium supplementation for prevention of bone loss and a trend toward reduction of vertebral fractures, but it is unclear whether calcium intake reduces the incidence of nonvertebral fractures [71,72]. In another meta-analysis, vitamin D plus calcium was superior to no therapy or calcium alone in the management of glucocorticoid-induced osteoporosis [73]. Because of low toxicity and cost, all patients being started on glucocorticoids should receive prophylactic therapy with calcium and vitamin D in the absence of any contraindications, including nephrolithiasis, hypercalciuria, or hypocalcemia. Adult SLE patients on glucocorticoid therapy should receive 1500 mg per day of oral calcium supplementation [74]. Vitamin D at the generally recommended amount of 400 to 800 IU can aid in absorption of dietary calcium and may assist in maintaining BMD and reduce risk of fractures and therefore should be taken with calcium supplementation [71,75,76]. Currently, there is insufficient information on any protective benefits of calcium with or without vitamin D supplementation in SLE patients who are premenopausal or not receiving glucocorticoids.

*Hormone therapy*

Hormone replacement therapy (HRT) has proven benefits for increasing BMD both in younger perimenopausal and older postmenopausal non-SLE women [71]. Kung and coworkers [77] assessed the efficacy of calcitriol and HRT in 28 hypogonadal women who have SLE having a history of chronic steroid use of more than 10 mg per day. Women were randomized to receive either HRT consisting of conjugated conjugated estrogen (0.625 mg)–progesterone combination or calcitriol 0.5 μg daily. All women also were given 1 g of calcium carbonate per day. After 2 years, the HRT-treated women had a 2.0% increase in lumbar spine BMD, whereas the calcitriol group experienced 1.7% reduction in BMD. Additionally, whereas women given HRT had no change in BMD at the distal radius, those in the calcitriol group were found to have a 2.3% loss in BMD at this site. There were no adverse effects of HRT on disease activity [77]. Similarly, results of a 1-year randomized, double-blind, placebo-controlled trial suggested that transdermal estradiol may prevent bone loss in postmenopausal SLE women at the lumbar spine and femur without increasing disease activity [28]. The use of hormones in SLE is controversial despite its benefits for bone health. In addition to lupus being a disease of young women of reproductive age, estrogen exposure causes worsening of disease in murine models of lupus, and there have been case reports of disease flares in SLE patients receiving hormones [78]. Additionally, in a large prospective cohort study (part of the Nurses' Health Study) the incidence of SLE—defined as those meeting ACR criteria for SLE and a diagnosis of SLE by an ACR member—showed an approximate twofold increase (RR = 1.9, 95% CI: 1.1 to 3.3) in women who used oral contraceptives compared with those who never did [79]. A more recent population-based, case-control study, however, failed to find an increased risk of SLE with estrogen exposure [80].

Exogenous estrogen can increase hypercoagulability, therefore HRT and oral contraceptive use is contraindicated in SLE patients who have antiphospholipid syndrome [81]. Additionally, data from the Women's Health Initiative indicated HRT reduced hip and vertebral fractures, but the study was prematurely halted due to adverse events in cardiovascular-related mortality and breast cancer endpoints [82]. With accumulating evidence of increased cardiovascular risk in SLE, there is added concern over the potential cardiovascular risk posed by use of hormone therapy in SLE patients. Nevertheless, the bone benefits of hormones may be gained by SLE patients who require HRT for menopausal symptoms severe enough to interfere with their quality of life, as well as in those individuals who cannot take other bone protective agents. Any plans to initiate hormone therapy in SLE patients should be done only after the risks and benefits of HRT have been thoroughly discussed between patient and physician.

*Selective estrogen receptor modulators*

Selective estrogen receptor modulators (SERMs), such as raloxifene and tamoxifene, interact with the estrogen receptor to induce selective agonist or antagonist action in estrogen-responsive target tissues. Raloxifene is approved for treatment of postmenopausal osteoporosis. Raloxifene given at 60 mg per day has been shown to increase BMD in the spine and femoral neck, decrease vertebral, but not nonvertebral fractures, and is currently approved for the prevention and treatment of postmenopausal osteoporosis [83]. Similar to HRT, women receiving raloxifene had increased risk of venous thromboembolus compared with women taking placebo (RR = 3.1; 95% CI: 1.5 to 6.2). Unlike HRT, raloxifene has not been associated with any increased risk for cardiovascular events [84]. Physicians should consider bone protective agents other than SERMs for SLE patients who have antiphospholipid syndrome or underlying hypercoagulopathy. However, raloxifene may be an alternative option for SLE patients requiring bone protective agents who are not ideal candidates for HRT and have no risk factors for hypercoagulopathy as it modestly improves BMD in non-SLE patients.

*Bisphosphonates*

Bisphosphonates possess a high affinity for bone hydroxyapatite and are potent inhibitors of osteoclastic bone resorption. The ability of bisphosphonates to increase BMD and reduce vertebral and nonvertebral fractures has been demonstrated in randomized controlled trials. Additionally, bisphosphonates can also preserve BMD in patients receiving long-term glucocorticoid therapy [85]. In the absence of contraindications, bisphosphonates should be considered for use in SLE patients who have osteoporosis or prior fragility fractures, as well as for prevention of glucocorticoid-induced osteoporosis because of their proven efficacy for reducing fractures.

Of the clinically used bisphosphonates, only alendronate and residronate are approved by the US Food and Drug Administration (FDA) for use in osteoporosis and glucocorticoid-induced osteoporosis. Both agents are taken orally, and daily and weekly doses are available for prevention and treatment of osteoporosis. Alendronate increases spine and hip BMD and significantly lowers the risk of vertebral, hip, and forearm fractures a compared with placebo in postmenopausal women [86,87]. Alendronate (10 mg/day or 70 mg/week) is approved for prevention and treatment of postmenopausal osteoporosis, whereas lower doses (5 mg/day or 35 mg/week) may be used in the prevention and treatment of glucocorticoid-induced osteoporosis. Similar to alendronate, residronate has been shown to increase spine and hip BMD and reduce fracture risk at the spine and hip [88,89]. Risedronate is approved for use at 5 mg per day, and 35 mg per week is for treatment of postmenopausal osteoporosis; same dosages may be used in the management of glucocorticoid-induced osteoporosis.

Etidronate is a cyclically administered bisphosphonate, which is a non-FDA–approved therapy for treatment of osteoporosis. Etidronate given orally at a dose of 400 mg per day for 14 days followed by 76 days of elemental calcium (500 mg/day) and then repetition of this cycle four times a year for 2 years has been demonstrated to increase spine BMD by up to 2.2% and maintain hip BMD while reducing rate of vertebral fractures in postmenopausal women and in subjects taking glucocorticoids in placebo-controlled trials [90,91]. Pamidronate is an intravenously administered bisphosphonate, and it is currently approved for treatment of hypercalcemia of malignancy and Paget's disease, but not for osteoporosis. Yet, pamidronate has been used off-label to treat postmenopausal and corticosteroid-induced osteoporosis and prevent postmenopausal osteoporosis. Pamidronate is administered intravenously in most cases with initial dose of 90 mg and subsequently 30 mg every 3 months [92]. Zoledronic acid is also given intravenously and has been used in the treatment of hypercalcemia of malignancy in multiple myeloma and bone metastasis. Like etidronate and pamidronate, zoledronic acid is not approved for use in the treatment of osteoporosis. Zoledronic acid, however, has been shown to improve BMD at the spine and hip up to 5.1% and 3.5% higher than placebo, respectively, while suppressing markers of bone resorption, even in those given a single dose of 4 mg in a 1-year study [93]. Current study is ongoing to evaluate the potential use of zoledronic acid in postmenopausal women who have osteoporosis.

*Calcitonin*

Calcitonin, an endogenous peptide that inhibits osteoclast activity, is available in nasal, subcutaneous, and intramuscular form and may be offered as an alternative for SLE patients who are unable to take HRT, raloxifene, or bisphosphonates. It has been shown to increase BMD in the spine and femoral neck [94] and decrease vertebral fractures, but convincing data for nonvertebral fractures are lacking. In light of the limited information on fracture prevention, calcitonin should be regarded as second-line therapy in managing osteoporosis in SLE patients. Additionally, calcitonin may relieve acute pain resulting from vertebral fractures [85] and therefore may be of benefit in pain reduction in SLE patients sustaining vertebral fractures.

*Parathyroid hormone*

Human parathyroid hormone or (hPTH) is an endogenous, 84-amino-acid peptide with anabolic properties that can promote bone formation. Although primary hyperparathyroidism or conditions of endogenous sustained excess hPTH have been known to contribute to cortical bone loss, intermittent administration of hPTH can increase BMD to a greater extent than can other available agents, restore the microarchitecture, and increase bone size [95,96]. hPTH given at the 40-$\mu$g dose has been shown to reduce both vertebral fractures (RR = 0.35; 95% CI: 0.22 to 0.55) and nonvertebral fragility fractures (RR = 0.47; 95% CI: 0.25 to 0.88) [97]. hPTH is being evaluated as a potential therapeutic agent for glucocorticoid-induced osteoporosis, but at present, no data exist to recommend its use either for prevention or treatment of glucocorticoid-induced osteoporosis in the setting of SLE or otherwise. Among its contraindications, hPTH is not approved for use in children and young adults with open epiphyses or women during pregnancy. Notably, long-term hPTH at high doses has been associated with an increased risk of osteosarcoma in rats, but no cases of osteosarcoma have been reported in human trials [85]. hPTH should be viewed as second-line therapy and reserved for SLE patients at greatest risk for fractures or with prior or current fragility fractures in whom bisphosphonate therapy is poorly tolerated or contraindicated. Due to limited data on the long-term effects, hPTH administration should be limited to no more than 1 to 2 years.

*Combination therapies and potential future treatments*

HRT combined with alendronate appears to improve BMD to a greater extent than either agent used alone. Risedronate and estrogen used together have demonstrated small increases in BMD at the spine, hip, and wrist after 1 year. However, there is rapid bone loss after withdrawal of HRT. Similarly, raloxifene combined with alendronate appears to modestly improve BMD at the spine, hip (femoral neck), and wrist compared with either agent used alone. Studies have suggested that gains in BMD achieved with PTH treatment can be preserved when followed by alendronate or estrogen therapy [85]. On the other hand, there is no evidence of synergy between PTH and alendronate, and concurrent use of alendronate may reduce the anabolic effects of PTH [98]. Similarly, the use of alendronate has been shown to impair the ability of PTH to increase BMD at the lumbar spine and the femoral neck in men [99].

The benefits of hydroxychloroquine in SLE are well recognized, but there are minimal data on bone health. Hydroxychloroquine use has been associated with higher BMD of the hip and spine in women who have SLE [17], but additional studies are needed to validate these findings and to determine whether any benefit exists for lowering fracture occurrence. Thiazide diuretics have been shown to improve gastrointestinal absorption and decrease urinary excretion of calcium, which can help minimize hypercalciuria associated with glucocorticoid use. In the setting of low urinary calcium, SLE patients receiving glucocorticoid therapy may benefit from thiazide diuretics as a means to prevent bone loss [48]. Dehydroepiandrosterone (DHEA) or prasterone, a weak androgen used to control lupus activity, may be useful in preserving BMD in SLE patients receiving glucocorticoids [100], but further study is ongoing. Other agents, including fluoride, insulin growth factor type 1 (IGF-I), and statins may have some benefit in improving BMD in SLE patients, but results of active clinical trials will shed greater light on their clinical utility. Finally, other potential future therapies for reducing bone loss in SLE may include biologic agents involving monoclonal antibodies directed against specific cytokine targets, such IL-1, IL-6, and RANK-L. An initial placebo-controlled study of a fully human monoclonal antibodies to RANK-L appears to reduce both serum and urine markers of bone turn over in postmenopausal women may hold promise for future use in populations at risk for bone loss, such as SLE [101].

## Summary

Bone loss and fractures are emerging as important lupus-related conditions paralleling increased SLE incidence and survival. Bone loss in SLE is likely a multifactorial process involving both traditional and SLE-related risk factors for osteoporosis. Improved recognition of these risk factors is essential for early identification and prompt initiation of preventive measures to minimize further bone loss and fracture risk. Currently available knowledge on agents used in the prevention and treatment of osteoporosis in SLE is largely derived from studies performed in the non-SLE population. Therefore, awareness of specific caveats in the use of bone protective agents germane to SLE is important to optimize bone health and minimize therapeutic toxicity in the SLE patient.

## References

[1] Gordon C. Long-term complications of systemic lupus erythematosus. Rheumatology (Oxford) 2002;41(10):1095–100.
[2] Urowitz MB, Gladman DD, Abu-Shakra M, Farewell VT. Mortality studies in systemic lupus erythematosus. Results from a single center. III. Improved survival over 24 years. J Rheumatol 1997;24(6):1061–5.
[3] Uramoto KM, Michet Jr CJ, Thumboo J, et al. Trends in the incidence and mortality of systemic lupus erythematosus, 1950–1992. Arthritis Rheum 1999;42(1):46–50.

[4] Trager J, Ward MM. Mortality and causes of death in systemic lupus erythematosus. Curr Opin Rheumatol 2001;13(5):345–51.

[5] Sacks JJ, Helmick CG, Langmaid G, et al. Trends in deaths from systemic lupus erythematosus—United States, 1979–1998. MMWR Morb Mortal Wkly Rep 2002;51(17):371–4.

[6] Cervera R, Khamashta MA, Font J, et al. European Working Party on systemic lupus erythematosus. morbidity and mortality in systemic lupus erythematosus during a 10-year period: a comparison of early and late manifestations in a cohort of 1,000 patients. Medicine (Baltimore) 2003;82(5):299–308.

[7] Kalla AA, Fataar AB, Jessop SJ, Bewerunge L. Loss of trabecular bone mineral density in systemic lupus erythematosus. Arthritis Rheum 1993;36(12):1726–34.

[8] Formiga F, Moga I, Nolla JM, et al. Loss of bone mineral density in premenopausal women who have systemic lupus erythematosus. Ann Rheum Dis 1995;54(4):274–6.

[9] Houssiau FA, Lefebvre C, Depresseux G, et al. Trabecular and cortical bone loss in systemic lupus erythematosus. Br J Rheumatol 1996;35:244–7.

[10] Trapani S, Civinini R, Ermini M, et al. Osteoporosis in juvenile systemic lupus erythematosus: a longitudinal study on the effect of steroids on bone mineral density. Rheumatol Int 1998;18:45–9.

[11] Sinigaglia L, Varenna M, Binelli L, et al. Determinants of bone mass in systemic lupus erythematosus: a cross sectional study on premenopausal women. J Rheumatol 1999;26(6): 1280–4.

[12] Pons F, Peris P, Guanabens N, et al. The effect of systemic lupus erythematosus and long-term steroid therapy on bone mass in pre-menopausal women. Br J Rheumatol 1995;34(8): 742–6.

[13] Kalla AA, van Wyk Kotze TJ, Meyers OL. Metacarpal bone mass in systemic lupus erythematosus. Clin Rheumatol 1992;11(4):475–82.

[14] Kipen Y, Buchbinder R, Forbes A, et al. Prevalence of reduced bone mineral density in systemic lupus erythematosus and the role of steroids. J Rheumatol 1997;24(10):1922–9.

[15] Gilboe I, Kvien TK, Haugeberg G, Husby G. Bone mineral density in systemic lupus erythematosus: comparison with rheumatoid arthritis and healthy controls. Ann Rheum Dis 2000; 59(2):110–5.

[16] Jardinet D, Lefebvre C, Depresseux G, et al. Longitudinal analysis of bone mineral density in pre-menopausal female systemic lupus erythematosus patients: deleterious role of glucocorticoid therapy at the lumbar spine. Rheumatology (Oxford) 2000;39(4):389–92.

[17] Lakshminarayanan S, Walsh S, Mohanraj M, Rothfield N. Factors associated with low bone mineral density in female patients with systemic lupus erythematosus. J Rheumatol 2001;28(1): 102–8.

[18] Becker A, Fischer R, Scherbaum WA, Schneider M. Osteoporosis screening in systemic lupus erythematosus: impact of disease duration and organ damage. Lupus 2001;10(11):809–14.

[19] Leong NM, Shamiyeh E, Chung AH, et al. Longitudinal analysis of bone mineral density in women with recent onset systemic lupus erythematosus. J Bone Miner Res 2003;18(2):S398.

[20] Swaak AJ, van den Brink HG, Smeenk RJ, et al. Systemic lupus erythematosus: clinical features in patients with a disease duration of over 10 years, first evaluation. Rheumatology (Oxford) 1999;38(10):953–8.

[21] Redlich K, Ziegler S, Kiener HP, et al. Bone mineral density and biochemical parameters of bone metabolism in female patients with systemic lupus erythematosus. Ann Rheum Dis 2000;59(4):308–10.

[22] Kipen Y, Briganti E, Strauss B, et al. Three year followup of bone mineral density change in premenopausal women with systemic lupus erythematosus. J Rheumatol 1999;26(2):310–7.

[23] Uaratanawong S, Deesomchoke U, Lertmaharit S, Uaratanawong S. Bone mineral density in premenopausal women with systemic lupus erythematosus. J Rheumatol 2003;30(11):2365–8.

[24] Teichmann J, Lange U, Stracke H, et al. Bone metabolism and bone mineral density of systemic lupus erythematosus at the time of diagnosis. Rheumatol Int 1999;18(4):137–40.

[25] Petri M. Musculoskeletal complications of systemic lupus erythematosus in the Hopkins Lupus Cohort: an update. Arthritis Care Res 1995;8(3):137–45.

[26] Formiga F, Nolla JM, Mitjavila F, et al. Bone mineral density and hormonal status in men with systemic lupus erythematosus. Lupus 1996;5(6):623–6.

[27] Hansen M, Halberg P, Kollerup G, et al. Bone metabolism in patients with systemic lupus erythematosus. Effect of disease activity and glucocorticoid treatment. Scand J Rheumatol 1998;27(3):197–206.

[28] Bhattoa HP, Kiss E, Bettembuk P, Balogh A. Bone mineral density, biochemical markers of bone turnover, and hormonal status in men with systemic lupus erythematosus. Rheumatol Int 2001;21(3):97–102.

[29] Li EK, Tam LS, Young RP, et al. Loss of bone mineral density in Chinese pre-menopausal women with systemic lupus erythematosus treated with corticosteroids. Br J Rheumatol 1998; 37(4):405–10.

[30] Cummings S, Melton III LJ. Epidemiology and outcomes of osteoporotic fractures. Lancet 2002;359(9319):1761–7.

[31] Chadha A, Shamiyeh E, Manzi S, et al. Race may not protect against low bone mineral density in women with lupus. J Bone Miner Res 2003;18(2):S154.

[32] Boyanov M, Robeva R, Popivanov P. Bone mineral density changes in women with systemic lupus erythematosus. Clin Rheumatol 2003;22(4–5):318–23.

[33] Dhillon VB, Davies MC, Hall ML, et al. Assessment of the effect of oral corticosteroids on bone mineral density in systemic lupus erythematosus: a preliminary study with dual energy x-ray absorptiometry. Ann Rheum Dis 1990;49(8):624–6.

[34] Ramsey-Goldman R, Dunn JE, Huang CF, Dunlop D, et al. Frequency of fractures in women with systemic lupus erythematosus: comparison with United States population data. Arthritis Rheum 1999;42(5):882–90.

[35] Melton III LJ, Thamer M, Ray NF, et al. Fractures attributable to osteoporosis: report form the National Osteoporosis Foundation. J Bone Miner Res 1997;12:16–23.

[36] Kanis JA, Melton 3rd LJ, Christiansen C, et al. The diagnosis of osteoporosis. J Bone Miner Res 1994;9(8):1137–41.

[37] International Society for Clinical Densitometry Position Development Conference. Position statement: diagnosis of osteoporosis in men, pre-menopausal women, and children. The writing group for the ISCD position development conference. J Clin Densitometry 2004;7(1): 17–26.

[38] Hannan MT, Felson DT, Dawson-Hughes B, et al. Risk factors for longitudinal bone loss in elderly men and women: the Framingham Osteoporosis Study. J Bone Miner Res 2000; 15(4):710–20.

[39] Lunt M, Masaryk P, Scheidt-Nave C, et al. The effects of lifestyle, dietary dairy intake and diabetes on bone density and vertebral deformity prevalence: the EVOS study. Osteoporos Int 2001;12(8):688–98.

[40] Albrand G, Munoz G, Sornay-Rendu E, et al. Independent predictors of all osteoporosis-related fractures in healthy postmenopausal women: the OFELY study. Bone 2003;32(1): 78–85.

[41] Bainbridge KE, Sowers M, Lin X, Harlow SD. Risk factors for low bone mineral density and the 6-year rate of bone loss among premenopausal and perimenopausal women. Osteoporos Int 2004;15(6):439–46.

[42] Schapira D, Kabala A, Raz B, Israeli E. Osteoporosis in murine systemic lupus erythematosus– a laboratory model. Lupus 2001;10(6):431–8.

[43] Al-Janadi M, Al-Dalaan A, al-Balla S, et al. Interleukin-10 (IL-10) secretion in systemic lupus erythematosus and rheumatoid arthritis: IL-10-dependent CD4 + CD45RO + T cell-B cell antibody synthesis. J Clin Immunol 1996;16(4):198–207.

[44] Tanaka Y, Watanabe K, Suzuki M, et al. Spontaneous production of bone-resorbing lymphokines by B cells in patients with systemic lupus erythematosus. J Clin Immunol 1989;9(5): 415–20.

[45] Linker-Israeli M, Deans RJ, Wallace DJ, et al. Elevated levels of endogenous IL-6 in systemic lupus erythematosus. A putative role in pathogenesis. J Immunol 1991;147(1):117–23.

[46] MacDonald BR, Gowen M. Cytokines and bone. Br J Rheumatol 1992;31(3):149–55.

[47] Stolina M, Guo J, Faggioni R, et al. Regulatory effects of osteoprotegerin on cellular and humoral immune responses. Clin Immunol 2003;109(3):347–54.

[48] Pasoto SG, Mendonca BB, Bonfa E. Menstrual disturbances in patients with systemic lupus erythematosus without alkylating therapy: clinical, hormonal and therapeutic associations. Lupus 2002;11(3):175–80.

[49] Medeiros MC, Silveira VL, Menezes AT, Carvalho RC. Risk factors for ovarian failure in patients with systemic lupus erythematosus. Braz J Med Biol Res 2001;34(12):1561–8.

[50] Kemmler W, Lauber D, Weineck J, et al. Benefits of 2 years of intense exercise on bone density, physical fitness, and blood lipids in early postmenopausal osteopenic women: results of the Erlangen Fitness Osteoporosis Prevention Study (EFOPS). Arch Intern Med 2004; 164(10):1084–91.

[51] Sen D, Keen RW. Osteoporosis in systemic lupus erythematosus: prevention and treatment. Lupus 2001;10(3):227–32.

[52] Hooyman JR, Melton 3rd LJ, Nelson AM, et al. Fractures after rheumatoid arthritis. A population based study. Arthritis Rheum 1984;27(12):1353–61.

[53] Cooper C, Coupland C, Mitchell M. Rheumatoid arthritis, corticosteroid therapy and hip fracture. Ann Rheum Dis 1995;54(1):49–52.

[54] Kanis JA, Johansson H, Oden A, et al. A meta-analysis of prior corticosteroid use and fracture risk. J Bone Miner Res 2004;19(6):893–9.

[55] Weinstein RS, Jilka RL, Parfitt AM, Manolagas SC. Inhibition of osteoblastogenesis and promotion of apoptosis of osteoblasts and osteocytes by glucocorticoids. Potential mechanisms of their deleterious effects on bone. J Clin Invest 1998;102(2):274–82.

[56] Boumpas DT, Austin 3rd HA, Vaughan EM, et al. Risk for sustained amenorrhea in patients with systemic lupus erythematosus receiving intermittent pulse cyclophosphamide therapy. Ann Intern Med 1993;119(5):366–9.

[57] Huong du L, Amoura Z, Duhaut P, et al. Risk of ovarian failure and fertility after intravenous cyclophosphamide. A study in 84 patients. J Rheumatol 2002;29(12):2571–6.

[58] Cueto-Manzano AM, Konel S, Crowley V, et al. Bone histopathology and densitometry comparison between cyclosporine a monotherapy and prednisolone plus azathioprine dual immunosuppression in renal transplant patients. Transplantation 2003;75(12):2053–8.

[59] Cranney AB, McKendry RJ, Wells GA, et al. The effect of low dose methotrexate on bone density. J Rheumatol 2001;28(11):2395–9.

[60] Ruiz-Irastorza G, Khamashta MA, Nelson-Piercy C, Hughes GR. Lupus pregnancy: is heparin a risk factor for osteoporosis? Lupus 2001;10(9):597–600.

[61] Pettila V, Leinonen P, Markkola A, et al. Postpartum bone mineral density in women treated for thromboprophylaxis with unfractionated heparin or LMW heparin. Thromb Haemost 2002; 11:680–2.

[62] Brey RL, Escalante A. Neurological manifestations of antiphospholipid antibody syndrome [review]. Lupus 1998;7(Suppl 2):S67–74.

[63] Marcus R, Feldman D, Kelsey J. Osteoporosis. In: Jergas M, Genant HK, editors. Imaging of osteoporosis. 2nd edition. vol. 2. San Diego: Academic Press, Harcourt Science and Technology Co; 2001. p. 411–31.

[64] Pineau CA, Urowitz MB, Fortin PJ, et al. Osteoporosis in systemic lupus erythematosus: factors associated with referral for bone mineral density studies, prevalence of osteoporosis and factors associated with reduced bone density. Lupus 2004;13(6):436–41.

[65] Siris ES, Chen YT, Abbott TA, et al. Bone mineral density thresholds for pharmacological intervention to prevent fractures. Arch Intern Med 2004;164(10):1108–12.

[66] Espallargues M, Sampietro-Colom L, Estrada MD, et al. Identifying bone-mass-related risk actors for fracture to guide bone densitometry measurements: a systematic review of the literature. Osteoporos Int 2001;12(10):811–22.

[67] Cummings SR, Bates D, Black DM. Clinical use of bone densitometry: scientific review. JAMA 2002;288(15):1889–97.

[68] Farhat G, Yamout B, Mikati MA, et al. Effect of antiepileptic drugs on bone density in ambulatory patients. Neurology 2002;58(9):1348–53.

[69] Nordin BE. Calcium and osteoporosis. Nutrition 1997;13(7–8):664–86.

[70] Adachi JD, Bensen WG, Bianchi F, et al. Vitamin D and calcium in the prevention of corticosteroid induced osteoporosis: a 3 year followup. J Rheumatol 1996;23(6):995–1000.

[71] Shea B, Wells G, Cranney A, et al. Osteoporosis Methodology Group and The Osteoporosis Research Advisory Group. Meta-analyses of therapies for postmenopausal osteoporosis VII: meta-analysis of calcium supplementation for the prevention of postmenopausal osteoporosis. Endocr Rev 2002;23:552–9.

[72] Homik J, Suarez-Almazor ME, Shea B, et al. Calcium and vitamin D for corticosteroid-induced osteoporosis. Cochrane Database Syst Rev 2000;(2):CD000952.

[73] Amin S, LaValley MP, Simms RW, Felson DT. The role of vitamin D in corticosteroid-induced osteoporosis: a meta-analytic approach. Arthritis Rheum 1999;42(8):1740–51.

[74] Nishimura J, Ikuyama S. Glucocorticoid-induced osteoporosis: pathogenesis and management. J Bone Miner Metab 2000;18(6):350–2.

[75] Sambrook P, Birmingham J, Kelly P, et al. Prevention of corticosteroid osteoporosis. A comparison of calcium, calcitriol, and calcitonin. N Engl J Med 1993;328(24):1747–52.

[76] American College of Rheumatology Ad Hoc Committee on Glucocorticoid-Induced Osteoporosis. Recommendations for the prevention and treatment of glucocorticoid-induced osteoporosis: 2001 update. Arthritis Rheum 2001;44(7):1496–503.

[77] Kung AW, Chan TM, Lau CS, et al. Osteopenia in young hypogonadal women with systemic lupus erythematosus receiving chronic steroid therapy: a randomized controlled trial comparing calcitriol and hormonal replacement therapy. Rheumatology (Oxford) 1999;38(12): 1239–44.

[78] Askanase AD, Buyon JP. Reproductive health in SLE. Best Pract Res Clin Rheumatol 2002; 16(2):265–80.

[79] Sanchez-Guerrero J, Karlson EW, Liang MH, et al. Past use of oral contraceptives and the risk of developing systemic lupus erythematosus. Arthritis Rheum 1997;40(5):804–8.

[80] Cooper GS, Dooley MA, Treadwell EL, et al. Hormonal and reproductive risk factors for development of systemic lupus erythematosus: results of a population-based, case-control study. Arthritis Rheum 2002;46(7):1830–9.

[81] Lakasing L, Khamashta M. Contraceptive practices in women with systemic lupus erythematosus and/or antiphospholipid syndrome: what advice should we be giving? J Fam Plann Reprod Health Care 2001;27(1):7–12.

[82] Rossouw JE, Anderson GL, Prentice RL, et al. Writing Group for the Women's Health Initiative Investigators. Risks and benefits of estrogen plus progestin in healthy postmenopausal women: principal results From the Women's Health Initiative randomized controlled trial. JAMA 2002;288(3):321–33.

[83] Ettinger B, Black DM, Mitlak BH, et al. Reduction of vertebral fracture risk in postmenopausal women with osteoporosis treated with raloxifene: results from a 3-year randomized clinical trial. Multiple Outcomes of Raloxifene Evaluation (MORE) Investigators. JAMA 1999;282(7): 637–45.

[84] Barrett-Connor E, Grady D, Sashegyi A, et al. MORE Investigators (Multiple Outcomes of Raloxifene Evaluation). Raloxifene and cardiovascular events in osteoporotic postmenopausal women: four-year results from the MORE (Multiple Outcomes of Raloxifene Evaluation) randomized trial. JAMA 2002;287(7):847–57.

[85] Brown SA, Rosen CJ. Osteoporosis. Med Clin North Am 2003;87(5):1039–63.

[86] Liberman UA, Weiss SR, Broll J, et al. Effect of oral alendronate on bone mineral density and the incidence of fractures in postmenopausal osteoporosis. The Alendronate Phase III Osteoporosis Treatment Study Group. N Engl J Med 1995;333(22):1437–43.

[87] Cummings SR, Black DM, Thompson DE, et al. Effect of alendronate on risk of fracture in women with low bone density but without vertebral fractures: results from the Fracture Intervention Trial. JAMA 1998;280:2077–82.

[88] Reginster J, Minne HW, Sorensen OH, et al. Randomized trial of the effects of risedronate on vertebral fractures in women with established postmenopausal osteoporosis. Vertebral Efficacy with Risedronate Therapy (VERT) Study Group. Osteoporos Int 2000;11(1):83–91.

[89] McClung MR, Geusens P, Miller PD, et al. Hip Intervention Program Study Group. Effect of risedronate on the risk of hip fracture in elderly women. Hip Intervention Program Study Group. N Engl J Med 2001;344(5):333–40.

[90] Miller PD, Watts NB, Licata AA, et al. Cyclical etidronate in the treatment of postmenopausal osteoporosis: efficacy and safety after seven years of treatment. Am J Med 1997;103(6): 468–76.

[91] Adachi JD, Bensen WG, Brown J, et al. Intermittent etidronate therapy to prevent corticosteroid-induced osteoporosis. N Engl J Med 1997;337(6):382–7.

[92] Chan SS, Nery LM, McElduff A, et al. Intravenous pamidronate in the treatment and prevention of osteoporosis. Intern Med J 2004;34(4):162–6.

[93] Reid IR, Brown JP, Burckhardt P, et al. Intravenous zoledronic acid in postmenopausal women with low bone mineral density. N Engl J Med 2002;346(9):653–61.

[94] Cardona JM, Pastor E. Calcitonin versus etidronate for the treatment of postmenopausal osteoporosis: a meta-analysis of published clinical trials. Osteoporos Int 1997;7(3):165–74.

[95] Ejersted C, Andreassen TT, Oxlund H, et al. Human parathyroid hormone (1–34) and (1–84) increase the mechanical strength and thickness of cortical bone in rats. J Bone Miner Res 1993; 8(9):1097–101.

[96] Jilka RL, Weinstein RS, Bellido T, et al. Increased bone formation by prevention of osteoblast apoptosis with parathyroid hormone. J Clin Invest 1999;104(4):439–46.

[97] Neer RM, Arnaud CD, Zanchetta JR, et al. Effect of parathyroid hormone (1–34) on fractures and bone mineral density in postmenopausal women with osteoporosis. Engl J Med 2001; 344(19):1434–41.

[98] Black DM, Greenspan SL, Ensrud KE, et al. PaTH Study Investigators. The effects of parathyroid hormone and alendronate alone or in combination in postmenopausal osteoporosis. N Engl J Med 2003;349(13):1207–15.

[99] Finkelstein JS, Hayes A, Hunzelman JL, et al. The effects of parathyroid hormone, alendronate, or both in men with osteoporosis. N Engl J Med 2003;349(13):1216–26.

[100] Van Vollenhoven RF, Park JL, Genovese MC, et al. A double-blind, placebo-controlled, clinical trial of dehydroepiandrosterone in severe systemic lupus erythematosus. Lupus 1999;8(3): 181–7.

[101] Bekker PJ, Holloway DL, Rasmussen AS, et al. A single-dose placebo-controlled study of AMG 162, a fully human monoclonal antibody to RANKL, in postmenopausal women. J Bone Miner Res 2004;19(7):1059–66.

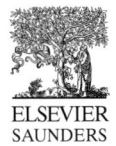

ELSEVIER
SAUNDERS

Rheum Dis Clin N Am 31 (2005) 387–402

RHEUMATIC
DISEASE CLINICS
OF NORTH AMERICA

# Exploring the Links Between Systemic Lupus Erythematosus and Cancer

Sasha Bernatsky, MD, MSc[a],
Rosalind Ramsey-Goldman, MD, DrPH[b],
Ann Clarke, MD, MSc[a],*

[a]Division of Clinical Epidemiology, Montreal General Hospital, 1650 Cedar Avenue, Room L10-520, Montreal, QC H3G 1A4, Canada
[b]Division of Rheumatology, Department of Medicine, Feinburg School of Medicine, Northwestern University, 240 East Huron Street, McGaw Pavilion 2300, Chicago, IL 60611, USA

For decades, concern has been mounting that individuals with systemic lupus erythematosus (SLE) have increased susceptibility to cancer. The first clinical evidence of an association between cancer and SLE came from case and case series reports [1–3]. Early cohort studies [4–10] produced various estimates of the cancer risk in SLE patients, and the conclusions have not been uniform [11–13]. Given the estimates and their confidence intervals, the findings of all studies could be compatible with an increased risk of cancer in SLE compared with the general population. Recent efforts have confirmed this increased risk [14].

## Review of cancer risk in systemic lupus erythematosus

Efforts to estimate cancer risk in SLE have most often been done with clinical cohorts [6–13], where subjects have a definite diagnosis of SLE, either by

The authors would like to acknowledge the following grant support: (S.B.) Canadian Institutes of Health Research (CIHR)/Lupus Canada Fellowship, Canadian Arthritis Network Fellowship, and Lupus Manitoba; R.R.-G) Arthritis Foundation, Clinical Science Grant, Arthritis Foundation Greater Chicago Chapter National Institutes of Health Grants AR 02138 and AR 48098, and Lupus Foundation of Illinois Chapter Grant; and (A.C.) National Cancer Institute of Canada grants CIHR 013135 and 10005, TAS 99105, Singer Family Fund for Lupus Research, and CIHR Investigator Award.

* Corresponding author.
E-mail address: ann.clarke@mcgill.ca (A. Clarke).

American College of Rheumatology (ACR) criteria [15] or by clinical judgment. As SLE is a rare condition [16], the sizes of these cohorts have been relatively small, ranging from 116 [13] to 724 [12]. Alternatively, attempts [5,17] have been made to generate much larger national cohorts, through assembling the names of individuals with a hospital-discharge diagnosis of SLE, and then linking these names to the national cancer registry. These cohorts were much greater in size than the clinical cohorts (for example, the cohort by Mellamkjaer et al [5] numbered 1585 subjects, and the cohort by Bjornadal et al [17] numbered 5715). These hospital-discharge studies may be biased, however, in that the subjects represent only a specific group of SLE patients (those admitted to hospital) and may not necessarily reflect the experience of the entire SLE population.

The parameter estimate presented in all cohort studies estimating cancer risk in SLE has been the standardized incidence ratio (SIR), which is the ratio of observed to expected cancers. The SIR estimates (for cancer overall) in these studies ranged from as low as 1.1 (95% confidence interval [CI] 0.7–1.6) [12] to as high as 2.6 (95% CI 1.5–4.4) [7]. All studies involved relatively small numbers of subjects, with resultant imprecise estimates, particularly for the clinical cohorts (Table 1).

The limitations of previous studies have recently been surmounted by a multisite international cohort study. It involves 23 centers from the Systemic Lupus International Collaborating Clinics (SLICC) and Canadian Network for Improved Outcomes in Systemic Lupus (CaNIOS) networks of lupus researchers [14] and draws from academic and community-based practices to produce a study sample representative of the general SLE population. This study showed, for all cancers combined, an SIR estimate of 1.15 (95% CI 1.05–1.27). This is consistent with

Table 1
Standardized incidence ratios of overall cancer occurrence in systemic lupus erythematosus with 95% confidence interval–clinical cohort studies

| Study [Ref.] | Location | Calendar years | N | Total cancer SIR (95% CI) |
|---|---|---|---|---|
| *Clinical cohort studies* | | | | |
| Pettersson et al [7] | Helsinki, Finland | 1967–1987 | 205 | 2.6 (1.5–4.4) |
| Ramsey-Goldman et al [8] | Chicago, United States | 1985–1995 | 616 | 2.0 (1.4–2.9) |
| Cibere et al [6] | Saskatoon, Canada | 1985–1995 | 297 | 1.6 (1.1–2.3) |
| Nived et al [13] | Lund, Sweden | 1981–1998 | 116 | 1.5 (0.8–2.6) |
| Sweeney et al [11] | Pittsburgh, United States | 1981–1991 | 219[a] | 1.4 (0.5–3.0) |
| Sultan et al [10] | London, United Kingdom | 1978–1999 | 276 | 1.2 (0.5–2.1) |
| Abu Shakra et al [12] | Toronto, Canada | 1970–1994 | 724 | 1.1 (0.7–1.6) |
| | | | | |
| *Hospital discharge database studies* | | | | |
| Bjornadal et al [17] | Stockholm, Sweden | 1964–1995 | 5715 | 1.4 (1.3–1.5) |
| Mellemkjaer et al [5] | Copenhagen, Denmark | 1977–1989 | 1585 | 1.3 (1.1–1.6) |

[a] Cohort was updated in 1998 to total 412 persons with 1157 years of follow-up. The SIR estimate is unchanged although the CI has narrowed (0.9, 2.2).

earlier estimates, although vastly more precise than earlier studies. Thus, the data do support a small increased risk for SLE patients in cancer overall.

The next question of interest is whether specific types of cancers increased in SLE. Several of the cohort studies of malignancy in SLE (mentioned previously) have suggested an increased risk of particular cancer types; hematologic malignancies (particularly non-Hodgkin's lymphoma [NHL]) have been implicated most often. In addition, increased incidence rates of lung, hepatobiliary, and other kinds of nonhematologic tumors have been variously suggested.

*Hematologic malignancies*

Most of the data from earlier cohort studies strongly suggested an increased incidence of hematologic malignancies, generally estimating that the risk for patients who have SLE is increased twofold compared with the general population [6–9,11–13]. Because the SIR estimates were generally based on small numbers, the confidence intervals for these earlier estimates were almost always wide.

The results from the recent multicenter international cohort study demonstrated almost a fourfold increased risk for NHL in SLE [14]. This is consistent with previous estimates, though the results from the multicenter international effort are vastly more precise than previous studies using clinical cohorts [6–9, 11–13].

NHL includes a heterogeneous group of subtypes, including both indolent and more aggressive types [18]. There is some suggestion that more aggressive NHL histologic subtypes predominate in SLE [19,20]. Preliminary data suggest a poorer prognosis in SLE patients that develop NHL compared with the general population [21]. However, it is not known if this may be related to more aggressive presentation, delayed cancer diagnosis, decreased survival related to SLE or other comorbidity, or other factors. Some therapeutic measures, particularly radiation therapy, may be inappropriately withheld from SLE patients who develop cancer [22]. Ongoing collaborative efforts of clinical research networks SLICC and CaNIOS should provide much-needed insight into the patterns of presentation, prognosis, and cause of NHL in SLE.

*Other tumors*

In contrast to hematologic malignancy, the findings of cohort studies regarding other specific cancers types have not been uniform. In general, estimates from even the largest studies have yielded inconclusive results for most types of non-hematologic tumors. However, for lung cancer, there are some fairly consistent results suggesting a slightly increased risk for SLE patients compared with the general population. The recent multisite international cohort study showed this, with an SIR for lung cancer in SLE of 1.37 (95% CI 1.05–1.76) [14]. If this result is compared with earlier data, the SIR point estimates from five of the earlier clinical cohort studies [6,8,9,12,13] suggested an increased risk of lung cancer (SIR estimates of 1.1–4). The results of Ramsey-Goldman et al [8] produced the largest SIR; this was the only study of these five where the confidence interval did not include the null value (SIR 3.1, 95% CI 1.1–10.2). In the two studies that examined cancer risk in hospital-discharge SLE cohorts, both showed a definitely increased risk of lung cancer, with SIR estimates of 1.73 (95% CI 1.25–2.32) [17] and 1.9 (95% CI 1.1–3.1) [5].

Another nonhematologic cancer type where there seems to be some evidence for an increased risk in SLE is primary hepatobiliary cancer. The results of the large multicenter cohort study supported this increased risk, with an SIR estimate of 2.60, (95% CI 1.25–4.78) [14]. Mellemkjaer et al [5], in a Danish hospital-discharge SLE cohort, found an increased risk of liver cancer (SIR 8.0, 95% CI 2.6–18.6). The estimate by Bjornadal et al [17] for primary liver cancer, using the same method of cohort assembly in Sweden, was 1.6 (0.93–2.6).

There is little that is definitive regarding other nonhematologic cancers. The recent multicenter cohort study suggested that this sample overall had less occurrence of breast cancer than in the general population (SIR 0.76; 95% CI 0.60–0.95) [14]. This is intriguing because there has been some suggestion (based on earlier clinical cohorts) of increased breast cancer risk in SLE, with a Chicago-based study published in 1998 which found increased occurrence of breast cancer in white women with SLE (SIR 2.9; 95% CI 1.4–6.4) [8]. At least one other study was supportive of this magnitude of risk, although the confidence limits included the null value (SIR 3.4; 95% CI 0.9–8.7) [23]. The SIR point estimates for breast cancer risk in several other cohorts (1.2–2.8) could be consistent with a small increased risk of breast cancer in SLE [7–11], but the confidence intervals for these estimates were quite wide and included the possibility of a small protective effect. On the other hand, two clinical cohort studies whose SIR point estimate was below 1 [6,12] also had wide confidence intervals, with upper limits that included the possibility of about a twofold increased risk. One of the studies in a hospital-discharge SLE cohort provided evidence of a decreased risk of breast cancer in SLE (SIR 0.72; 95% CI 0.54–0.95) [17], whereas the SIR point estimate of the other hospital-discharge cohort was 1.0 (95% CI 0.5–1.7) [5]. Thus, there appears to be some inhomogeneity of published results with respect to breast cancer in SLE.

Because SLE is a disease predominantly of women, there is a natural interest in the incidence of cancers of the female genital tract (including vulvar and vaginal, invasive cervical, ovarian, and endometrial cancers). Even the international cohort study recorded only a few of these rare events. In all but one of the published cohort studies [6,9,11,12,17] the SIR estimates for cervical neoplasms have been imprecise; Cibere et al [6] was the only study that produced a clearly increased risk of cervical cancer (SIR 8.2; 95% CI 1.6–23.8). Cibere et al [6] was also the only single-center cohort study that included both in situ and invasive cervical neoplasms, which was possibly one reason why they were able to produce precise estimates; the other studies, including the international study, focused only on invasive lesions, hence finding fewer cervical cancers and less precise SIR estimates. Data suggest that women with SLE have an increased prevalence of cervical dysplasia and atypia on Pap testing, compared with the general population [24–27].

With respect to ovarian malignancy, the results from the international multi-center cohort study showed a trend suggesting decreased risk for ovarian cancer (SIR 0.62; 95% CI 0.28–1.18). This protective effect for ovarian cancer was demonstrated in Bjornadal's [17] cohort assembled through hospital discharge (SIR 0.48; 95% CI 0.19–0.99), although for the category of *unspecified female cancer* the SIR was greater than 1 (2.70; 95% CI 1.09–5.57), which raises the question as to whether some of these unspecified female cancers in SLE were ovarian malignancies, hence explaining the low numbers of ovarian cancers recorded in their SLE sample. The results from the clinical cohort studies [7–12] have been variable and imprecise.

Endometrial cancer occurrence in clinical cohort studies of malignancy in SLE [6–8,10–12] has been reported very rarely. The recent international cohort study estimated a decreased incidence of endometrial cancer in SLE (SIR 0.36; 95% CI 0.13–0.78) [14].

The decreased risk of colorectal cancer seen in rheumatoid arthritis (RA) [28] and other rheumatic populations [29–31] has not been demonstrated in SLE. On the other hand, research in SLE has also not shown the same dramatic increased risk of bladder cancer as has been demonstrated in oral cyclophosphamide-treated vasculitis patients [32,33].

To summarize, patients who have SLE are at particular risk for certain types of cancer, notably NHL, and likely lung and hepatobiliary cancers. Quite variable results have been found for other tumors; the relative inhomogeneity of published results suggests a complex interplay of risk factors that differ across centers or calendar time.

## Is surveillance bias a concern?

There are strong reasons to believe that surveillance bias does not entirely explain the findings of an increased risk of malignancy in SLE. Breast cancer, a neoplasm amenable to screening, is not consistently increased in SLE cohort studies, in contrast to the striking increase in hematologic cancers, where there is no formal screening strategy for early detection. Bias could still operate in that cancers may be uncovered sooner in a lupus patient (during a periodic clinic visit) than in the general population. This might create *lead time* in diagnosis but not an increased cancer incidence and thus would not bias the incidence rate or SIR, providing the follow-up time in the cohort under study is adequate.

Additionally, in a study of 1193 women who have SLE, the proportion of cancer cases presenting at a localized stage did not appear to differ from the general population, suggesting that increased scrutiny does not explain an observed increased risk of cancer in SLE [34]. As well, recent data suggest that cancer mortality (not just incidence) is increased in SLE, which also argues for a true increased risk of cancer in SLE [35].

## Etiology of cancer risk in systemic lupus erythematosus

Because the association between malignancy and SLE seems to be substantiated, what are the pathogenic pathways linking SLE and cancer? Possibilities include an increased prevalence of traditional *lifestyle* risk factors influencing cancer incidence, putative links between medication use and cancer in SLE, or potential interactions between medications and viral exposures. Also of interest are clinical characteristics, such as secondary Sjogren's or other overlap syndromes; geographic and race or ethnic factors; and intrinsic abnormalities of the immune system. Different factors are probably of varying importance in different types of malignancies. For example, there is evidence of a common genetic predisposition to autoimmunity and hematologic malignancy [36,37], but it is unknown whether these genetic factors, or other forces, drive the risk of non-hematologic cancers in SLE. Links between lung and hepatobiliary cancer have been reported for other autoimmune disorders, including RA and systemic sclerosis [38,39]. Again, it is not known what drives the observed associations; it may be the autoimmune state, or it may be other factors, such as medication exposures.

## Lifestyle cancer risk factors in systemic lupus erythematosus: smoking and obesity

Important lifestyle factors associated with cancer development in the general population include smoking and obesity. Tobacco use, particularly cigarette smoking, is an important cause of lung and other cancers [40]. The prevalence of smoking in SLE has been estimated in several cohorts [41–45], but comparable figures for the population have often not been presented. Several small studies [6,45,46] have suggested that the proportion of smokers in SLE is similar to that of the general population. In one study among current smokers, however, the mean pack-years was higher in patients who had SLE [47] than in the age- and sex-matched general population.

Obesity is associated with greater risk of endometrial, prostate, colorectal, gallbladder, and postmenopausal breast cancer [48–51]. Obesity prevalence has been determined in SLE cohort studies [6,42,47], although a comparison with 207 population figures has been provided only by two investigators [6,47]. In one cohort of men and women who have SLE, obesity prevalence was identical to population figures [6] (although a slightly higher value of body mass index for the definition of obesity was used for the SLE population) [52]. In another age-adjusted cohort study women who had SLE had an increased prevalence of obesity compared with the general population [47].

The above factors seem unlikely to completely explain the association between increased cancer risk and SLE, particularly with respect to the association
between SLE and NHL. Other putative determinants of an increased cancer risk
in SLE include medication exposures.

## Medications and cancer in systemic lupus erythematosus

Although there are several case reports of malignancies associated with either
azathioprine [53,54] or cyclophosphamide [55–57] in SLE, the striking association of azathioprine with lymphoreticular malignancies in the NZB/NZW
mouse model of SLE [58] and in organ transplant recipients [59,60] (where
cyclosporin also seems culpable) has not been clearly demonstrated in human
populations with SLE [61]. There is also no convincing evidence that cancer
occurrence is a common outcome after intravenous (IV) cyclophosphamide therapy in SLE [62–65]. In these studies, not only was the duration of follow up
likely too short to adequately capture the cancer experience of these patients, but
also the mean duration of exposure was rather low and might not reflect the
experience of SLE patients treated as per the early (circa 1980s) National Institutes of Health cyclophosphamide nephritis protocol [64]. An increased risk of
cervical dysplasia in SLE patients treated with cyclophosphamide has been noted,
however. Also, there is evidence that at least some of the increased burden of
cancer seen in RA and other rheumatic diseases is mediated by medication exposure [38,66].

To date, no study has been designed to specifically evaluate the relative
importance of alkylating agents and immunosuppressive drugs in SLE-related
malignancies, although some of the low-powered cohort studies have attempted
to look at the issue. Cibere et al [6] did not believe that use of immunosuppressive or cytotoxic agents was linked to the cancer cases in their cohort, as only 2 of
27 (7%) patients who have SLE and cancer had been exposed to any of these
agents. Other investigators reported similar findings and drew the same conclusions [7,8,10–12]. The moderately low rate of exposure to these agents compounded by the relatively infrequent occurrence of malignancy within observed
cohorts make it difficult to establish the effect of these drug exposures on malignancy risk in SLE.

Although it has been observed that women who have SLE have an increased
prevalence of cervical dysplasia and atypia on peroxidase–antiperoxidase (pap)
testing, compared with the general population of women [24–27], the determinants of this association are not clear. However, immunosuppressive medication exposure may be an etiologic factor [24–27], possibly related to the resultant
decreased ability to clear human papilloma virus (HPV), which is a causative
agent in cervical dysplasia.

In the multicenter international cohort study of cancer incidence in SLE [14],
the data showed an increased cancer risk (for all cancers combined, as well as for
the hematologic cancer group) even early in the course of SLE. This may suggest

that cumulative drug exposure is not the primary cause of the association between cancer and SLE.

On the other hand, nonsteroidal anti-inflammatories (NSAIDs) and aspirin have been suggested as a factor potentially protective against colorectal, breast, lung, and other tumors in the general population [67–69]. Interestingly, recent evidence suggests that NSAIDs may not have as important an effect as aspirin [70]. One might suspect that aspirin and NSAIDs might be used more in SLE than in the general population and actually confer some protection against certain types of nonhematologic tumors. Some evidence supports a protective effect of aspirin against cancer development in SLE [23].

As stated earlier, research in SLE has not shown the same dramatic increased risk of bladder cancer as has been demonstrated in vasculitis patients treated with oral cyclophosphamide [32,33]. This may be due to the fact that patients who have SLE receive more moderate cyclophosphamide doses, usually by the IV route, which is believed to decrease the carcinogenic potential of this agent (at least in the bladder), although this is not definitively known.

The recent international cohort study [14] estimated a decreased incidence of endometrial cancer, breast cancer, and possibly ovarian cancer in SLE. The relative inhomogeneity of published results [4–14] suggests a complex interplay of risk factors for breast cancer in SLE that differ across centers or calendar time. Possible risk factors for breast cancer in SLE in some populations might include exposure to alklyating agents (ie, cyclophosphamide). Conversely, the use of aspirin (and potentially NSAIDs) in some patients who have SLE may confer protection against the development of breast and other cancers [23]. Also of interest are data suggesting that women who develop SLE enter menopause earlier than women who do not have SLE [71]. At the same time, because of clinical concern that exogenous estrogens may cause lupus flares [72], some samples of women who have SLE may be less likely to be maintained on hormone replacement therapy (HRT) than women in the general population. These factors (more aspirin use or less endogenous–exogenous estrogen exposure) potentially could explain the overall decreased risk of breast cancer seen in the large international cohort study of cancer in SLE [14].

Endometrial cancer, like breast (and probably ovarian) cancer, is an estrogen-sensitive malignancy [73–75]. As mentioned previously, it is possible that some female SLE study populations, being at risk for early ovarian failure [71,76], tend overall to have less endogenous estrogen exposure than women who do not have SLE [71]. And, as also mentioned previously, in the past some clinicians avoided HRT in SLE as it has been suspected of causing lupus flares [72]. These factors might also have mediated a decreased risk of endometrial (and possibly ovarian) cancer seen in the recent international multicenter cohort study.

Although these hypotheses are interesting, in general, there are currently insufficient data on the role of medication exposures and cancer risk in SLE. It is on this basis that members of the SLICC and CaNIOS networks have initiated an extension of the multicenter cohort study of cancer and SLE, in a case-cohort study, to determine how medication exposures affect the risk of cancer. The results of this work will shed much-needed light on the extent to which medications influence cancer incidence in SLE.

## Potential interactions between medications and viral exposures

As well as potentially relevant exposures of immunosuppressive agents, one might also invoke viral exposures [77–80] or an interaction between immuno-suppressive agents and viral exposures. It is possible that infectious exposures, particularly viruses such as the Epstein-Barr virus (EBV), may both trigger SLE [81] and create a predisposition to malignancy [82]. Although this hypothesis is intriguing, EBV infection is not likely to entirely explain the increased risk of cancer in SLE, particularly with respect to the increased risk of NHL in SLE, as EBV infection is not believed to play as primary a role in most types of NHL as it does in Hodgkin's lymphoma [83].

Use of immunosuppressive agents may predispose patients who have lupus to infection (or delay the clearance of infectious agents) and thus allow viral and other infectious triggers to initiate abnormal cell differentiation conferring malignant potential. This may be true with respect to HPV and cervical dysplasia [84], and some work suggests that women who have SLE have increased prevalence of HPV infection [85]. Whether this is due to medication exposure or to a baseline abnormality in the immunology of patients who have SLE [86] is unknown. Some have suggested that the increased risk of heptobiliary cancers in SLE may be related to increased susceptibility for (or a decreased ability to clear) hepatic viral infections [5], but at present this is only a hypothesis.

## Possible clinical characteristics important in systemic lupus erythematosus–related malignancy

One factor that has been postulated as a potential mediator of cancer incidence in patients who have SLE is the secondary occurrence of Sjögren's syndrome. Because of the striking association between primary Sjögren's and NHL [87], it has been proposed that secondary Sjögren's may explain some of the increased cancer risk in SLE [88,89] However, the few studies assessing the relationship between secondary Sjögren's syndrome in SLE and cancer have not definitively established this link. The lymphoma types that arise in primary Sjögren's appear to be quite different from lymphomas that arise in other autoimmune conditions. In primary Sjögren's, marginal-cell lymphomas appear to dominate, whereas in RA [90] and possibly in SLE [19,20], more aggressive types of lymphomas may predominate. This suggests more than one etiologic pathway in the occurrence of hematologic malignancies in autoimmune diseases.

Scleroderma can coexist with SLE in overlap syndromes [91], and there is evidence of a link with scleroderma and nonhematologic tumors, including lung cancers [92,93]. Hepatobiliary cancer is strongly associated with autoimmune liver disease (eg, primary biliary cirrhosis [94]), which can coexist in SLE [95]. Thus, perhaps those patients who have SLE and specific overlap features may be the most likely to develop lung and hepatobiliary tumors. The unifying process may be that neoplasia arises as a consequence of inflammation or fibrosis in involved organs.

## Geographic variations and race/ethnicity in cancer risk

There are, of course, important worldwide variations [96] in the baseline population cancer rates that are, in part, dependent not just on the country where one lives, but also on the racial or ethnic mix (as different race or ethnic groups have different baseline cancer risk [40,96–98]). There has been some preliminary work within the multicenter SLE cohort established by members of SLICC and CaNIOS with respect to the effect of geographic factors and race/ethnicity on cancer incidence. For example, cohort members from North American countries were more likely to have a cancer than those from other countries (odds ratio [OR] 2.0; 95% CI 1.5–2.7) [99]. This may represent a mix of effects, including clinical features, race/ethnicity, and differences in completeness of cancer registration [100–103].

Controlling for age, sex, SLE duration, and geographic location (that is, country and continent), investigators found that white subjects who have SLE were associated with the occurrence of cancer (OR 2.9; 95% CI 2.3–3.8) [99]. In terms of comparisons for specific cancer type, the possibility of an increased risk of cancer in white subjects who have SLE compared with subjects of all other races/ethnicities may be related more to nonhematologic tumors such as breast cancer, than for hematologic tumors such as NHL [8,99].

## Genetic factors and their place in the pathways between autoimmunity and non-Hodgkin's lymphoma

The genetic abnormalities that may underlie the association between SLE and NHL are unknown. An important feature of NHL is the presence of chromosomal abnormalities (Table 2), such as translocations where an oncogene is juxtaposed

Table 2
Selected chromosomal abnormalities seen in specific subtypes of non-Hodgkin's lymphoma

| Molecular events | Translocation | Oncogene affected | Example of NHL subtype |
|---|---|---|---|
| Apoptosis inhibition | t(14;18)(q32;q21) | bcl-2 | Follicular |
|  | t(1;14)(p22;q32) | bcl-10 | Marginal zone MALT |
| Lymphocyte proliferation | t(3;16)(q27;p11) | bcl-6 | Diffuse large B cell |
|  | t(8;14)(q24;q32) | c-myc | Burkitt's lymphoma |

Abbreviation: MALT, mucosal-associated lymphoid tissue.

next to a gene important in immune cell function [104]. These chromosomal abnormalities are of interest in terms of being possible common pathways linking SLE and lymphoproliferative malignancies.

## Recommendations for cancer screening

With respect to what recommendations can be made to clinicians for suggested cancer screening of patients who have SLE, there is no evidence that any formal strategies be used, aside from following age and specific recommendations for the general population [105]. Caveats to this include the following suggestions for patients exposed to immunosuppressive agents: (1) specific screening for cyclophosphamide-related bladder cancer and (2) recommendations for the frequency of pap testing in any women receiving immunosuppressive agents. These are discussed later.

Because hematuria may be the first manifestation of bladder cancer, it has been recommended that all patients treated with cyclophosphamide have a urinalysis every 3 to 6 months, even after cyclophosphamide therapy is discontinued [106]. These recommendations stem from experience with the use of oral, not IV, cyclophosphamide in the rheumatic diseases. Caution would advise, however, the extension of these suggestions to patients receiving cyclophosphamide regardless of the route. Talar-Williams et al [106] further suggest that patients who have cyclophosphamide-induced cystitis should also undergo cytologic examination of the urine every 6 to 12 months and that any atypia or dysplasia be followed up with cystoscopic evaluation. The authors add that as urine cytology is relatively insensitive for detecting lower-grade malignant lesions, routine cystoscopy every 1 or 2 years should be considered for all patients who have cyclophosphamide-induced hematuria.

In addition, recent guidelines published by the American College of Obstetricians and Gynecologists (ACOG) [107] recommend that all women receiving immunosuppressive agents should be screened at least annually for cervical cancer with pap smears.

As a final point, Bruce et al [45] found that physicians providing care for patients who have SLE tended not to provide advice regarding cessation of smoking. Rectification of this would assist in limiting the damage done to individuals who have SLE, not only in coronary heart disease but presumably with respect to malignancies as well.

## Summary

Recent data confirm that certain cancers, particularly hematologic, occur more frequently in SLE than in the general population. Numerous pathogenic mechanisms are possible, but hypotheses remain largely speculative. In particular, data are inadequate on how cancer risk in SLE may be related to medication exposures. To evaluate the impact of medication exposures on cancer risk in SLE, cooperative efforts of SLICC and CaNIOS are currently in progress. This should provide much-needed insight into the pathogenesis of the association between cancer and SLE.

## References

[1] Black KA, Zilko PJ, Dawkins RL, et al. Cancer in connective tissue disease. Arthritis Rheum 1982;25:1130–3.

[2] Canoso JJ, Cohen AS. Malignancy in a series of 70 patients with systemic lupus erythematosus. Arthritis Rheum 1974;17:383–90.

[3] Dupla ML, Khamashta M, Garcia VP, et al. Malignancy in SLE: a report of five cases in a series of 96 patients. Lupus 1993;2:177–81.

[4] Bjornadal L, Lovstrom B, Lundberg I, et al. Patients with SLE have an increased cancer risk [abstract]. Arthritis Rheum 2000;43:S165.

[5] Mellemkjaer L, Andersen V, Linet MS, et al. Non-Hodgkin's lymphoma and other cancers among a cohort of patients with systemic lupus erythematosus. Arthritis Rheum 1997;40: 761–8.

[6] Cibere J, Sibley J, Haga M. Systemic lupus erythematosus and the risk of malignancy. Lupus 2001;10:394–400.

[7] Pettersson T, Pukkala E, Teppo L, et al. Increased risk of cancer in patients with systemic lupus erythematosus. Ann Rheum Dis 1992;51:437–9.

[8] Ramsey-Goldman R, Mattai SA, Schilling E, et al. Increased risk of malignancy in patients with systemic lupus erythematosus. J Investigative Med 1998;46:217–22.

[9] Ramsey-Goldman R, Clarke A. Double trouble: are lupus and malignancy associated? Lupus 2001;10:388–91.

[10] Sultan SM, Ioannou Y, Isenberg DA. Is there an association of malignancy with SLE? An analysis of 276 patients under long-term review. Rheumatol 2000;39:1147–52.

[11] Sweeney DM, Manzi S, Janosky J, et al. Risk of malignancy in women with SLE. J Rheumatol 1995;22:1478–82.

[12] Abu-Shakra M, Gladman DD, Urowitz MB. Malignancy in systemic lupus erythematosus. Arthritis Rheum 1996;39:1050–4.

[13] Nived O, Bengtsson A, Jonsen A, et al. Malignancies during follow-up in an epidemiologically defined SLE inception cohort in southern Sweden. Lupus 2001;10:500–4.

[14] Bernatsky S, Ramsey-Goldman R, Boivin J-F, et al. Cancer in systemic lupus erythematosus: an international multi-centre cohort study. Arthritis Rheum 2005, in press.

[15] Tan EM, Cohen AS, Fries JF, et al. The 1982 revised criteria for the classification of SLE. Arthritis Rheum 1982;25:1271–7.

[16] Stahl-Hallengren C, Jonsen A, Nived O, Sturfelt G. Incidence studies of systemic lupus erythematosus in Southern Sweden: increasing age, decreasing frequency of renal manifestations and good prognosis. J Rheumatol 2000;27:685–91.

[17] Bjornadal L, Lofstrom B, Yin L, et al. Increased cancer incidence in a Swedish cohort of patients with systemic lupus erythematosus. Scand J Rheumatol 2002;31(2):66–71.

[18] Fisher R. Overview of non-Hodgkin's lymphoma: biology, staging, and treatment. Semin Oncol 2003;30(2):3–9.

[19] Pettersson T, Pukkala E, Teppo L, et al. Increased risk of cancer in patients with systemic lupus erythematosus. Ann Rheum Dis 1992;51:437–9.

[20] Mellemkjaer L, Andersen V, Linet MS, et al. Non-Hodgkin's lymphoma and other cancers among a cohort of patients with systemic lupus erythematosus. Arthritis Rheum 1997;40(4): 761–8.

[21] Bernatsky S, Ramsey-Goldman R, Rajan R, et al. Non-Hodgkin's lymphoma in systemic lupus erythematosus. Arthritis Rheum 2004;50(9 Suppl):S1850.

[22] Benk VM, Al Herz A, Gladman D, et al. Role of radiation therapy in patients with both a diagnosis of lupus and cancer. Int J Radiation Oncol Biol Phys 2003;57(2 Suppl 1): S421–2.

[23] Leung M. Analysis of a ten-year prospective cohort of multi-ethnic systemic lupus erythematosus patients—focusing on mortality, malignancy and organ damage [dissertation]. University of Birmingham: Birmingham (UK); 2001.

[24] Dhar J, Kmak D, Bhan R, et al. Abnormal cervicovaginal cytology in women with lupus: a retrospective cohort study. Gynecol Oncol 2001;82(1):4–6.

[25] Blumenfeld Z, Lorber M, Yoffe N, et al. Systemic lupus erythematosus: predisposition for uterine cervical dysplasia. Lupus 1994;3(1):59–61.

[26] Bateman H, Yazici Y, Leff L, et al. Increased cervical dysplasia in intravenous cyclophosphamide-treated patients with SLE: a preliminary study. Lupus 2000;9(7):542–4.

[27] Nyberg G, Eriksson O, Westberg N. Increased incidence of cervical atypia in women with SLE treated with chemotherapy. Arthritis Rheum 1981;24(5):648–50.

[28] Mellemkjaer L, Linet MS, Gridley G, et al. Rheumatoid arthritis and cancer risk. Eur J Cancer 1996;32(10):1753–7.

[29] Signorello LB, Ye W, Fryzek JP, et al. Nationwide study of cancer risk among hip replacement patients in Sweden. JNCI Cancer Spectrum 2001;93(18):1405–10.

[30] Paavolainen P, Pukkala E, Pulkkinen P, et al. Cancer incidence in Finnish hip replacement patients from 1980 to 1995: a nationwide cohort study involving 31,651 patients [published erratum appears in J Arthroplasty 2000;15(1):136–7]. J Arthroplasty 1999;14(3): 272–80.

[31] Olsen J, McLaughlin J, Nyren O, et al. Hip and knee implantations among patients with osteoarthritis and risk of cancer: a record-linkage study from Denmark. Int J Cancer 1999; 81(5):719–22.

[32] Knight A, Askling J, Ekbom A. Cancer incidence in a population-based cohort of patients with Wegener's granulomatosis. Int J Cancer 2002;100(1):82–5.

[33] Talar-Williams C, Hijazi Y, Walther M, et al. Cyclophosphamide-induced cystitis and bladder cancer in patients with Wegener granulomatosis. Ann Intern Med 1996;124(5):477–84.

[34] Bernatsky S, Clarke A, Ramsey-Goldman R, et al. Breast cancer stage at time of detection in women with systemic lupus erythematosus (SLE). Lupus 2004;13(6):469–72.

[35] Moss KE, Ioannou Y, Sultan SM, et al. Outcome of a cohort of 300 patients with systemic lupus erythematosus attending a dedicated clinic for over two decades. Ann Rheum Dis 2002;61(5): 409–13.

[36] Yoshitomo H, Sachiko H, Akinori I, et al. Susceptibility alleles for aberrant B-1 cell proliferation involved in spontaneously occurring B-cell chronic lymphocytic leukemia in a model of New Zealand white mice. Blood 1998;92:3772–9.

[37] Straus SE, Jaffe ES, Puck JM, et al. The development of lymphomas in families with autoimmune lymphoproliferative syndrome with germline Fas mutations and defective lymphocyte apoptosis. Blood 2001;98(1):194–200.

[38] Thomas E, Brewster D, Black R, et al. Risk of malignancy among patients with rheumatic conditions. Int J Cancer 2000;88(3):497–502.

[39] Rosenthal A, McLaughlin J, Gridley G, et al. Incidence of cancer among patients with systemic sclerosis. Cancer 1995;76(5):910–4.

[40] International Agency for Research on Cancer. Facts and figures of cancer in the European community. Lyon (France): World Health Organization; 1993.

[41] Ward MM, Studenski S. Clinical prognostic factors in lupus nephritis. The importance of hypertension and smoking. Arch Intern Med 1992;152:2082–8.

[42] Petri M, Perez-Gutthann S, Spence D, et al. Risk factors for coronary artery disease in patients with SLE. Am J Med 1992;93:513–9.

[43] Rahman P, Urowitz MB, Gladman DD, et al. Contribution of traditional risk factors to coronary artery disease in patients with SLE. J Rheumatol 1999;26:2363–8.

[44] McAlindon T, Giannotta L, Taub N, et al. Environmental factors predicting nephritis in systemic lupus erythematosus. Ann Rheum Dis 1993;52:720–4.

[45] Bruce IN, Gladman DD, Urowitz MB. Detection and modification of risk factors for coronary artery disease in patients with systemic lupus erythematosus: a quality improvement study. Clin Exp Rheumatol 1998;16:435–40.

[46] Bruce IN, Urowitz MB, Gladman DD, et al. Risk factors for coronary heart disease in women with systemic lupus erythematosus: the Toronto Risk Factor Study. G Arthritis Rheum 2003; 48(11):3159–67.

[47] Bernatsky S, Boivin J, Joseph L, et al. The prevalence of factors influencing cancer risk in lupus: social habits reproductive issues and obesity. J Rheumatol 2002;29(12):2551–4.

[48] Garfinkel L. Overweight and cancer. Ann Intern Med 1985;103:1034–6.

[49] Moller H, Mellemgaard A, Lindvig K, et al. Obesity and cancer risk: a Danish record-linkage study. Eur J Cancer 1994;30A(3):344–50.

[50] Austoker J. Diet and cancer. BMJ 1994;308:1610–4.

[51] Levi F, La Vecchia C, Negri E, et al. Body mass at different ages and subsequent endometrial cancer risk. Int J Cancer 1992;50:567–71.

[52] Reeder BA, Angel A, Ledoux M, et al. Obesity and its relation to cardiovascular disease risk factors in Canadian adults. Canadian Heart Health Surveys Research Group. CMAJ 1992; 146:2009–19.

[53] Cras P, Franckx C, Martin J. Primary intracerebral lymphoma in systemic lupus erythematosus treated with immunosuppressives. Clin Neuropathol 1989;8:200–5.

[54] Hehir ME, Sewell JR, Hughes GRV. Reticulum cell sarcoma in azathioprine-treated systemic lupus erythematosus. Ann Rheum Dis 1979;38:94–5.

[55] Elliott RW, Essenhigh DM, Morley AR. Cyclophosphamide treatment of systemic lupus erythematous: risk of bladder cancer exceeds benefits. BMJ 1982;284:1160–1.

[56] Ortiz AM, Gonzalez-Parra E, Alvarez-Costa G, et al. Bladder cancer after cyclophosphamide therapy for lupus nephritis. Nephron 1992;60:378–9.

[57] Thrasher JB, Miller GJ, Wettlaufer JN. Bladder leiomyosarcoma following cyclophosphamide therapy for lupus nephritis. J Urol 1990;143:119–21.

[58] Casey TP. Azathioprine (Imuran) administration and the development of malignant lymphoma in NZB mice. Clin Exp Immunol 1968;3:305–12.

[59] Kyllonen L, Salmela K, Pukkala E. Cancer incidence in a kidney-transplanted population. Transpl Int 2000;13(Suppl 1):S394–8.

[60] Opelz G, Henderson R. Incidence of non-Hodgkin lymphoma in kidney and heart transplant recipients. Lancet 1993;342(8886–7):1514–6.

[61] Nossent H, Koldingsnes W. Long-term efficacy of azathioprine treatment for proliferative lupus nephritis. Rheumatol 2000;39(9):969–78.

[62] Martin F, Lauwerys B, Lefebvre C, et al. Side-effects of intravenous cyclophosphamide pulse therapy. Lupus 1997;6(3):254–7.

[63] Belmont HM, Storch M, Buyon J, et al. New York University/Hospital for Joint Diseases experience with intravenous cyclophosphamide treatment. Lupus 1997;4(2):104–8.

[64] Boumpas DT, Austin 3rd HA, Vaughan EM, et al. Severe lupus nephritis: controlled trial of pulse methylprednisone versus two different regiments of pulse cyclophosphamide. Lancet 1992;340:741–4.

[65] Austin H, Klippel J, Balow J, et al. Therapy of lupus nephritis. Controlled trial of prednisone and cytotoxic drugs. N Engl J Med 1986;314(10):614–9.

[66] Asten P, Barrett J, Symmons D. Risk of developing certain malignancies is related to duration of immunosuppressive drug exposure in patients with rheumatic diseases. J Rheumatol 1999; 26(8):1705–14.

[67] Williams C, Smalley W, DuBois R. Aspirin use and potential mechanisms for colorectal cancer prevention. J Clin Invest 1997;100(6):1325–9.

[68] Baron J, Sandler R. Nonsteroidal anti-inflammatory drugs and cancer prevention. Annu Rev Pharmacol Toxicol 2000;51:511–23.

[69] Garcia-Rodriguez LA, Huerta-Alvarez C. Reduced risk of colorectal cancer among long-term

users of aspirin and nonaspirin nonsteroidal antiinflammatory drugs. Epidemiology 2001;12: 88–93.

[70] Perron L, Bairati I, Moore L, et al. Dosage, duration and timing of nonsteroidal antiinflammatory drug use and risk of prostate cancer. Int J Cancer 2003;106(3):409–15.

[71] Cooper G, Dooley M, Treadwell E, et al. Hormonal and reproductive risk factors for development of systemic lupus erythematosus: results of a population-based, case-control study. Arthritis Rheum 2004;46(7):1830–9.

[72] Mok CC, Lau CS, Ho CT, et al. Safety of hormonal replacement therapy in postmenopausal patients with systemic lupus erythematosus. Scand J Rheumatol 1998;27:342–6.

[73] Xu W, Xiang Y, Ruan Z, et al. Menstrual and reproductive factors and endometrial cancer risk: results from a population-based case-control study in urban Shanghai. Int J Cancer 2004; 108(4):613–9.

[74] Beresford SAA, Weiss NS, Voigt LF, et al. Risk of endometrial cancer in relation to use of oestrogen combined with cyclic progestagen therapy in postmenopausal women. Lancet 1997; 349:458–61.

[75] Pike MC, Peters RK, Cozen W, et al. Estrogen-progestin replacement therapy and endometrial cancer. J Natl Cancer Inst 1997;89:1110–6.

[76] Takada K, Illei G, Boumpas D. Cyclophosphamide for the treatment of systemic lupus erythematosus. Lupus 2001;10(3):154–62.

[77] Abu-Shakra M, Ehrenfeld M, Shoenfeld Y. Systemic lupus erythematosus and cancer: associated or not? Lupus 2002;11(3):137–44.

[78] Bernatsky S, Clarke A, Ramsey-Goldman R. Malignancy and systemic lupus erythematosus. Curr Rheumatol Rep 2002;4(4):351–8.

[79] Ehrenfeld M, Abu-Shakra M, Buskila D, et al. The dual association between lymphoma and autoimmunity. Blood Cells Mol Dis 2001;27(4):750–6.

[80] Trejo O, Ramos-Casals M, Lopez-Guillermo A, et al. Hematologic malignancies in patients with cryoglobulinemia: association with autoimmune and chronic viral diseases. Semin Arthritis Rheum 2003;33(1):19–28.

[81] Pender MP. Infection of autoreactive B lymphocytes with EBV, causing chronic autoimmune diseases. Trends Immunol 2003;24:584–8.

[82] Hummel M, Anagnostopoulos I, Korbjuhn P, et al. Epstein-Barr virus in B-cell non-Hodgkin's lymphomas: unexpected infection patterns and different infection incidence in low-and high-grade types. J Pathol 1995;175:263–71.

[83] Jarrett RF, MacKenzie J. Epstein-Barr virus and other candidate viruses in the pathogenesis of Hodgkin's disease. Semin Hematol 1999;36(3):260–9.

[84] Schiffman MH, Bauer HM, Hoover RN, et al. Epidemiological evidence showing that human papillomavirus infection causes most cervical intraepithelial neoplasia. J Natl Can Inst 1993; 1993:958–64.

[85] Berthier S, Mougin C, Vercherin P, et al. Does a particular risk associated with papillomavirus infections exist in women with lupus? Rev Med Interne 1999;20(2):128–32.

[86] Kigawa J, Kanamori Y, Takeuchi Y, et al. Involvement of the local immune response in a case of advanced cervical cancer in a patient with systemic lupus erythematosus. Gynecol Obstet Invest 1993;36(1):62–4.

[87] McCurley TE, Collins RD, Ball E. Nodal and extranodal lymphoproliferative disorders in Sjögren's syndrome: a clinical and immunopathological study. Hum Pathol 1990;21: 482–92.

[88] Valesini G, Priori R, Bavoillot D, et al. Differential risk of non-Hodgkin's lymphoma in Italian patients with primary Sjogren's syndrome. J Rheumatol 1997;24(12):2376–80.

[89] Ioannidis J, Vassiliou V, Moutsopoulos H. Long-term risk of mortality and lymphoproliferative disease and predictive classification of primary Sjogren's syndrome. Arthritis Rheum 2002; 46(3):741–7.

[90] Baecklund E, Sundstrom C, Ekbom A, et al. Lymphoma subtypes in patients with rheumatoid arthritis—increased proportion of diffuse large B cell lymphoma. Arthritis Rheum 2003;48(6): 1543–50.

[91] Pope J. Scleroderma overlap syndromes. Curr Opin Rheumatol 2002;14(6):704–10.

[92] Hill CL, Nguyen AM, Roder D, et al. Risk of cancer in patients with scleroderma: a population based cohort study. Ann Rheum Dis 2003;62(8):728–31.

[93] Pearson JE, Silman AJ. Risk of cancer in patients with scleroderma. Ann Rheum Dis 2003; 62(8):697–9.

[94] Findor J, He XS, Sord J, et al. Primary biliary cirrhosis and hepatocellular carcinoma. Autoimmun Rev 2002;1(4):220–5.

[95] Abraham S, Begum S, Isenberg D. Hepatic manifestations of autoimmune rheumatic diseases. Ann Rheum Dis 2004;63(2):123–9.

[96] Parkin D, Whelan S, Ferlay J, et al, editors. Cancer incidence in five continents, vol. VI. IARC Scientific Publication no. 143. Lyon (France): International Agency for Research on Cancer; 1997.

[97] Landis S, Murray T, Bolden S, et al. Cancer statistics, 1999. CA Cancer J Clin 1999;49(1):8–31.

[98] Henson D, Chu K, Levine P. Histologic grade, stage, and survival in breast carcinoma: comparison of African American and Caucasian women. Cancer 2003;98(5):908–17.

[99] Bernatsky S, Ramsey-Goldman R, Boivin J-F, et al. Racial factors relating to cancer occurrence in systemic lupus [Abstract]. Arthritis Rheum 2003;(9 Suppl):S1821.

[100] Izquierdo J, Schoenbach VJ. The potential & limitations of data from population-based state cancer registries. Am J Public Health 2000;90:695–8.

[101] Brewster D, Crichton J, Muir C. How accurate are Scottish cancer registration data? Br J Cancer 1994;70:954–9.

[102] Rawson NS, Robson DL. Concordance on the recording of cancer in the Saskatchewan Cancer Agency Registry, hospital charts and death registrations. Can J Public Health 2000;91:390–3.

[103] Swerdlow AJ, Douglas AJ, Vaughan HG, Vaughan HB. Completeness of cancer registration in England and Wales. Br J Cancer 1993;67:326–9.

[104] Freedman A, Nadler L. Non-Hodgkin's lymphomas. In: Bast R, Kufe W, Pollock R, et al, editors. Cancer medicine. Section 134. Hamilton (Canada): BC Decker Inc; 2000.

[105] Bowles KE, Wynne C, Baime MJ. Screening for cancer in the patient with rheumatic disease. Rheum Dis Clin North Am 1999;25(3):719–44.

[106] Talar-Williams C, Hijazi YM, Walther MM, et al. Cyclophosphamide-induced cystitis and bladder cancer in patients with wegener granulomatosis. Ann Intern Med 1996;124(5):477–84.

[107] ACOG Committee on practice bulletins. ACOG Practice Bulletin: clinical management guidelines for obstetrician-gynecologists. Number 45, August 2003. Cervical cytology screening (replaces committee opinion 152, March 1995). Obstet Gynecol 2003;102(2):417–27.

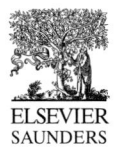

**ELSEVIER
SAUNDERS**

Rheum Dis Clin N Am 31 (2005) 403–409

RHEUMATIC
DISEASE CLINICS
OF NORTH AMERICA

# Index

*Note:* Page numbers of article titles are in **boldface** type.

# Changing Your Address?

Make sure your subscription changes too! When you notify us of your new address, you can help make our job easier by including an exact copy of your Clinics label number with your old address (see illustration below.) This number identifies you to our computer system and will speed the processing of your address change. Please be sure this label number accompanies your old address and your corrected address—you can send an old Clinics label with your number on it or just copy it exactly and send it to the address listed below.

We appreciate your help in our attempt to give you continuous coverage. Thank you.

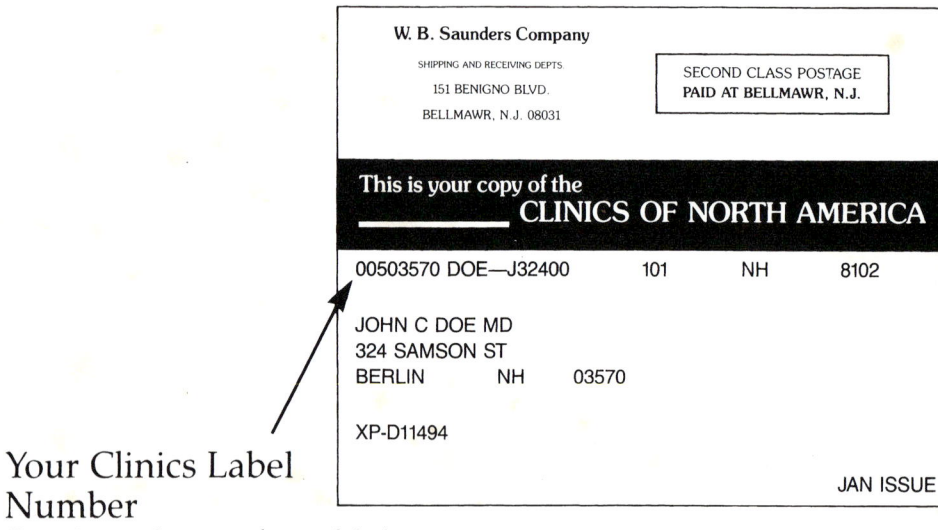

**W. B. Saunders Company**

SHIPPING AND RECEIVING DEPTS.
151 BENIGNO BLVD.
BELLMAWR, N.J. 08031

SECOND CLASS POSTAGE
PAID AT BELLMAWR, N.J.

This is your copy of the
_____ CLINICS OF NORTH AMERICA

00503570 DOE—J32400       101        NH        8102

JOHN C DOE MD
324 SAMSON ST
BERLIN        NH        03570

XP-D11494

JAN ISSUE

## Your Clinics Label Number

Copy it exactly or send your label along with your address to:
**W.B. Saunders Company, Customer Service**
Orlando, FL 32887-4800
Call Toll Free 1-800-654-2452

Please allow four to six weeks for delivery of new subscriptions and for processing address changes.